John Gray Hunter M.D.
Resident in Surgery
N.Y.U - Bellevue Medical Center

Nov. 13, 1950

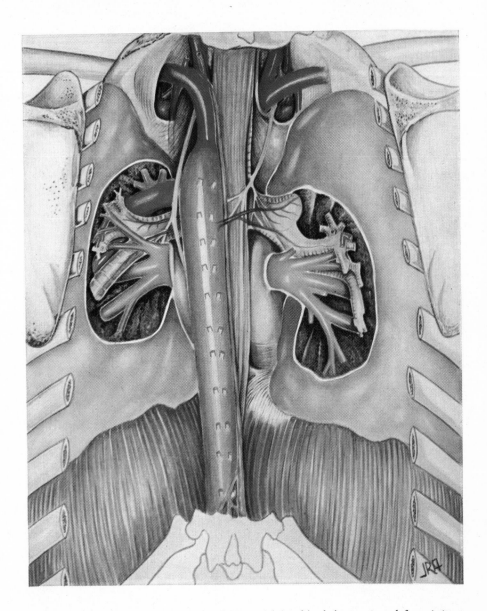

Fig. 1. The structures in the mediastinum and hili of both lungs viewed from behind after removal of a portion of the vertebral column and the medial portions of the ribs except the first and twelfth, which are shown. Illustrated are: the aorta with the severed ends of the intercostal arteries; the subclavian, common carotid and internal mammary arteries; the subclavian veins; the vagus nerves; the right recurrent laryngeal nerve; the posterior pulmonary plexuses; the esophagus; the right margin of the trachea; the major bronchi with some of their lobar and segmental branches; the pulmonary arteries and veins; the pericardium; the inferior vena cava; and the diaphragm.

THORACIC SURGERY

BY RICHARD H. SWEET, M.D.

Associate Clinical Professor of Surgery

Harvard University Medical School

Illustrations by

JORGE RODRIGUEZ ARROYO, M.D.

Assistant in Surgical Therapeutics

University of Mexico Medical School

PHILADELPHIA & LONDON

W. B. SAUNDERS COMPANY

1950

PREFACE

The present volume is based upon the concept that any properly qualified surgeon can acquire with relative ease a satisfactory proficiency in thoracic surgery by employing the technics herein described. The subject matter has been chosen carefully to include every aspect of the specialty. It is arranged upon a regional anatomic basis, starting with a chapter on the surgical anatomy of the thorax and proceeding, after introductory chapters on general technical considerations and thoracic incisions, through the surgery of the chest wall, the pleural cavity, the lungs, and the mediastinum including the heart and great vessels, the thoracic duct, and the esophagus. A separate chapter is devoted to the subject of abdominal operations performed through thoracic incisions. The final chapter deals with the surgery of the diaphragm.

Although the emphasis is placed upon operative technic, there are large sections which deal with the appropriate application of the methods described, the prevention and overcoming of difficulties which may be encountered, the variations of technic which must be made to suit the pathologic processes dealt with, and finally, in some detail, the postoperative care of the patient.

The wide scope of the material presented necessitates the description of procedures which involve a familiarity not only with the thorax but also with the neck and abdomen. This fact serves to illustrate the oneness of all surgery and to emphasize the concept that competence in the special field of thoracic surgery demands a thorough familiarity with the surgery of these other regions as well.

In an effort to keep the volume practical, only those operations which I have found to be useful in everyday practice are given thorough consideration. Many procedures which are obsolete or which have been supplanted by better methods, or which are still in the phase of trial and development and therefore not well established, are omitted or are merely mentioned. Those operations which are described and illustrated, however, are presented with great thoroughness in the belief that the relative success or failure of any surgical procedure lies in attention to what may on first thought appear to be unimportant small details.

It would be impossible to enumerate all the surgeons both living and deceased to whom credit should be given for originating many of the technics and modifications of procedures which have been described or to acknowledge the authorship of innumerable concepts which have influenced the formulation of many of the ideas expressed. Because of the fear of inadvertent failure to mention some, I have intentionally, with few exceptions, refrained from naming any.

The majority of the illustrations consist of original drawings made by Dr. Jorge Rodriguez Arroyo whose knowledge of surgery and native ability as an artist make him unusually well fitted to execute this important part of the work. The anatomic drawings were developed from original sketches made by Dr. Rodriguez Arroyo from dissections done in collaboration with Dr. Luis Gerez Maza and Dr. Ignacio Purpon at the Juarez Hospital in Mexico City. The drawings of surgical technics are from sketches made from actual operations observed by Dr. Rodriguez Arroyo while he was acting in the capacity of Fellow in Thoracic Surgery at the Massachusetts General Hospital.

Mrs. Muriel McLatchie Miller, Head of the Department of Medical Art at the Massachusetts General Hospital, contributed helpful advice concerning the technical details of the illustrations. Several of the drawings are from her hand. Acknowledgment is made also to the J. B. Lippincott Company for permission to reproduce from the Annals of Surgery the illustrations included here as Figures 57 and 58, 95 and 96.

Finally, sincere thanks are due to Miss Dorothy N. Saunders for her superlative skill and untiring patience in the typing of the manuscript and for the innumerable helpful suggestions and textual corrections which she made during the course of the work.

Boston   RICHARD H. SWEET
August, 1950

CONTENTS

Chapter 1

SURGICAL ANATOMY OF THE THORAX

Chapter 2

GENERAL TECHNICAL CONSIDERATIONS

Chapter 3

THORACIC INCISIONS

Chapter 4

OPERATIONS ON THE THORACIC WALL

Chapter 5

OPERATIONS CONCERNING THE PLEURAL CAVITY

Chapter 6

OPERATIONS ON THE LUNG

Chapter 7

OPERATIONS WITHIN THE MEDIASTINUM

Chapter 8

OPERATIONS ON THE ESOPHAGUS

Chapter 9

OPERATIONS ON THE ESOPHAGUS (*Continued*)

Chapter 10

ABDOMINAL OPERATIONS PERFORMED THROUGH
THORACIC INCISIONS

Chapter 11

SURGERY OF THE DIAPHRAGM

CHAPTER 1

SURGICAL ANATOMY OF THE THORAX

The thorax comprises that portion of the body which lies between the neck and the abdomen. It consists of a skeletal framework which is covered by important muscles beneath the common integument, and contains the principal organs of circulation and respiration. The esophagus and certain vital nerves and blood vessels pass through it. The bones of the chest are the sternum, the ribs and the thoracic vertebrae, all of which are a part of the axial portion of the skeleton.

The shape of the chest is conical, with the large diameter at the bottom. In infancy the transverse and anteroposterior diameters are approximately equal. As development progresses the transverse diameter enlarges at the expense of the anteroposterior so that by the second year of life the chest is ovoid in shape. In adults it is kidney-shaped in transverse section, and the transverse diameter exceeds the anteroposterior by approximately one fourth.

All degrees of variation in the size and shape of the thorax exist, from the very slight and insignificant to the severe and crippling. Some of these are developmental and congenital; others are acquired as the result of disease. Thus there may be a protrusion of the sternum ("pigeon breast"), a series of prominences along the costochondral junctions ("rachitic rosary"), or a groove extending outward from the xiphoid cartilage along the lower costal cartilages ("Harrison's groove"), all the result of rickets in infancy. The funnel-shaped depression of the lower end of the sternum (pectus excavatum) sometimes observed has an etiology which is still obscure, but it is probably developmental in origin.

Structural abnormalities of the spine usually induce changes in the shape of the chest. Outstanding examples of this are the kyphosis produced by caries of the dorsal vertebrae (Pott's disease) and the complex distortion of the entire thorax which accompanies scoliosis.

Noticeable alterations in the contour of the chest also result from diseases of the lungs and pleurae. The flattening of the rib cage over an area of advanced phthisical involvement is well known. This change is also observed when the respiratory motions of the thoracic wall become impaired by fixation of the pleura from exudation and fibrosis in chronic empyema, and in untreated, unabsorbed hemothorax. The rounded, overexpanded appearance of the chest observed in chronic pulmonary emphysema should be mentioned.

These considerations relative to the size and shape of the chest are of great importance to the thoracic surgeon in the choice of the site and kind of incision to make in operations on any of the thoracic viscera.

The interior of the thorax comprises a large space which is subdivided into the two pleural cavities with the mediastinal space between. The anterior, lateral and posterior limits of each pleural cavity are determined by the bones of the thorax. Medially lies the mediastinum. The inferior boundary is fixed by the diaphragm which gives this portion of the pleural space a concave configuration. The contour of the superior limit of the pleural cavity is conical, ending in a small dome-shaped projection of the pleura which extends above the level of the first rib. In this small area, therefore, a portion of the thoracic cavity on each side lies within the neck. Operations which require deep dissection in the lower cervical region immediately above the clavicle may be complicated by the accidental opening of the pleural cavity, with resultant pneumothorax. There is likewise danger of puncturing the apex of the lung while injecting a local anesthetic into the cords of the brachial plexus in this area. Tension pneumothorax may develop as a result of this accident.

BONES OF THE THORAX

The sternum consists of three portions: the manubrium (upper), the gladiolus (central) and the xiphoid cartilage (lower). The manubriogladiolar junction is a semirigid articulation which is capable of slight degrees of motion. The anterior projection caused by this joint is known as the "angle of Ludwig." It is the most frequent site of fracture of this bone.

There are normally twelve pairs of ribs. Sometimes on one or both sides there may be an extra rib, either in the cervical or in the lumbar region. The former is the more frequent. The first seven ribs are called true ribs because they articulate with the sternum. The eighth, ninth and tenth ribs articulate each with the costal cartilage of the rib above. The tenth rib is usually the lowermost fixed rib, although it is frequently unattached. The ninth and tenth ribs are sometimes not firmly attached to the costal arch; in this case four of the five false ribs are actually free or floating. Usually only the eleventh and twelfth have this characteristic. A knowledge of these variations is of importance in the making of an abdominothoracic incision or in enlarging a thoracotomy incision by extending it into the abdomen.

The ribs slope downward and forward. The first is the most nearly horizontal in direction. Beginning with the second, the obliquity increases until the ninth when it decreases with each succeeding rib. The relative obliquity varies considerably from person to person. In some persons the ribs are small and fragile; in others they are large, broad and strong. In childhood and during early adult years the ribs are strong and pliable; fractures are relatively infrequent both as a result of external violence in injuries and also from forcible retraction with the rib spreader during a thoracic operation. With advancing age the ribs lose their strength as a result of cortical atrophy and become fragile, so that fractures may follow the application of minor forces such as the strain of coughing, the pressure of the surgeon's fingers or the gentle retraction of wound edges during thoracotomy. Each rib ends in a cartilaginous portion which, in the case of the seven true ribs, unites directly with the sternum, and in the first three false ribs with the superjacent rib cartilage.

The intercostal spaces are wider in front than behind. They are also wider in the upper portion of the thorax than in the lower. The size of these spaces is much influenced by the position of the body. They are narrowed by forward bending and widened by backward extension of the trunk. Lateral bending tends to narrow those on the side to which the body inclines and widens those of the opposite side. Advantage is taken of this phenomenon in the making and closing of thoracic incisions.

The groove on the inner aspect of the lower edge of the ribs holds the intercostal nerve, artery and vein. Posterior to the rib angle there is no groove for these structures which at that point traverse the middle of the intercostal space.

Orientation on the surface of the chest wall for the purpose of placing thoracotomy incisions and identifying the rib which is to be resected is made by counting the ribs from some known point. This may be done by counting upward from the twelfth rib or, during the making of a major thoracotomy incision, by counting downward from the first rib after the latissimus dorsi muscle has been severed. Enumeration of the ribs anterolaterally is easily accomplished by counting down from the second rib which lies at the manubriogladiolar junction (Ludwig's angle) (Fig. 2). If the arm is not abducted, the seventh rib can be identified posteriorly because it ordinarily lies beneath the tip of the scapula (inferior angle) (Fig. 3). However, with the change in position of the scapula which results from motions of the shoulder girdle, this observation is unreliable.

The thoracic vertebrae are of importance to the thoracic surgeon principally because of their relations to the ribs. Two articulations exist; one is between the head of the rib and the body of the vertebra, and the other between the tubercle of the rib and the vertebral transverse process. A knowledge of these articulations is necessary in the total removal of a rib for sarcoma and in the performance of thoracoplastic rib resections, with excision of the correlative transverse processes.

SOFT PARTS OF THE THORACIC WALL

The intercostal spaces are occupied by two layers of intercostal muscle, with their fascial investments, and the intercostal nerve, artery and vein (Fig. 5). The external intercostal muscle fibers extend downward and forward, beginning at the tubercles of the ribs posteriorly and ending at the costal cartilages anteriorly. From this point to the sternum they are in continuity with the anterior intercostal membrane. The internal intercostal muscle fibers extend downward and backward, beginning at the edge of the sternum and ending at the angles of the ribs, whence they are in continuity with the posterior intercostal membrane which extends to the spine (Fig. 2).

This knowledge of the obliquity of the insertions of the external intercostal muscles into the ribs should be considered during the stripping of the periosteum from the rib edges for rib resection. A forward sweep of the periosteal elevator along the superior margin and a backward motion along the inferior margin of the rib favor the free passage of the instrument along the bone, whereas the stripping is difficult if the directions are reversed.

The intercostal arteries arise anteriorly from the internal mammary arteries and posteriorly from the aorta (Fig. 5). The anterior portions of these arteries may be single or double, arising as superior and inferior branches. If single, they soon divide into two branches. At their origin they lie between the pleura and the internal intercostal muscle, but they soon penetrate the muscle and then extend posteriorly between the internal and external muscles. The posterior portion of each intercostal artery arises as a single trunk from the aorta, extending between the pleura and the external intercostal muscle as far as the angles of the ribs; there it divides into superior and inferior branches which anastomose with the corresponding branches of internal mammary origin. Between the vertebra and the angle of the rib the posterior vessel lies approximately midway between the adjacent ribs. At this point it can be injured during the performance of a thoracentesis or during the making of an intercostal incision. Perforating branches arise from the intercostal arteries posteriorly close to their origin from the aorta, at several points along their lateral course in the intercostal spaces, and anteriorly close to their connections with the internal mammary arteries. The majority of these branches are encountered in making an intercostal incision (Fig. 5). The intercostal veins follow the course of the arteries. They communicate anteriorly with the internal mammary veins and posteriorly with the azygos and hemiazygos veins. The intercostal nerve passes forward beside the posterior intercostal artery and comes to occupy the intercostal groove on the inferior edge of the corresponding rib along with the superior branch of the artery.

The origins and insertions of the muscles of the thorax are well known and need no description. It is important at both extremities of the chest to conceive of these muscles as they lie in planes or layers which are intimately related to, or at least in functional continuity with, the muscles of the neck and shoulder girdle above and those of the abdominal wall below. Thus the pectoralis major lies in the same plane with the sternocleidomastoid and trapezius muscles through their sternal and clavicular attachments. Posteriorly the trapezius, the rhomboids and the levator scapulae lie partly in the neck as well as over the thorax. At a deeper level the serratus posterior superior, the splenius capitis and the posterior scalene muscles are in a contiguous plane. In the lower aspect of the thorax the thoracic and abdominal muscles and the diaphragm have an important relation to one another. Anteriorly the pectoralis major muscle and the rectus abdominis muscle, each lying in the same plane, insert into the lower end of the sternum and the sixth, seventh and eight costal cartilages. Further laterally the external oblique muscle of the abdominal wall lies in continuity with the serratus anterior muscle by means of its interdigitating insertions into the ribs. These interdigitations are always encountered in the making of major thoracotomy incisions at the usual levels. Further posteriorly along the lower ribs the fibers of the external oblique muscle bear a similar relation to those of the latissimus dorsi muscle by way of their costal insertions. The interdigitations of these muscles are seen when the incision is made low on the chest wall, as when a combined abdominothoracic approach is used for splenectomy or nephrectomy (Figs. 2, 3 and 4).

At the costal margin the insertions of the internal oblique muscle of the abdominal wall have no counterpart in the chest unless it be the lower intercostal muscles which insert from above. The transversalis muscle, on the other hand, has an interesting and important relation to the chest wall because by means of its insertion into the inner surfaces of the lower ribs it lies in the same plane and in direct continuity with the insertions of the diaphragm on the same rib surfaces. The transversus thoracis muscle represents the intrathoracic continuation of the muscle plane in which the transversus abdominis lies. The deepest layer is the peritoneum which passes from the inner surface of the transversalis muscle to the inferior surface of the diaphragm as a continuous membrane; on the other side of the diaphragm lies the pleura.

It is convenient, therefore, from the structural point of view to consider the abdomen and thorax not as isolated portions of the trunk but as a single continuous expanse of muscle, fascia, subcutaneous tissue and skin, lined with a serous membrane and separated into two compartments by the diaphragm. This concept is useful in the understanding of the spread of sepsis from one cavity to the other and especially in the planning of thoracoabdominal incisions which are now so important in the management of conditions involving certain upper abdominal organs (Figs. 2, 3 and 4).

From the topographical viewpoint also it should be remembered that because of the dome-shaped contour of the diaphragm and to some extent the configuration of the lower portion of the chest wall, portions of the abdominal viscera are actually within the thoracic cage. If it were not for the presence of the diaphragm to separate the pleural cavities from the abdominal cavity, the liver, the spleen, the major portion of the stomach, and also the suprarenal glands and kidneys would actually be thoracic organs. The topography of this area is shown in Figure 6.

With certain variations which are characteristic of the anatomy at different levels, thoracotomy incisions obviously involve the transection of several groups of muscles. Anteriorly, cutting across the middle section of the pectoralis major muscle can be avoided by using a curved submammary incision. Posteriorly and laterally, in the upper portion of the chest, the large muscles of the shoulder girdle must be divided. Thus in the operation of thoracoplasty and in upper major thoracotomy incisions such as those used for upper lobectomy, the latissimus dorsi muscle must be completely divided and a large portion of the trapezius and rhomboid muscles must be severed. In the anterior portion of such an incision a considerable division of the serratus anterior muscle must be made.

In low thoracotomy incisions, on the other hand, the extent of division of muscles is considerably less because of their anatomic relations. Thus for an incision over the ninth rib, although a wide section of the latissimus dorsi must be transected, only small areas of the serratus anterior and trapezius muscles lie in the course of the incision. With incisions which are midway between the upper and lower extremes, relatively large portions of all the important muscles must be divided. In this area there is a small triangular-shaped space which is not crossed by any muscle (the so-called "auscultatory triangle" of the older textbooks). This space is bounded superiorly by the rhomboid major muscle, inferiorly by the latissimus dorsi muscle, and medially by the trapezius muscle. In its depths a small surface of the seventh rib lies exposed (Fig. 4).

THE MEDIASTINUM

The mediastinum is that portion of the interior of the chest which lies between the pleural membranes laterally and is bounded in front by the sternum and behind by the vertebral column. The arbitrary division of this space into superior, anterior, middle and posterior areas is artificial and unimportant. It is better to think of the mediastinum as a single space which is in direct continuity superiorly with the deep subfascial spaces of the neck and is limited inferiorly by the diaphragm excepting for the apertures through which the inferior vena cava, the aorta and the esophagus pass; there it has continuity with the retroperitoneal tissues of the abdomen. This concept is important when it comes to the interpretation of extensions of extravasated blood, accumulations of pus and infiltrations of air from the mediastinum upward into the neck or downward into the retroperitoneal tissues of the abdomen. Because of the effects of gravity, fluid accumulations in the deep fascial spaces of the neck are prone to extend down into the mediastinum; those originating in the mediastinum may pass into the retroperitoneal area. Conversely, infiltrations of air such as exist in mediastinal emphysema may extend upward into the neck because of the tendency of gases to rise to the uppermost regions with the patient in the usual semirecumbent posture.

Structures Within the Mediastinum

A thorough knowledge of the topographical relations of the many vital structures which lie within the mediastinum is essential to the thoracic surgeon because of the numerous operations which are now regularly performed on mediastinal organs such as the heart and great vessels, the esophagus, the thymus, the thoracic duct and others. Some of these relations are illustrated in Figure 1 (frontispiece in color) which depicts the posterior aspect of the mediastinum as exposed by the removal of the spinal column and the medial ends of all the ribs except the first. Further evidence of the importance of a knowledge of the anatomy of this region rests in the fact that a large portion of the dissection in the performance of a pneumonectomy and also, in some cases, a lobectomy, according to the modern technic, is carried out within the mediastinum. This applies particularly to the removal of a lung for carcinoma, with radical extirpation of the subcarinal and other mediastinal lymph nodes.

The standard textbooks of anatomy should be consulted for detailed descriptions, but mention should be made at this point of certain anatomic facts which have a surgical bearing.

The Thymus Gland. The thymus gland, which is easily exposed through a sternum–splitting incision, is mostly a thoracic organ but extends a short distance into the neck. It lies within the areolar tissues of the mediastinal space between the sternum anteriorly and the pericardium, the ascending aorta and the left innominate vein posteriorly. On each side it touches the pleural sac. It is shaped like the letter H. The two large downward extensions lie over the aorta and pericardium. They may extend posteriorly on either side of the ascending aorta, sometimes as far as the phrenic nerves. A few small blood vessels enter the gland in this area. There are usually two principal arteries which arise from the internal mammary vessels and enter the gland laterally near the central portion. The upward extension of each lobe of the gland ascends a short distance into the neck beneath the corresponding sternothyroid muscle. There is always a small artery which enters each upper pole of the gland. It arises from the inferior thyroid artery. The venous return from the thymus converges principally in one or two small veins which enter the left innominate vein from the posterior surface of the gland. From the upper poles one or two small veins accompany the arteries, there to empty into the thyroid veins. All these vessels are readily identified during the operation of thymectomy.

The Heart and Pericardium. The heart and pericardium lie directly beneath the lower portion of the sternum and the lower left costal cartilages from the third to the sixth. The right chambers are most anteriorly placed. Because of the rotation of its long axis to the left, access to the left side of the heart may require the use of special incisions to be described later. The relations of the great vessels at the base of the heart and of the reflection of the pericardium in this area are of importance. It should be remembered that the pulmonary veins have a short course through the pericardial sac before they enter the left atrium. This makes it possible, in certain cases of carcinoma of the lung, to excise sections of the pericardium after ligating the veins close to the heart and actually within the pericardial sac (Figs. 7 and 8). Posteriorly the pericardium is reflected around the superior and inferior venae cavae, the pulmonary veins, and superiorly around the aorta and pulmonary artery before it divides. Between these two reflections there is a space behind the latter two vessels near the heart where there is no pericardium. This is known as the transverse sinus (Fig. 9).

The Esophagus. The intrathoracic portion of the esophagus lies upon the anterior surfaces of the vertebral bodies behind the trachea above and the aortic arch, the left main bronchus and the pericardium below. As it passes behind the aortic arch it deviates to the right. This displacement is sharply accentuated by pathologic enlargement of the aorta in this area. Behind the pericardium it lies almost in the center of the mediastinum behind the left atrium (auricle) from which it is separated by the posterior portion of the pericardium. In enlargements of the left auricle, however, the esophagus may be pushed far to the right, although occasionally the displacement is to the left. In the lowermost portion of its course within the mediastinum it lies slightly to the left of the midline where it passes through its hiatus in the diaphragm close to the descending aorta. In general the thoracic segment of the esophagus is more easily reached for surgical operations through a right transthoracic approach, but for reasons to be described elsewhere the left side is usually chosen. The principal anatomic difficulty from the left side is the fact that a portion of the organ lies to the right of the aortic arch.

A condition of considerable surgical importance is the congenitally short esophagus in which the cardia and a portion of the stomach are located in the lower mediastinum. The cardia in this condition is often 3 or 4 inches above the diaphragm. The intrathoracic portion of the stomach either is like an inverted cone or is actually cylindrical in shape. The true nature of such an arrangement can usually be determined by a skilled roentgenologist, but sometimes it is discovered only at the operating table.

BLOOD SUPPLY OF THE ESOPHAGUS. The blood supply of the esophagus is segmental in origin and distribution. The arteries are as follows: The cervical and superior mediastinal portions are supplied by branches from the inferior thyroid and the right highest intercostal arteries. Just below the aortic arch there are branches from the bronchial arteries and sometimes from the inferior surface of the aortic arch itself. From this point downward there are from two to five aortic esophageal branches. In the region of the hiatus in the diaphragm there are branches from the inferior phrenic, the pericardiophrenic, the left gastric and the left superior suprarenal arteries (Fig. 105).

The esophageal veins empty in the upper portion into the thyroid veins. Below this area they join the azygos and hemiazygos veins. In the lower end close to the cardia there are anastomotic venous communications with the left gastric and splenic veins which empty into the portal system. It is this communication which is responsible for the varicose dilatations of the lower esophageal veins observed in portal venous hypertension.

Muscular attachments between the esophagus and the left main bronchus are sometimes encountered and musculofascial strands extending to the vertebral column are usually observed in the midthoracic portion of the esophagus during the performance of an esophagectomy.

The Thoracic Duct. The thoracic duct enters the mediastinum from the retroperitoneal area by way of the aortic hiatus in the diaphragm and extends upward close to the spine in a groove between the aorta and the esophagus. In this area it is well concealed, but as it emerges from behind the aortic arch, it becomes subpleural where it can be seen through the mediastinal pleural reflection. At this level it swings forward to ascend into the neck beside the subclavian artery (Fig. 1).

Nerves. THE PHRENIC NERVES. The phrenic nerves enter the mediastinum from the neck after they leave the anterior surface of the anterior scalene muscles and descend anterior to the hilus of each lung to the pericardium, along which they pass to the diaphragm. Throughout their course in the chest they lie immediately beneath the mediastinal reflection of the pleura. The right phrenic nerve in the upper portion of its course in the mediastinum lies upon the anterolateral surface of the superior vena cava. The left nerve lies in front of the subclavian vein and crosses the aortic arch as it passes in front of the hilus of the left lung to reach the pericardium. Each nerve is accompanied by the pericardiophrenic artery and its associated veins. This vessel is a branch of the internal mammary artery. A knowledge of the location and course of the phrenic nerves assists the surgeon in orientation when the relations of the viscera may be distorted by the pressure of tumors or obscured by inflammatory infiltrations. The nerve may be approached at any level in the mediastinum for the purpose of crushing it to produce paralysis of the diaphragm. This is done usually after pneumonectomy or during the repair of a hiatus hernia, or as a part of the operation for transthoracic gastrectomy or esophagectomy. The short segment of nerve between the point where it leaves the pericardium and the diaphragm is usually the most convenient for this purpose.

THE VAGUS NERVES. The vagus nerves are of considerable importance to the surgeon. They pass behind the hili of the lungs, and in the lower portion of the mediastinum lie close to the esophagus. The *right vagus nerve* enters the superior portion of the mediastinum from the carotid sheath, passing between the right subclavian artery and the right innominate vein. At this point the right recurrent branch comes off and winds around beneath the subclavian artery to ascend toward the larynx. The main trunk then descends beside the trachea to the posterior surface of the bronchus where it gives off the branches which form a plexus in the posterior portion of the pulmonary hilus. From this point on it lies upon the esophagus, over the lower portion of which it divides to form the esophageal plexus with corresponding branches from the left nerve. From the plexus one or more trunks pass into the abdomen through the esophageal hiatus to join the celiac plexus and to be distributed over the posterior surface of the stomach.

The *left vagus nerve* enters the mediastinum between the left common carotid and subclavian arteries behind the left innominate vein. As it crosses the left side of the aortic arch it gives off its recurrent laryngeal branch which passes around beneath the ligamentum arteriosum or around the ductus arteriosus, when patent, to ascend to the larynx. Below the aortic arch it sends off branches which form the posterior pulmonary plexus. It then courses along the anterolateral surface of the esophagus to the esophageal plexus where it divides into several branches which unite with those from the right side. From this plexus it enters the abdomen through the esophageal hiatus and is distributed over the fundus and anterior surface of the stomach.

The anatomic characteristics of the vagus nerves below the level of the pulmonary plexus are exceedingly variable. Sometimes there is a single trunk; more often each nerve consists of several large fibers, one of which is frequently larger than the others. From the esophageal plexus down they vary markedly from person to person. In some instances two large nerve trunks can be identified. In others there are multiple smaller trunks. On the right side two distinct trunks are often observed. One of these leaves the lower esophagus or cardiac region of the stomach and extends along the gastrohepatic ligament to the celiac plexus where it lies close to the left gastric artery and vein (Fig. 138). An understanding of the variations which may be encountered is essential in the performance of a vagotomy for peptic ulcer, whether by the supradiaphragmatic or the abdominal approach.

The vagus nerves must be divided during the performance of an esophagectomy or a proximal gastrectomy. The branches of the posterior pulmonary plexus are always interrupted during a pneumonectomy and usually during a lobectomy. Some of these fibers likewise have to be cut to expose the pulmonary artery for anastomosis with the aorta or one of its major branches. The nerves of the left pulmonary plexus must also be severed to some extent during the operations for interruption of a patent ductus, excision of a coarctation of the aorta, and division of one of the components of a double aortic arch to release the constriction of the trachea and esophagus.

THE RECURRENT LARYNGEAL NERVES. The *left* recurrent laryngeal nerve must be identified and retracted during the performance of these operations. It may be injured or deliberately sacrificed during a wide excision of the lymph nodes as a part of the operation of pneumonectomy for carcinoma of the lung on the left side. Care must be exerted also when retracting the left vagus nerve above the aortic arch to avoid injury to the laryngeal fibers before they come off the main trunk. The *right* recurrent nerve is rarely injured during the course of a thoracic operation except in the removal of superior mediastinal tumors and the type of intrathoracic goiter which descends posteriorly.

ADDITIONAL NERVES. The thoracic portion of the *sympathetic trunk* can be seen lying beneath the pleura in the costovertebral gutter on each side of the chest. The ganglia lie on the heads of the ribs. The greater and lesser *splanchnic nerves* arise in this area and descend through the crura of the diaphragm to enter the abdomen. The ease of access to these nerves through the open thorax has led to the adoption by certain surgeons of the transpleural approach for the operation of splanchnicectomy.

Lymph Nodes. Large numbers of lymph nodes are located in the mediastinum. These are grouped principally around the trachea and primary bronchi, the roots of the lungs and the lower portion of the esophagus. A large group lies behind the pericardium in the subcarinal triangle. There are rich lymphatic connections with these nodes from the lungs and the esophagus. Primary carcinoma in either of these organs is a frequent source of malignant metastases in them. It is incumbent upon the surgeon, therefore, to include the removal of as many of these regional nodes as is technically possible in the operations of pneumonectomy or esophagectomy when applied to cases of carcinoma.

Inflammatory diseases of the lungs give rise to inflammatory changes in the lymphatic vessels and nodes which make extirpative surgery difficult and hazardous. This is seen in a pronounced degree in chronic bronchiectasis and lung abscess. Tuberculous lymphadenitis in the mediastinum may also occasionally cause difficulties in the performance of mediastinal operations.

The Trachea. The total length of the trachea in the adult is variable, averaging approximately 11 cm. It ends in the right and left major bronchi at the level of the manubriogladiolar joint which lies opposite the fifth thoracic vertebra. The shortness of the trachea is of concern to the anesthetist because of the ease with which the intratracheal anesthesia tube may be inserted beyond the level of the carina into one bronchus or the other. This accident would interfere seriously with the respiratory exchange and if not discovered in time might lead to an alarming degree of anoxia of the patient. This danger is particularly important in children.

The Pleura. The pleura is the serous membrane which invests each lung and lines the thoracic cavity on the corresponding side. Because of the interposition of the mediastinum there are two separate pleural sacs. Inferiorly the parietal pleura covers the superior surface of the diaphragm except for the central portion on which the pericardium rests. The cone-shaped superior reflection rises several centimeters above the inner margin of the first rib into the base of the neck.

THE LUNGS

Surgery of the lungs has progressed to the point where it is necessary for the surgeon to be familiar not only with the lobes and the larger structures of the hilus, but also with the intricate anatomy of the bronchopulmonary segments. Although the right and left lungs differ in several unimportant respects, there is a striking similarity between them so far as the segmental arrangement is concerned. Each segment has its separate bronchus and its own branches of the pulmonary artery and veins. The parenchymal substance of each segment is distinct from that of the adjacent segments. The presence of these independent areas of which the lobes of the lung are composed is sometimes indicated by the occurrence of indentations on the surface of the lung which delineate partially the location of one or more intersegmental planes. Occasionally such a cleavage is so deep that it actually represents an anomalous fissure. These supernumerary intersegmental partial or complete fissures may be observed in any of the lobes of each lung, but they are most frequently found between the superior and basal segments of the lower lobes and between the superior lingular segment and the upper segments of the left upper lobe.

On the other hand, although the interlobar fissures are complete in the majority of cases, there may be wide variations from the usual arrangement. On the right side, the fissure between the upper and middle lobes is frequently absent or only partially complete. In fact, it is unusual to find these lobes completely separate. On both sides, also, the superior segment of the lower lobe, especially in its posterior aspect, is often anatomically fused with the adjacent portion of the upper lobe. The normal direction and the topographical relations of the fissures of each lung to the chest wall, particularly the ribs, are illustrated in Figures 10, 11, 12 and 13.

Although the right lung has three lobes and the left lung has only two, the detailed anatomy of each is similar. Actually, if it were not for the fact that the lingular bronchus of the left lung usually arises from the upper lobe bronchus, the arrangement of both lungs would be essentially the same.

Occasionally the lingular bronchus arises from the main bronchus below the upper lobe orifice, in which case the lingular portion of the lobe is the homologue of the middle lobe of the right side. This is not to be confused with the state of affairs which exists in situs inversus, where the right or three-lobed lung is actually in the left side and the left or two-lobed lung is in the right. In such cases the apex of the heart points to the right and the abdominal viscera are also transposed.

In rare instances one or more lobes of either lung or even the entire lung may be congenitally absent (agenesis).

There are normally ten segments in each lung. In some classifications, as will be described, two pairs on the left side are grouped as one, making the total number of segments on that side only eight. Each segment extends to the pleural surface, expanding in volume from its central to its peripheral portion. The surface of each lobe of each lung, therefore, is composed of continuous but independent segmental areas which have a more or less constant and characteristic arrangement and a fairly typical relation to the overlying ribs. Schematic three-dimensional representations of the segments of each lung are shown in Figures 14 and 15. These should be consulted in conjunction with the ensuing description.

The Right Lung. On the right side the upper lobe contains three segments. In the upper part of the lobe is the apical segment, which occupies the dome-shaped apex of the lung and presents on all four sides (anterior, lateral, posterior and medial). Beneath this are the anterior segment, which presents on the anterior and medial surfaces of the lobe, and the posterior segment, which presents posteriorly and laterally. The inferior surfaces of these segments are the lower boundaries of the lobe. The anterior segment lies along the fissure next to the middle lobe and the posterior segment along the fissure between the upper lobe and the superior segment of the lower lobe.

The middle lobe is divided almost equally into two segments: the lateral, which presents on its anterolateral aspect, and the medial, which occupies its anteromedial aspect. As will be observed from the diagrams (Figs. 10, 11 and 12) the surface of the middle lobe does not reach the chest wall posteriorly. Its largest surface lies anteriorly, but triangular-shaped surfaces present laterally against the chest wall beneath the fourth and fifth ribs and medially against the pericardium. The inferior surface of the medial segment rests upon the diaphragm.

The right lower lobe contains five segments. The largest single segment in this lobe is the superior which on the posterior surface lies against the pleura beneath portions of the fourth, fifth, sixth, seventh and eighth ribs (Fig. 11). Medially and laterally this segment extends around to the fissure where its surface lies against the inferior surface of the posterior segment of the upper lobe, as mentioned before. Thus the superior segment has a surface which presents against the mediastinum and one which lies against the lateral thoracic wall. The basal or inferior portion of the lower lobe consists of four segments which together comprise the largest portion of this lobe which, in turn, is the largest of the three. These are the posterior, which also contributes to a portion of the mediastinal surface of the lower lobe, the lateral whose surface is actually partially posterior as well, the anterior which is also partly lateral, and the medial which presents entirely on the medial and diaphragmatic surfaces of the lobe (Fig. 14). To the name of each of these segments should be added the term "basal" when each is spoken of separately. The inferior surfaces of all four basal segments lie upon the diaphragm (Figs. 10, 11 and 12).

A peculiar abnormality which occurs occasionally in the right lung consists of an anomalous longitudinal cleavage of the upper lobe in the anteroposterior diameter, at the bottom of which lies the arch of the azygos vein. The portion of lung which is medial to this cleft is called the azygos lobe although it does not have any distinctive bronchial or vascular components.

The Left Lung. On the left side the upper lobe is composed of five segments. By some authors the apical and posterior segments are sometimes grouped together as one, which they call the apico-posterior segment. This alternative classification is based upon the fact that there are only two large bronchial divisions of the upper lobe bronchus beyond the lingular branch. But the upper of these two bronchi subdivides promptly to form apical and posterior branches, each of which can be identified separately. Each of these bronchi supplies an independent area. It is proper, therefore, to consider that the so-called apico-posterior segment is in fact two distinct segments like those in the right upper lobe (Fig. 15). In front of these lies the anterior which presents anteriorly, laterally, and also medially in very much the same way as its counterpart on the right side. The two remaining segments of the left upper lobe are those which make up the lingular portion. They are the superior lingular and the inferior lingular segments. Both of these have lateral, anterior and medial surfaces. The tip or lower extremity of the inferior lingular segment rests upon the diaphragm close to the pericardium (Figs. 11, 12 and 13).

The left lower lobe, except for its smaller size, is almost the exact counterpart of the corresponding lobe on the right. The same five segments exist although, as in the upper lobe, two are sometimes grouped together and classified as one. The large superior segment is identical in extent and relations with that on the right side. The basal segments are likewise actually the same as on the right. They are the posterior, which presents partly on the medial surface of the lobe, the lateral, the anterior and the medial. Because their bronchi usually arise as a single trunk from the lower lobe bronchus before subdivision into two branches, the anterior and medial segments are sometimes spoken of as the anteromedial segment. As in the case of the so-called apico-posterior segment of the upper lobe, it is preferable to maintain a consistent point of view regarding the separate existence of these segments even though the bronchi do not arise independently from the principal lobar trunk (Figs. 10, 11, 13 and 15).

Each bronchopulmonary segment is supplied by one or more branches of the pulmonary artery which can be identified during the dissection of the hilus in preparation for the excision of that particular segment. It is necessary, however, in many instances to carry the dissection partway into the lung itself in order to find these vessels. Anomalous vessels and abnormal distribution of vessels which arise in the usual manner are frequently encountered, making it necessary for the surgeon to make himself familiar with these peculiarities. Each segment likewise has its veins which find their way into the larger pulmonary veins, usually in a characteristic manner. Anomalous venous channels, however, are also sometimes found. The segmental branches of the pulmonary veins lie principally along the intersegmental planes and receive tributaries frequently from the adjacent segment. Advantage is taken of this fact in the operation of excision. By following the veins the limits of the segment which is being removed can be more readily delineated.

The segmental arteries, on the other hand, tend to occupy a more nearly central position in the corresponding segment, their smallest branches ending along the intersegmental planes. This explains the fact that there is relatively little pulmonary arterial bleeding when the dissection is accurately done along these planes.

It is important also to observe that the segmental bronchus and its larger subdivisions occupy a central location within the segment, with the smallest branches nearest the segmental limits. Thus it is that dissection along an intersegmental plane does not result in much leakage of air because there are no bronchi of any appreciable caliber to be cut across.

The Hili of the Lungs. In a general way the hili of the two lungs are identical. They both contain the major bronchi with their primary subdivisions, the branches of the pulmonary artery and the pulmonary veins, the bronchial arteries and lymphatic vessels, numerous lymph nodes and the nerve fibers of the pulmonary plexuses, enveloped by a reflection of the pleura as it passes from the surface of the mediastinum to the surface of the lung. The topographical relations of the bronchi, arteries and veins, however, vary markedly between the sides and must therefore be given detailed consideration.

THE RIGHT HILUS. Figures 16, 17, 18 and 19 comprise a series of illustrations of the anatomy of the hilus of the right lung based upon an actual dissection. They depict the relations of the various structures at several depths as seen from in front. Figure 20 illustrates structures seen only from within the fissures. Figure 21 presents some of the more frequent anomalies of the pulmonary vessels on the right side.

The right main bronchus is shorter, wider, and more vertical in direction than the left. About 2 cm. from its origin at the carina it gives off the upper lobe branch. This branch assumes an almost horizontal direction but soon subdivides into its three segmental branches, apical, anterior and posterior. Immediately distal to the origin of the upper lobe bronchus on the anterior surface of the main bronchus there is a groove or sulcus in which the pulmonary artery rests. From the anterolateral aspect below this groove, the middle lobe bronchus arises. Close to its origin this bronchus divides into its medial and lateral segmental branches. Beyond this point all of the bronchi are distributed to the segments of the lower lobe. The superior segmental branch of the lower lobe bronchus arises posteriorly and pursues a horizontal course to give off its various subdivisions. The exact point of origin of this bronchus varies greatly in relation to the origin of the middle lobe bronchus from the other side of the principal trunk. Although it usually arises at a slightly more distal level than the middle lobe branch, it may come off exactly opposite or even slightly proximal to it. These variations are of great importance in the operation of middle or lower lobectomy or of segmental excisions involving the lower lobe. In the performance of a lower lobectomy it may be necessary to remove the middle lobe as well if the origin of the superior segmental branch is too far proximal in relation to the middle lobe bronchus. In some cases, however, the middle lobe can be preserved by dividing independently the superior segment bronchus and the remainder of the lower lobe bronchus. Below the superior segment branch the bronchus terminates in the four basal segmental branches.

Only the bronchial arrangement most frequently encountered has been described, but anomalies of the various segmental branches of any of the three lobes are sometimes seen.

The right pulmonary artery differs markedly from the left. From its point of origin it follows a short horizontal course in front of the main bronchus until it reaches the anterior surface of the upper lobe bronchus, where it gives off its first branch to the upper lobe. This branch soon divides into two trunks, one for the apical and one for the anterior segment of the upper lobe. Occasionally these branches arise from the main vessel separately. Below the first upper lobe branch the artery curves downward where it lies in the groove on the anterior surface of the bronchus below the upper lobe branch. At this level the artery to the posterior segment of the upper lobe comes off. This vessel enters the lobe beneath the fissure and cannot be seen unless the depths of the fissure between the upper and middle and to some extent that between the upper and the lower lobes are exposed by dissection (Fig. 20). This vessel is somewhat smaller in caliber than the others. Anomalies of this artery are sometimes seen, the principal one being its origin from the segmental artery which supplies the superior segment of the lower lobe (Fig. 21, *D*). When this occurs, this artery is encountered during the dissection of the fissure between the upper lobe and the superior segment of the lower. Other anomalies of the right upper lobe arteries are the occurrence of two separate branches to the posterior segment, the origin of all three segmental branches from a common trunk, and the occurrence of only two branches to the upper lobe instead of the usual three (Fig. 21, *A*, *B* and *C*).

The middle lobe is usually supplied by two branches of the pulmonary artery which arise close together at the base of the confluence of the fissures in the hilus below the posterior segmental branch to the upper lobe (Fig. 20). They pass into the lobe close to the superior and posterior surfaces of the middle lobe bronchus. Sometimes there is only one branch to this lobe. Occasionally there are three middle lobe branches. Another anomaly seen occasionally is a branch of the distal middle lobe artery which passes into the lower lobe (Fig. 21, *E*, *F* and *G*).

Distal to the origin of the middle lobe branches the artery terminates in the lower lobe divisions. The superior segmental artery arises first. It passes downward and posteriorly into its particular segment. This branch may arise close to or occasionally above the point of origin of the middle lobe branches. Not infrequently two separate vessels are observed (Fig. 21, *H*). The basal segmental branches come off a common trunk below the origin of the superior segmental branch. The first portion of the medial segmental branch can usually be seen immediately beneath the surface of the lobe, in the fissure between the middle and lower lobes. These vessels tend to lie in front of their corresponding bronchi.

The veins which lead off from the various segments of each lobe on the right converge into larger trunks which end in two principal pulmonary veins, the superior and inferior. The veins are the most anteriorly located of the hilar structures, lying in front of the arteries. The superior pulmonary vein receives the apical, posterior and anterior segmental veins and usually two or more veins from the middle lobe. However, the number and distribution of the branches is exceedingly variable, making it difficult to identify the exact segmental arrangement in some cases. The middle lobe veins sometimes enter the left auricle as separate vessels. Occasionally there is only one vein from this lobe; sometimes there are more than two. The lowermost middle lobe vein frequently empties into the inferior pulmonary vein (Fig. 21, *I*).

The inferior pulmonary vein receives branches from all of the lower lobe segments. The branch from the superior segment is easily identified as it passes in front of and beneath the corresponding segmental bronchus. The preservation of this vein in segmental excision of the basal portion of the lung, leaving the superior segment, is important and relatively easily accomplished. This vein occasionally enters the left atrium independently of the main inferior trunk. The inferior vein as it enters the pericardial sac is a large short vessel situated at the upper limit of the pulmonary ligament. Accidental injury to the vein during division of the pulmonary ligament is avoided by observing two important landmarks which signify the close proximity of the vessel. These are a prominent lymph node at the upper limit of the ligament and a small systemic artery which courses along the inferior surface of the vein. When these structures are encountered, the vein will be found immediately beneath them. These relations apply also in the case of the left inferior vein.

In rare instances on the right side all the pulmonary veins end in one large single trunk which enters the left atrium as one vessel.

THE LEFT HILUS. Figures 22, 23, 24 and 25 comprise a series of illustrations of the anatomy of the hilus of the left lung based, as with those of the right side, upon an actual dissection. They depict the relations of the various structures at several depths as seen from in front. Figures 26 and 27 illustrate the structures seen best from within the fissure. Figure 28 presents some of the more frequent anomalies of the pulmonary vessels on the left side.

The left main bronchus is longer and less oblique in its downward inclination than the right. The upper lobe bronchus on this side arises from the superior margin of the main bronchus; in the average case this promptly divides into the lingular bronchus and another stem which further subdivides into a branch to the anterior segment and another branch which supplies the apical and posterior segments. This branch is sometimes supplanted by two separate bronchi which arise from the main upper lobe stem beyond the origin of the lingular branch. Because these two segmental branches so frequently arise together as one bronchus, the portions of the upper lobe which they supply are sometimes called the apico-posterior segment, although actually there are two segments in this region exactly as in the corresponding portion of the right upper lobe. The lingular bronchus usually arises from the upper lobe bronchus a short distance away from the origin of the latter from the primary bronchus. It may come off, however, close to the base of the upper lobe bronchus or even from the main bronchus itself below the upper lobe orifice. Such a relationship bears an obvious similarity to the arrangement of the bronchi of the right side. Occasionally also the lingular bronchus arises from the anterior segmental branch. Two subdivisions of the lingular bronchus supply the superior and inferior lingular segments.

The lower lobe bronchus on the left side gives off first the superior segmental branch which arises from its posterior surface like its counterpart on the right. The basilar branches are usually three in number, one for the posterior, one for the lateral, and one for the anterior and medial basal segments. The latter bronchus promptly subdivides to supply the two segments mentioned, but because these two subdivisions usually arise as a single stem the corresponding segments are sometimes classified jointly as the anteromedial basal segment.

The left pulmonary artery has a longer main trunk proximal to its first branches than the right. For this reason it can usually be ligated independently in doing a pneumonectomy, whereas on the right side it is frequently necessary to tie the first upper lobe branch separately and then ligate the remainder of the main trunk (Chap. 6). The artery arches upwards, inclining posterolaterally above the bronchus. At this point it usually gives off its first upper lobe branch which is distributed to the apical and posterior segments. This branch passes medial and anterior to the upper branches of the upper lobe bronchus and is crossed by the corresponding apical and posterior segmental veins which lie in front of it. The main vessel rises over and curves behind the upper lobe bronchus. Along this curved portion it gives off one or more branches to the apical, posterior and anterior segments. The number, site of origin and distribution of these branches is exceedingly variable. There may be from three to seven separate upper lobe branches including those to the lingula. The lingular branch arises from the main artery in the interlobar fissure. It is usually a single trunk which soon subdivides into superior and inferior segmental branches. These may, however, arise separately from the main artery or one may arise from a branch destined primarily to the anterior segment. Occasionally a branch to the lingula arises from one of the lower lobe branches, often the superior segmental branch, sometimes from the anteromedial basal branch. It would be unprofitable to enter into a detailed presentation of all the possible variations. The principal anomalies are illustrated in Figure 28, *A–G.*

The left lower lobe arteries are similar to those on the right side. They arise from the interlobar portion of the artery. The superior segmental branch frequently arises at a somewhat further proximal level than the lingular branch, but the reverse may be true. There are sometimes two independent branches (Fig. 28, *H*). The basal segment branches arise at more distal levels close to the bronchi of the segments which they supply.

There is frequently a tough fibrous band which passes from the left pulmonary artery soon after its origin to the aorta near the beginning of the descending portion. This is the ligamentum arteriosum which represents the remains of the ductus arteriosus of fetal life. In certain cases the ductus remains patent so that some of the aortic blood flows back into the pulmonary artery, producing enlargement of that vessel and increased pressure within it. The upper portion of the pericardium is usually reflected over this vessel, sometimes as far as the aortic arch. The left recurrent laryngeal nerve passes beneath it at its junction with the aorta. The size of a patent ductus varies greatly, but it tends to be relatively longer in children than in adults.

In the latter it is often so short that there is sometimes hardly more than a foramen between the two larger vessels.

The superior pulmonary vein receives the tributaries which arise in the various upper lobe segments. These are grouped in patterns which vary from person to person but in general they conform roughly to the segmental arrangement. The lingular veins (or vein) are easily identified because they usually run very close to the visceral pleura on the inferior medial aspect of the lingula and can be clearly seen. One or more lingular veins may occasionally join the inferior pulmonary vein in the same way as the middle lobe veins may do on the right side (Fig. 28, *I*). The inferior pulmonary vein is formed from tributaries from the lower lobe segments. The superior segment branch is relatively constant, but the basal branches are variable in size and distribution. There is no appreciable difference from the corresponding system of veins on the right side.

As on the right side, there may be a single pulmonary vein into which all the branches from both the upper and the lower lobes empty.

Bronchial Arteries and Veins. The bronchial arteries are systemic, arising from the aorta, usually in common with an aortic intercostal artery, just beyond the arch. There are numerous variations in number and course. The most frequent arrangements are (1) two branches to the left side and one to the right which branches promptly into two; (2) one branch only for each lung; and (3) two branches for each lung. Other arrangements are much less frequent. Occasionally on either side one branch descends from the subclavian artery. There are superior and inferior branches which arborize over the surface of the bronchus posteriorly, with ramifications extending around to the anterior surface. Each bronchial subdivision has its concomitant bronchial arteries. Important anastomoses exist between these arteries and other vessels such as the pericardiophrenic, the internal mammary, the superior intercostal and the aortic mediastinal branches. In addition to their major distribution to the bronchi, the bronchial arteries send branches to the intrahilar and tracheobronchial lymph nodes, the pericardium, the pulmonary plexuses and the esophagus.

In disorders requiring surgery, such as chronic inflammatory lesions of the lung, pulmonary cysts, congenital pulmonary stenosis and others, the bronchial vessels are frequently enormously dilated and, if not ligated promptly, may be responsible for an appreciable degree of blood loss during surgical procedures.

The bronchial veins empty into the azygos and hemiazygos veins.

THE DIAPHRAGM

The diaphragm, which separates the thoracic from the abdominal cavity, is of enormous importance both physiologically and anatomically. It is of concern to the surgeon chiefly when there are herniations of abdominal viscera through it. The most frequent site of herniation is the esophageal hiatus through which the stomach and sometimes the colon and omentum may pass. The cause of this condition is rarely obvious, but there is undoubtedly a congenital laxity of the diaphragmatic crura which is the predisposing factor. Two other apertures through which herniation may develop should be mentioned. The more frequent is the space along the inner surface of the costochondral margin near the sternum between the costal and the sternal insertions of the diaphragm. This is variously referred to as the sinus of Morgagni or the space of Larrey. Normally there is only a potential aperture at this point, but in some persons there is a congenital weakness there which permits the development of a hernia. The colon is the abdominal organ usually found in these hernias. The other opening through which abdominal viscera may pass is the pleuroperitoneal sinus, sometimes called the sinus of Bochdalek. This is a small oval defect in the lateral area of the muscular portion of the diaphragm close to the costal insertion. It is of congenital origin. Unlike the others, this aperture is usually not covered by peritoneum and pleura so that in herniations through it there is no hernia sac. The misplaced abdominal viscera, therefore, lie uncovered within the pleural cavity.

Another developmental anomaly of the diaphragm which is worthy of mention is the condition known as eventration. This represents an agenesis of one half or less of the diaphragm which allows the abdominal viscera beneath that area to assume a higher position in the body. Although there is no muscular action of such an area, there is a pleural and a peritoneal reflection as usual and between these layers a thin film of tissue which corresponds to the atrophied or absent muscle. The condition may occur on either side.

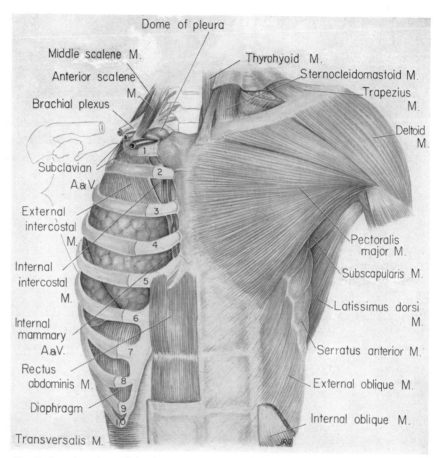

Fig. 2. Anterior view of the thorax and contiguous portions of the base of the neck and the anterior abdominal wall. The left half illustrates the superficial layer of muscles and fascia. The right half illustrates the relations of the deep muscles of the neck and abdomen to the rib cage; the intercostal muscles; the diaphragm; the internal mammary vessels; the relations of the muscles, nerves and vessels with the first rib; and the anterior relations of the lung.

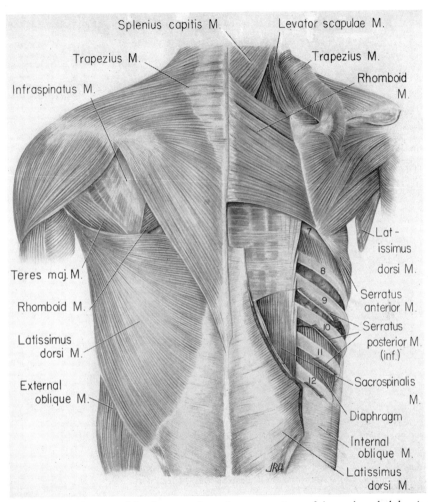

Fig. 3. Posterior view of the thorax and contiguous portions of the neck and abdominal wall. The left half illustrates the superficial muscles. The right half illustrates the deeper muscles and topographic relations of the lung and diaphragm.

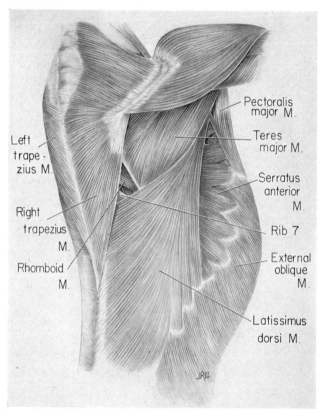

Fig. 4. Lateral view of the thorax showing the superficial muscle layer.

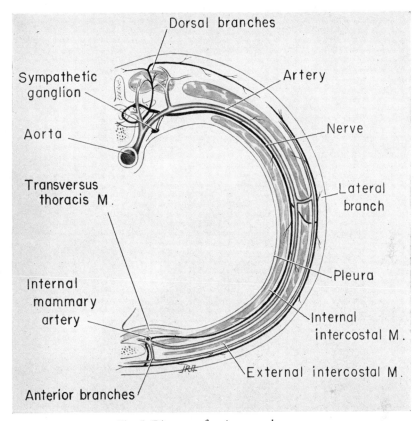

Fig. 5. Diagram of an intercostal space.

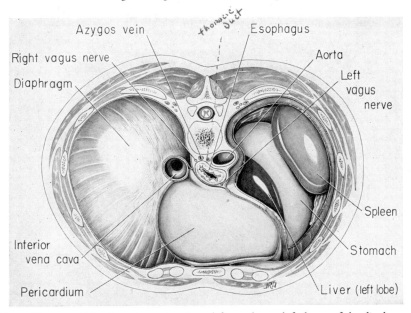

Fig. 6. Bottom of the thoracic cavity viewed from above; left dome of the diaphragm is removed to demonstrate the relations of the abdominal viscera beneath.

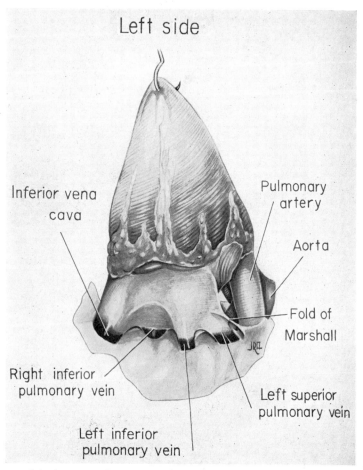

Fig. 7. Base of the heart seen from the left side to show the relations of the pericardium to the vessels on that side.

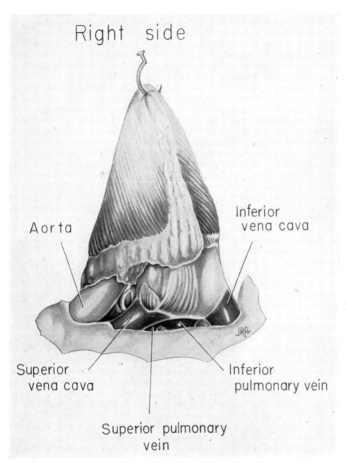

Fig. 8. Base of the heart seen from the right side to show the relations of the pericardium to the vessels on that side.

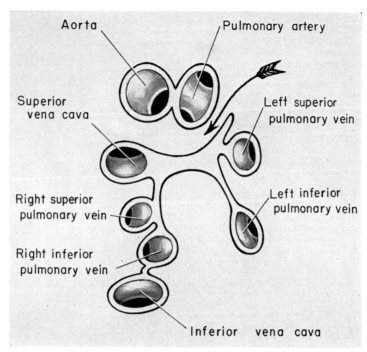

Fig. 9. Diagram of the reflections of the pericardium around the great vessels of the heart. Arrow is in the transverse sinus of the pericardium.

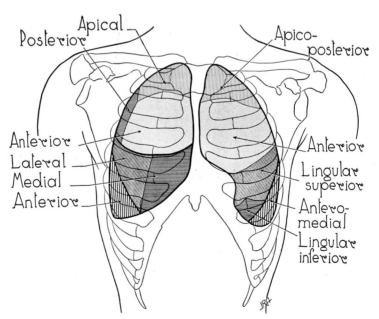

Fig. 10. Diagram of the segments of the lungs; anterior view.

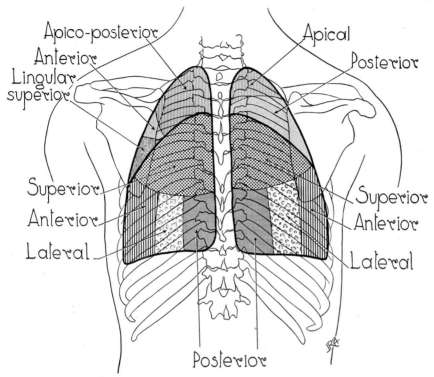

Fig. 11. Diagram of the segments of the lungs; posterior view.

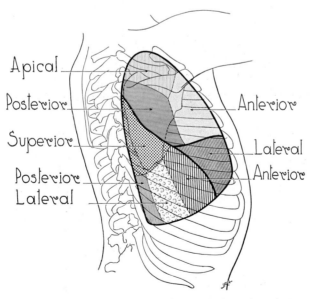

Fig. 12. Diagram of the segments of the right lung; lateral view.

3

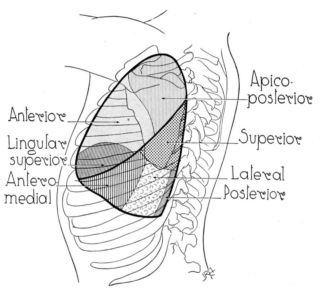

Fig. 13. Diagram of the segments of the left lung; lateral view.

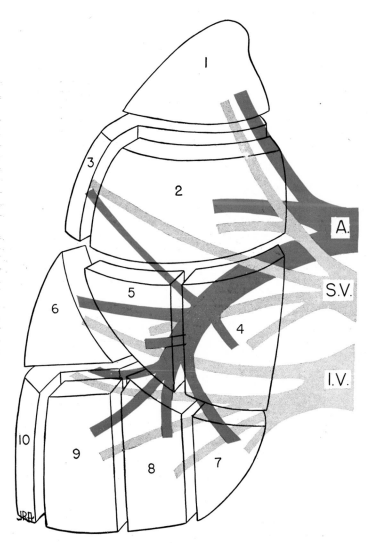

Fig. 14. Three dimensional diagram of the segments of the right lung, with schematic representation of the distribution of the pulmonary artery and veins. The segments of the right lung may be enumerated as follows: *Upper lobe:* (*1*) apical, (*2*) anterior, (*3*) posterior; *middle lobe:* (*4*) medial, (*5*) lateral; *lower lobe:* (*6*) superior, (*7*) medial basal, (*8*) anterior basal, (*9*) lateral basal and (*10*) posterior basal.

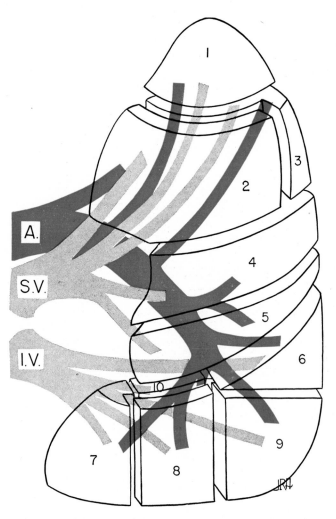

Fig. 15. Three dimensional diagram of the segments of the left lung, with schematic representation of the distribution of the pulmonary artery and veins. The segments of the left lung may be enumerated as follows: *Upper lobe:* (*1*) apical, (*2*) anterior, (*3*) posterior, (*4*) superior lingular, (*5*) inferior lingular (Note: Segments *1* and *3* are sometimes grouped together and called "apico-posterior"); *lower lobe:* (*6*) superior, (*7*) medial basal, (*8*) anterior basal, (*9*) lateral basal, (*10*) posterior basal. (Note: Segments *7* and *8* are sometimes grouped together and called "anteromedial.")

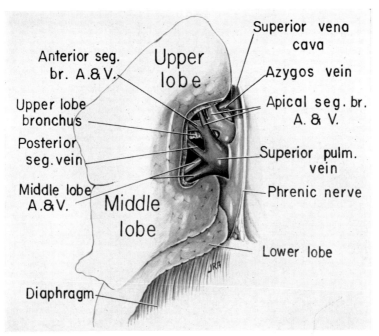

Fig. 16. Hilus of the right lung: partial dissection showing some of the upper and middle lobe vessels and bronchus; anterior view.

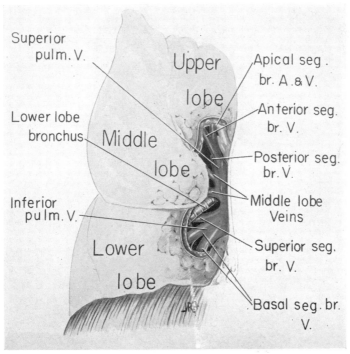

Fig. 17. Hilus of the right lung: dissection showing some of the vessels of all lobes; anterior view.

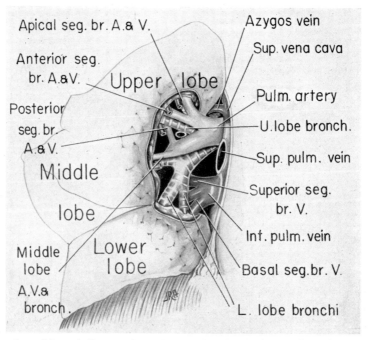

Fig. 18. Hilus of the right lung with superior pulmonary vein removed to show the deeper structures; anterior view.

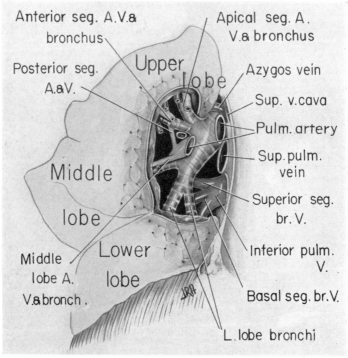

Fig. 19. Hilus of the right lung with superior pulmonary vein and a portion of the pulmonary artery removed to show the bronchus and its primary branches; anterior view.

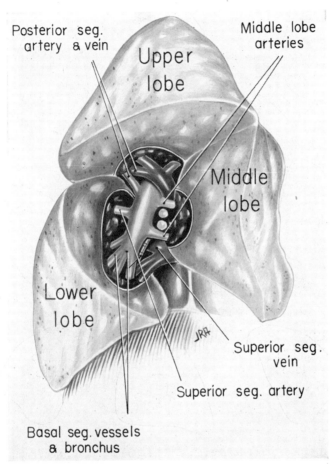

Fig. 20. Hilus of the right lung viewed from within the fissures to show the branches of the pulmonary artery and veins in that region.

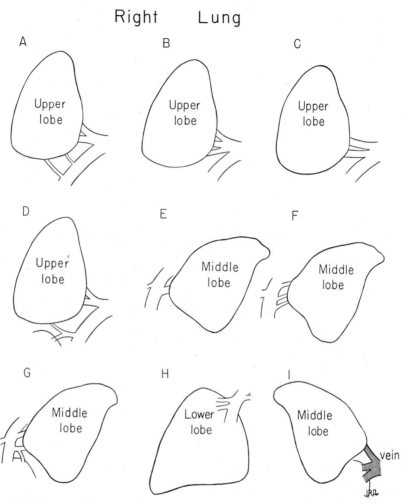

Fig. 21. Diagram of the more frequent vascular anomalies of the right lung. Upper lobe: A, three branches of the pulmonary artery; B, one branch of the artery; C, two branches of the artery; D, branch of the anterior segmental artery to the superior segment of the lower lobe. Middle lobe: E, one branch of the pulmonary artery; F, three branches of the artery; G, branch of one middle lobe artery to the basal segments of the lower lobe; H, lower lobe: two superior segmental branches of the pulmonary artery; I, middle lobe: middle lobe vein emptying into the inferior pulmonary vein.

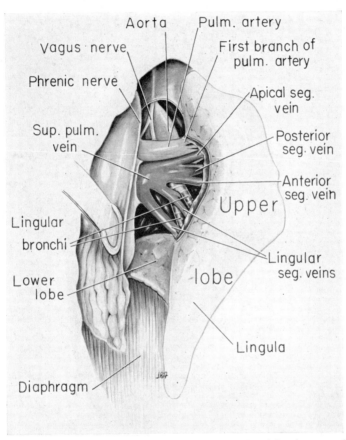

Fig. 22. Hilus of the left lung: partial dissection showing some of the elements of the upper lobe; anterior view.

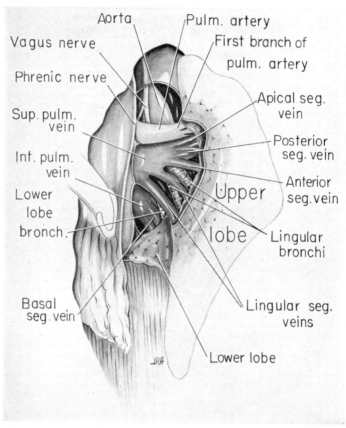

Fig. 23. Hilus of the left lung: completed dissection of the superficial aspect showing elements of both lobes; anterior view.

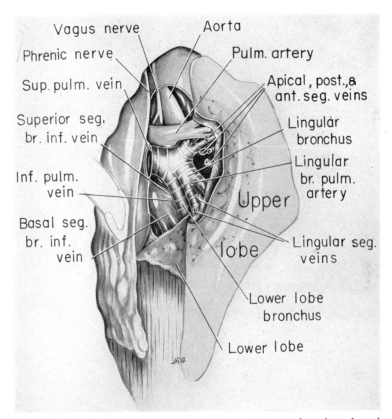

Vagus nerve

Phrenic nerve

Sup. pulm. vein

Superior seg.
br. inf. vein

Inf. pulm.
vein

Basal seg.
br. inf.
vein

Aorta

Pulm. artery

Apical, post.,&
ant. seg. veins

Lingular
bronchus

Lingular
br. pulm.
artery

Upper

lobe

Lingular seg.
veins

Lower lobe
bronchus

Lower lobe

Fig. 24. Hilus of the left lung: superior pulmonary vein removed to show branch of the artery and the bronchus beneath; anterior view.

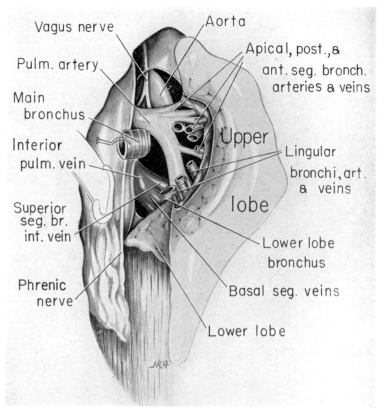

Fig. 25. Hilus of the left lung: superior pulmonary vein and section of bronchus removed to show the pulmonary artery; anterior view.

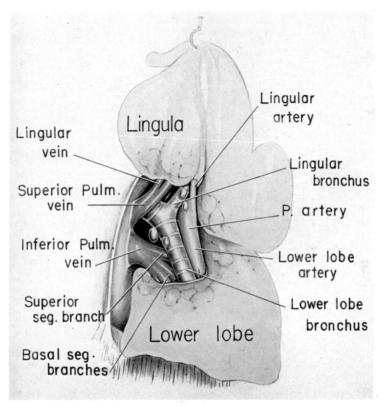

Fig. 26. Hilus of the left lung: anterior view of the structures seen in the dissection of the fissure.

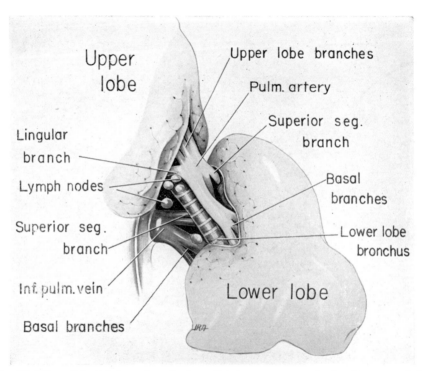

Fig. 27. Hilus of the left lung: lateral view of the structures seen in the dissection of the fissure.

Left   Lung

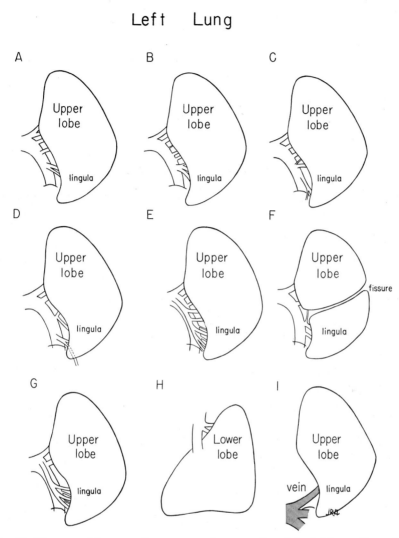

Fig. 28. Diagram of the more frequent vascular anomalies of the left lung. Upper lobe:
A, four branches of the pulmonary artery with lingular branch arising anteriorly instead of
beneath the fissure; *B*, six separate branches; *C*, five branches with branch from the lingular
artery to the lower lobe; *D*, four branches with branch of anterior segmental artery to the
lingula and a lingular branch to the lower lobe; *E*, six branches including anterior branch
with two subdivisions to the anterior segment and two to the lingula; *F*, complete fissure
making a separate lobe of the lingula with two lingular arteries; small branch of one of
these to the anterior segment; *G*, anterior origin of lingular artery with three branches.
Lower lobe: *H*, two separate superior segmental arteries; *I*, upper lobe vein emptying into
the inferior pulmonary vein.

CHAPTER 2

GENERAL TECHNICAL CONSIDERATIONS

ANESTHESIA

It is not within the scope of this book to present any detailed consideration of the physiologic, pharmacologic and technical aspects of the administration of anesthetics for thoracic surgery. For minor procedures, including the drainage of empyema or pulmonary abscess, local anesthesia with procaine hydrochloride is satisfactory. A 1 per cent solution should be introduced by a combination of regional block of the intercostal nerves and local infiltration. For all operations which involve a wide opening of the thoracic cavity, inhalation anesthesia (through a closed system with an inlying intratracheal tube) has become the standard procedure. This method is by far the safest means of securing anesthesia for major thoracic surgery if the anesthetic agent is administered with enough oxygen to maintain physiologically adequate oxygenation of the blood at all times. Attempts to perform open thoracotomies under local or spinal anesthesia are justifiable only under the most unusual circumstances.

The choice of anesthetic agent rests with the individual surgeon and the anesthetist, but accumulated experience suggests that a mixture of ether and oxygen is considerably safer than any of the other gases. Cyclopropane, which has the advantage of permitting a rapid recovery, is subject to the objections that there is a relatively small margin of safety between the light and the deep levels of anesthesia, and that it tends to slow the heart and in some cases to predispose to sudden cardiac arrest. Furthermore, there is the additional increased danger of explosion of the mixture which requires the observance of special precautions to prevent the occurrence of static electrical sparks in the operating room.

POSITION OF THE PATIENT ON THE OPERATING TABLE

Whenever an incision of any sort is made through the thoracic wall, it is important if at all possible to place the patient on an incline so that his head is lower than his chest. There are two important reasons for this: (1) to avoid the danger of air embolism to the cerebral vessels. This accident has been observed most frequently when operating in empyema or lung abscess cases with the patient in the sitting position. Such a position is allowable only when the patient is unable to lie down because of the tendency to cough or when there is serious impairment of the respiratory function because of a massive pleural effusion. (2) The danger of aspiration of secretions from the affected lungs into the other portions of the respiratory tract is lessened. This possibility is, of course, most marked in patients whose reflexes have been abolished by general anesthesia. The anesthetist must be ready at all times to empty the trachea and major bronchi by suction applied to a catheter which has been thrust down the intratracheal tube, or even to perform an emergency aspiration under direct vision through a bronchoscope. Such prompt action has saved the lives of many patients.

In general, three positions of the body are available for use. These are the lateral, the supine and the prone, with the patient lying respectively on his side, his back or face down.

The Lateral Position. The position which is most frequently employed by the majority of surgeons is the right or left lateral. This posture is more suitable for a wide variety of intrathoracic procedures, including operations upon the lung and the structures within the mediastinum, than either of the others. For pulmonary surgery it has this advantage: It gives ready access to both the anterior and the posterior surfaces of the hilus and makes adequate provision for the division of peripheral adhesions. It has these disadvantages: In pulmonary surgery the weight of the body rests upon the unaffected side, and the aspiration of secretions into the opposite lung is difficult to control. However, from the latter point of view, the alertness of an experienced anesthetist is all that is required to make the use of this position practicable.

To use the lateral recumbent position successfully the patient must lie squarely on the opposite side, with no tendency to lean either forward or backward. The arms are flexed in front of the face, with the uppermost extended somewhat and resting upon a pillow in a position convenient for the insertion of the intravenous infusion needle. This arm should not be suspended from the anesthetist's screen or strongly abducted in any direction because of the danger of injury resulting from traction upon the brachial plexus. The thighs should be flexed partially and a pillow inserted between the knees. A wide strap may be placed across the pelvis and fastened beneath the table to maintain the desired position once it has been obtained. The operating table should be inclined slightly so that the head of the patient is lower than his pelvis. In the majority of cases it is also helpful to place the patient in relation to the long axis of the table so that the lower portion of his chest lies over the point on the table from which the upper and lower halves can be made to slant (the so-called "break" in the table). This makes it possible to arch the patient's body slightly in order to facilitate the spreading

4

of the ribs on the side of operation. It is wise to place a pillow beneath the patient at that point. Figure 29 illustrates the correct use of the lateral position.

The Supine Position. For certain operations, notably those upon the heart and great vessels near the heart, for thymectomy, and for the removal of certain anterior mediastinal tumors, the supine position is necessary. Some

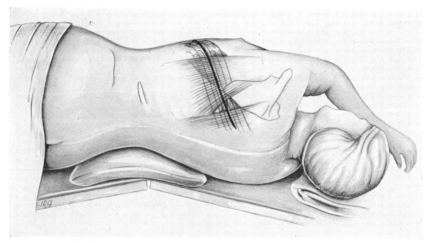

Fig. 29. Lateral thoracotomy position. Direction and location of standard thoracotomy incision over the seventh rib shown by dark line. Scapula and important muscles are shown in outline. Note the angulation of the table with pillow beneath the patient to arch the side of the operation so as to widen the intercostal spaces. The head is lower than pelvis.

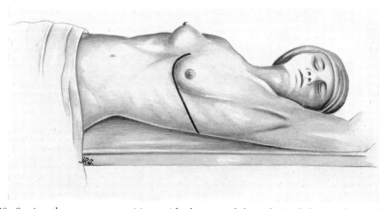

Fig. 30. Supine thoracotomy position with the arm abducted. Dark line indicates the site of the usual submammary incision.

surgeons employ this position for pulmonary surgery as well, especially with patients who have large amounts of secretions in the tracheobronchial tree as a result of suppurative or excavated lesions in the lung. No special description is required. One arm should be held in abduction for the purpose of administering the intravenous infusion. It should be laid on a nearby small table or a padded board or special arm rest extending out from the operating table at the shoulder level. Figure 30 serves to illustrate the supine position.

The Prone Position. The possibility of aspirating secretions into the opposite lung during the course of an operation may be diminished by using a prone position. This necessitates supporting the head and shoulders independently of the pelvis and lower extremities, leaving the chest free for manipulation. To accomplish this result an especially made operating table, such as that devised by Overholt, or some modification of the cerebellar attachment of the average table must be employed. The objections to this position, in addition to the necessity for special equipment, are (1) the anterior surface of the hilus of the lung is not readily accessible, and (2) certain procedures involving mediastinal viscera, particularly the esophagus, may not be so readily accomplished as with the lateral position. The principal

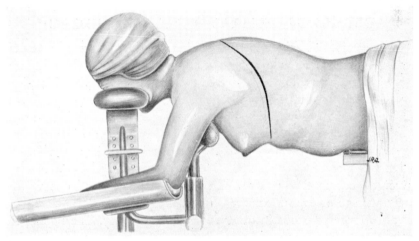

Fig. 31. Prone thoracotomy position. Note special support for the head and upper thorax, leaving the greater portion of the chest wall exposed for the making of the incision.

applicability of the prone position is in pulmonary surgery, especially in diseases such as bronchiectasis, lung abscess and tuberculosis with cavity formation in which there is an excess of secretions. Figure 31 demonstrates the appearance of the patient in the prone position.

No matter what position of the patient is used, however, whether lateral, supine or prone, the important consideration is to make certain what exposure is needed before the operation is started and to hold the patient in the position of choice by straps, sandbags, pillows or braces so that there will be no chance of shifting while the intrathoracic procedure is in progress.

ADMINISTRATION OF INTRAVENOUS INFUSIONS AND TRANSFUSIONS OF BLOOD

It is present established practice to administer saline or glucose solutions and blood during the progress of the operation in all major thoracotomy cases. Because the amount of blood lost in such operations is always considerable, varying by actual measurement from 300 to 1500 cc. or more, depending upon the type of case and the nature of the difficulties which may be encountered, it is wise to start a transfusion of whole blood concurrently with the making of the thoracotomy incision. For this purpose one of the ankle veins is used by many surgeons. It is preferable, however, to use a vein on the back of the hand or in the forearm of the side which lies uppermost. This is because experience has shown that there is less tendency for the transfusion to stop running if the arm is used and also because the functioning of the transfusion apparatus is more readily accessible to the anesthetist who should have the responsibility for its control along with his other duties. There is reason to believe, also, that infusions in the saphenous vein may predispose to the development of phlebothrombosis or thrombophlebitis of the leg veins during the early convalescent period.

DETAILS OF GENERAL OPERATIVE TECHNIC

It is convenient at this point to mention certain matters of a technical nature which have a wide application throughout the field of thoracic surgery and which need not be referred to again during the consideration of the specific operative procedures. In general, the sound principles of surgical technic which are used in other branches are equally applicable in the surgery of the chest. The minimization of trauma to tissues, the avoidance of mass ligatures, the maintenance of accurate hemostasis, and innumerable other small but important technical considerations which make the difference between an outstandingly successful surgical procedure and one which is of only average or even mediocre quality, apply as well to thoracic operations as to those practiced in other regions of the body. The fundamental principles are exactly the same.

Preservation of Asepsis. The maintenance of relative asepsis of the operative field is of just as much importance in thoracic surgery as in any other branch. The skin of the patient should be carefully cleansed by whatever method the surgeon may prefer. A thorough scrubbing with soap and water followed by the application of ether and finally of an antiseptic solution such as tincture of zephiran has proven to be a satisfactory routine procedure. With the exception of operations for the drainage of empyema or abscess, as soon as the incision has been made through the skin and subcutaneous fat, a sterile towel should be fastened to the skin edge on each side of the wound with a continuous suture or with towel clips. Michel skin clips are objectionable for this purpose because they may be lost in the wound. As soon as the chest has been opened through all layers, a protecting pad of gauze moistened in saline solution should be laid over each wound edge before the rib spreader is inserted. This tends to minimize trauma to the tissues of the wound edges and to prevent contamination of the wound in case an unsterile area should be entered during the course of the operation. In operations which require the opening of the esophagus or a bronchus, a second pair of gauze pads should be used to prevent soiling the wound itself and also the pleural cavity away from the immediate field of operation. In such cases, as soon as the unclean viscus has been closed and the field is once again relatively aseptic, the extra pair of gauze pads should be discarded and the members of the operative team should change their gloves before the closure of the incision is begun.

Prevention of Postoperative Empyema. It has been assumed without actual confirmation that the pleura is less resistant to the development of infection than the peritoneum. This impression is far from the truth. In fact, there is reason to believe that there is no significant difference in this respect between the two serous membranes. The apparent difference lies in the fact that accumulations of pus within the chest can be detected readily by physical examination, roentgenography and thoracentesis. Comparable accumulations in the abdominal cavity, on the other hand, can be discovered as a rule only with difficulty and sometimes, especially if localized among the loops of intestine, not at all. There is no doubt that many cases of localized peritonitis go undetected because of the impossibility of finding the focus, whereas in the chest the focus is nearly always readily discovered.

The incidence of postoperative empyema can be reduced in part by exerting special precautions to maintain relative asepsis in the field of operation as described above, but the utilization of penicillin and streptomycin in recent years has undoubtedly improved the results considerably. These important antibiotic agents should be administered in suitable doses preoperatively. The intramuscular administration of 100,000 units of penicillin four times a day and 0.5 gm. of streptomycin twice a day for two days before operation is an adequate preliminary preparation. This dosage is continued postoperatively for several days or until it is obvious that there is no further danger of the development of infection. If a lobectomy or pneumonectomy is performed, if the esophagus or stomach is opened, or if an abscess or bronchiectatic cavity is inadvertently entered during the course of the operation, a solution consisting of a mixture of 100,000 units of penicillin and 1 gm. of streptomycin in 30 cc. of saline solution should be instilled into the thoracic cavity before the wound is closed. In cases of carcinoma of the esophagus or stomach and in cases of diverticulum of the esophagus, it is wise to administer streptomycin, 0.25 gm. given four times a day by mouth in a gargle which is swallowed. This should be done for two days preceding operation in an attempt to reduce the bacterial content of the upper portion of the alimentary canal.

A further precaution which may be used in the prevention of postoperative infection of the pleural cavity is the employment of closed drainage during the first forty-eight hours or more after operation in any case in which the presence of contaminating bacteria may be suspected. It is well known that after almost every intrathoracic operation an effusion of serosanguineous fluid varying in amount from 200 to 500 cc. or more occurs, depending upon the type of case. This fluid comes in part from the division of vascular adhesions, from minute vessels in the mediastinum, from raw surfaces at

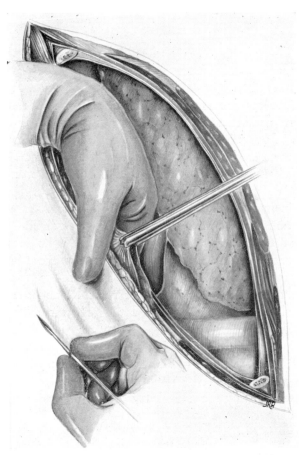

Fig. 32. First step in the insertion of a drainage catheter at the completion of a thoracic operation. The skin and muscle layers are drawn upward to their normal location so as to procure proper alignment for the short incision through which the catheter is to pass. The left hand of the surgeon is placed inside the chest wall to identify the correct intercostal space over which the skin incision is made as shown.

any point, and in a large measure from the edges of the thoracotomy incision itself. In pneumonectomy cases, because of the desirability of retarding the rapid shift of the mediastinum, and in the extirpative surgery of tuberculosis it is best not to drain the chest. If left alone the fluid will almost always disappear of itself. On the other hand, in cases in which contamination of the pleural cavity with pyogenic organisms may have occurred, especially when the esophagus or stomach has been opened or when a pulmonary procedure has been carried out because of a suppurative lesion, it is best to make provision for the egress of the effusion because it provides such a perfect culture medium for the growth of bacteria.

To accomplish this a short incision (0.5 cm.) is made through the skin over the posterolateral aspect of a lower intercostal space, such as the ninth. In order to be certain that the catheter will pass without angulation through the overlying muscle, fat and skin after the wound has been closed, these tissues are held in correct alignment by exerting traction on a tenaculum

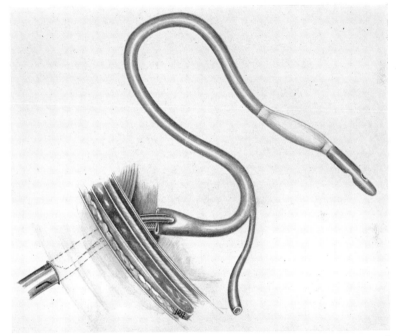

Fig. 33. Second step in the insertion of a drainage catheter. A curved hemostatic forceps inserted through the short intercostal incision is used to withdraw the catheter part way for the purpose of distending the balloon near its end.

forceps which is used to grasp the latissimus dorsi muscle. The jaws of a hemostatic forceps are then inserted through the intercostal space into the thoracic cavity and a catheter of suitable size (22 to 26) is grasped at its funnel-shaped open end and withdrawn through the chest wall, leaving its tip just inside the pleural cavity. A catheter of the Foley type made with a distensible balloon near its end makes a very satisfactory drain (Figs. 32, 33, 34). The catheter, whether of the plain or the Foley variety, is then held in place by means of a suture tied around it and attached to the skin. The outer end is closed temporarily by a ligature.

After the patient is returned to his room, the catheter is connected to a

long rubber tube which ends beneath the surface of a volume of water in a
large bottle placed on the floor, or it may be connected to a closed series of
three bottles which in turn are attached to a suction apparatus. The bottles

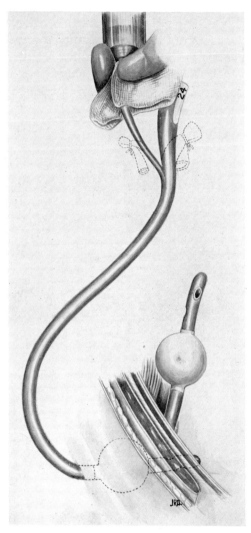

Fig. 34. Third step in the insertion of a drainage catheter. The balloon is distended by injecting it with saline solution. A fold of gauze is used to prevent the catheter slipping off
the syringe. The manner of occluding the ends of the catheter by ligatures is shown in
dotted lines. The ultimate position of the catheter in relation to the chest wall is shown by
the outline in dotted lines.

are arranged so that the first, to which the tube from the patient is attached,
provides a reservoir for the collection of fluid from the chest. This is in airtight continuity by means of a connecting link of tubing with a second
bottle which is half full of water. From the air space over the water a second

tube is connected to an empty bottle which in turn is in continuity with the source of suction. An air vent is provided in the second bottle in the form of a piece of glass tubing which passes deep beneath the surface of the water. Thus the purpose of the first bottle is to collect the fluid without having it mingle with the water. This makes it possible to make accurate measurements of the amount and to observe the characteristics of the fluid recovered. The second bottle makes it possible to control the degree of negative pressure exerted upon the chest by altering the depth of the air vent tube below the surface of the water. (Eight centimeters of negative pressure provides a satisfactory and safe degree of suction.) The third

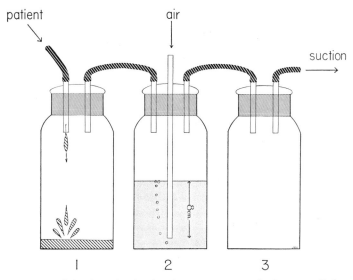

Fig. 35. Diagram of the three-bottle closed system to provide for controlled continuous suction on the chest drainage catheter with facilities for collecting the chest fluid (Bottle 1) and protection of the suction source (Bottle 3), as described in the text. The negative pressure in the catheter from the patient is the equivalent of the weight of the column of water expelled from the underwater length of the glass tube in Bottle 2 by the ingress of air in response to the negative pressure produced in the closed air chamber above the water. This is usually 8 cm. of water.

bottle provides a reservoir to collect water from the second bottle in case the incorrect adjustment of the apparatus might lead to its aspiration into the suction tubing. This protects the suction apparatus from injury (Fig. 35).

INSTRUMENTS REQUIRED FOR THORACIC SURGERY

As might be expected with a newly developed specialty such as thoracic surgery, innumerable specialized instruments have been devised for the performance of various technical procedures. Not all of these are necessary or even useful in the hands of the average surgeon. In general, it is best to avoid the use of unusual or complicated devices which have a limited field of applicability. Only those instruments which have been found particularly helpful will be mentioned. Many of those used in thoracic surgery are identical with those used in other fields or are adaptations of similar instruments. For the sake of convenience they are enumerated in groups as follows:

Group 1: Bone Instruments (Fig. 36). These include the costotomes, rongeurs, periosteal elevators, special bone-cutting instruments and rib approximators as follows:

1. Rongeur. Used for smoothing the ragged ends of rib after excision or fracture.

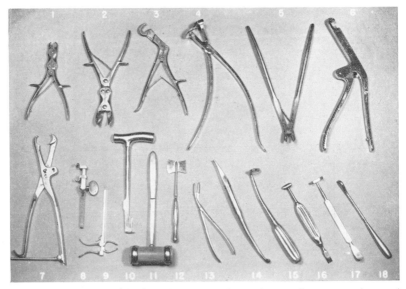

Fig. 36. Instruments used in thoracic surgery. Group 1: Bone instruments (see text).

2. Large Bone-cutting Forceps. For heavy work such as cutting the neck of the rib and tip of the transverse process in thoracoplasty; also for division of first rib cartilage. Various other uses as indicated.

3. Guillotine Type of Costotome. For cutting ribs at any point except the neck, where No. 5 is more useful.

4. Coryllos Costotome. For cutting the anterior portions of the ribs in the performance of a thoracoplasty. Its curved handles and transverse cutting jaws are a distinct advantage.

5. Bone-cutting Forceps of the Bethune Type. The instrument illustrated is actually a tack cutter which is used in the shoe manufacturing industry and has been adapted for use in thoracic surgery. It is used principally to cut across the neck of the rib.

6. First Rib Costotome, Sauerbruch Type. Rarely used nowadays. Was developed to divide the neck of the first rib.

7. Lambotte Bone-holding Forceps. Used in thoracic surgery as a rib approximator to facilitate closure of the incision (see Fig. 48).

8. Bailey Rib Approximator.

9. Rienhoff Rib Approximator.

10. Lebsche Sternum-cutting Knife.

11. Mallet. For use with sternum knife.

12. Saw. Used for transverse osteotomy of the sternum in the operation for correction of pectus excavatum.

13. Sequestrum Forceps. Used to hold small fragments of rib while they are being excised in order to prevent loss in thoracic cavity or the deep recesses of the incision.

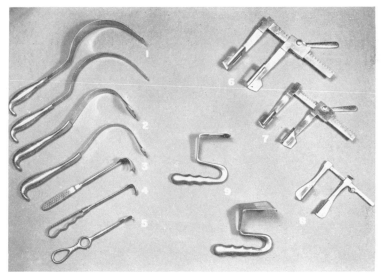

Fig. 37. Instruments used in thoracic surgery. Group 2: Retractors (see text).

14. Lewis Rib Periosteal Elevator. Valuable for general use.

15. Coryllos Modification of the Doyen Rib Periosteal Elevator.

16. Alexander Rib Periosteal Elevator. For general use.

17. Matson Rib Periosteal Elevator. Injury of the pleura is frequent with this instrument unless unusual care is exerted.

18. Sweet Rib Periosteal Elevator. Developed for use on the first rib during thoracoplasty.

Group 2: Retractors (Fig. 37).

1. Deaver Retractors. Used for retraction of the lung during esophagectomy in patients with a large chest. Two widths.

2. Harrington Retractors. For retraction of the lung during esophagectomy, repair of hiatus hernia, and similar operations. Two widths. The ferrule on the end tends to reduce the possibility of trauma to tissues.

3. Large Blunt Rake Retractor. For use on the muscles of the chest wall.

4. Small Richardson Type Retractor. Used in each end of thoracotomy incision to retract the muscles while the rib is being cut across.

5. Small Rake Retractor. Has many uses.

6 and 7. Finochietto Rib Retractors. Two sizes. A third and larger size is now available for patients with an unusually large chest. Other modifications with deeper blades, longer rack, curved bars, and so on are available for special uses. The two sizes shown are adequate for almost every occasion. The smaller size is intended for children but is too large for infants. It is the ideal size for separation of the edges of the sternum in anterior mediastinotomy sternum-splitting incisions.

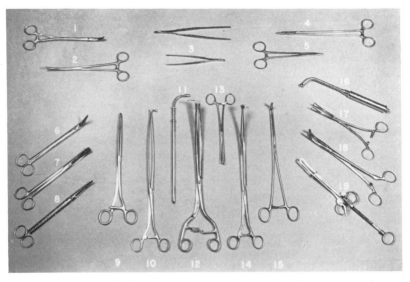

Fig. 38. Instruments used in thoracic surgery. Group 3: Special instruments for general use (see text).

8. Rienhoff Modification of the Tuffier Rib Retractor. For use in infants and small children. Three sizes are available. The set screw added by Rienhoff prevents slipping.

9. Davidson Scapula Retractors. Two widths. For retraction of the scapula during thoracoplasty. It is an unusually comfortable instrument for the assistant to hold.

Group 3: Special Instruments for General Use in Thoracic Surgery (Fig. 38).

1. Curved Hemostatic Forceps Having Long Handles and Short Pointed Jaws. This instrument, known ordinarily as the Moynihan cystic duct clamp, is invaluable in many thoracic operations, especially in pulmonary and esophageal surgery.

2. Full-length Hemostatic Forceps. This is the old-fashioned clamp developed originally for securing vessels in the broad ligament during

hysterectomy as performed in the early days of abdominal surgery. It is useful because of its length and slender jaws.

3. Thumb Forceps with Atraumatic Teeth. For grasping mucosa in anastomotic surgery of stomach and esophagus. Long and short sizes.

4. Wangensteen Needle Holder. This is invaluable in the performance of a high intrathoracic esophagogastric anastomosis.

5. Adson Needle Holder. For anastomotic work.

6. Sweet Bent Scissors. For division of the esophagus during esophagectomy.

7. Large Long Heavy Curved Scissors.

8. Long Mayo Type Dissecting Scissors.

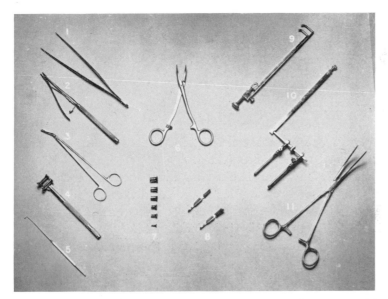

Fig. 39. Instruments used in thoracic surgery. Special instruments for surgery of the great vessels (see text).

9. Short Blade Fenestrated Gastric Clamp, Moynihan Type.

10. Straight Scudder Gastric Clamp. For closure of divided stomach by suture through the fenestrated blades.

11. Allen Aspirating Trocar. Shown with guard sheath in place. Used for aspirating fluid from the stomach during esophagogastric anastomosis.

12. Curved Kocher Crushing Gastric Clamp. Sometimes used in partial esophagectomy and gastrectomy.

13. Collin Type Mucosa Holding Forceps. Used chiefly to grasp the jejunum.

14. Curved Scudder Gastric Clamp. Otherwise same as 11.

15. Long Flexible Right Angle Clamp, Modified Mixter Type. Used to

grasp the esophagus distal to the level of transection during esophagectomy. Sometimes used to grasp the bronchus in the same manner during lobectomy or pneumonectomy.

16. Light. Can be sterilized along with other instruments, connected by sterilized wire cord to battery or rheostat. Used for transillumination of adhesions.

17. Large Duval Forceps. Used to grasp the portion of lung which is to be removed.

18. Curved Kidney Pedicle Clamp. To clamp the bronchus distal to the level of transection during pneumonectomy.

19. Bethune Lung Tourniquet. Now rarely used. Should be ready for emergencies.

Group 4: Instruments for Surgery of the Great Vessels (Fig. 39).

1. Long Delicate Smooth Thumb Forceps.
2. Needle Holder.
3. Bent Scissors (Lateral Angle).
4. Aorta Clamp. Three sizes available.
5. Suture Hook.

The above instruments were developed by Potts and his associate, Smith, for the performance of a lateral anastomosis between the left pulmonary artery and the descending aorta (Chap. 7).

6. Short Curved Forceps. Used for blunt dissection behind a patent ductus arteriosus in preparation for ligation or division.

7. Blakemore Vitallium Tubes. For blood vessel anastomosis.

8. Bulldog Clamps. For temporary occlusion of blood vessels.

9. Blalock Clamp. Used in blood vessel anastomosis for tetralogy of Fallot. Three sizes are available.

10. Bradshaw Clamp. Used for temporary occlusion of the aorta during excision of coarctation followed by end-to-end anastomosis.

11. Crafoord Aorta Occlusion Clamps. For coarctation operation.

Mention will be made of the uses of the majority of the instruments enumerated as the various operations are described.

CHAPTER 3

THORACIC INCISIONS

Thoracotomy incisions may be classified as minor or major according to their size and the purpose for which they are used. In the first category are those which are made to drain accumulations of pus in the pleural cavity, within the lung, or occasionally in the subdiaphragmatic space or the liver. Small thoracic incisions are sometimes used also to secure biopsy material from the chest wall itself or from intrathoracic tumors which have invaded it or become adherent to it. In the second category are those which are used for major operations upon the thoracic wall, such as thoracoplasty or excision of tumors of the ribs or sternum, and all those which are made for the purpose of performing surgical procedures on any part of the intrathoracic viscera. In each type accurate placement and adequate exposure are of fundamental importance.

MINOR THORACOTOMY INCISIONS

With the exception of closed thoracotomy for the continuous aspiration of air or fluid or the occasional performance of a biopsy of a tumor of the chest wall, short incisions through the structures of an intercostal space are inadequate for any purpose. In the majority of cases where a short thoracotomy incision is required, a segment of rib must be removed.

The relation between the inclination of the ribs and the direction of the incision through the skin, fat and muscles depends upon the purpose for which the incision is to be used. For the drainage of empyema the most important consideration is to have the drainage tube at the bottom of the cavity. In many cases an accurate determination of the rib which must be resected to accomplish this result can be made. In that event it is satisfactory to make the incision through the soft parts in the direction of the rib which is to be resected. When there is uncertainty as to the probable level of the deepest portion of the cavity, however, it is preferable to make the incision through the soft parts vertical in relation to the chest so that it lies across the long axis of the ribs beneath it. In this way, if the rib chosen for resection happens to lie too high, it is a simple matter to obtain dependent drainage by resecting a segment of the next rib below through the same incision, which can be enlarged downward for the purpose. Thus shelving edges and undermined pockets in the soft parts of the chest wall near the place of exit of the drainage tube are avoided.

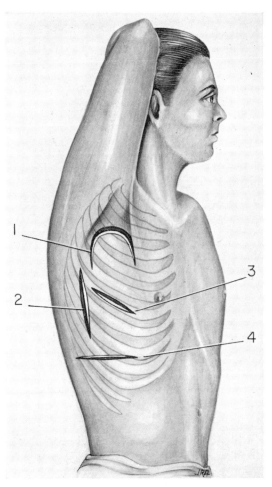

Fig. 40. Minor thoracotomy incisions for drainage of empyema and lung abscess. *1*, Inverted U-shaped axillary incision for drainage of abscesses in the upper lobe of the lung. *2*, Vertical incision over two or more adjacent ribs for drainage of empyema or abscess in the apex of the lung. For the latter it must be made between the medial border of the scapula and the spine. *3*, Oblique incision in the direction of a rib used in certain cases of empyema or pulmonary abscess where localization is accurate. *4*, Transverse incision used in transpleural drainage of subdiaphragmatic or liver abscesses.

In the drainage of lung abscess, on the other hand, localization of the focus can usually be made so accurate that a simple incision in the direction of the rib which has been chosen for resection is satisfactory. If the abscess is located in the anterior or posterior segment of the upper lobe, presenting on the axillary surface, an inverted U-shaped incision is often superior to a linear incision in the direction of the ribs or vertical in the midaxillary line. Furthermore, when a transthoracic approach is chosen for the drainage of a subdiaphragmatic or hepatic abscess, it is convenient to make the incision transversely across the lower chest wall so that a segment of rib anterior or posterior to that originally decided upon for resection can be removed. This is made necessary because of the great obliquity of the ribs in the lower part of the chest. Figure 40 illustrates the four types of short thoracic incision mentioned.

Technic of Rib Resection

After the direction and position have been decided upon, a short incision (3 to 5 inches in length) is made through the skin, fat and muscles. The blood vessels are ligated and the soft parts are retracted so as to expose the rib beneath. An incision of sufficient length is made through the periosteum

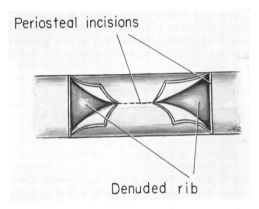

Fig. 41. Technic of rib resection. Correct placement of incisions in the periosteum to avoid necrosis of rib ends in empyema or abscess cases.

in the long axis of the rib. At each end of this incision the periosteum should be incised transversely across the rib (Fig. 41). If this is not done, the parting of the edges of the lengthwise periosteal incision leaves a V-shaped portion of the bone which is not covered by periosteum, and necrosis and sequestration of a small fragment of bone at the cut end may take place. The presence of these bony sequestra may not become known until years later when they may be the inciting cause of a recurrent abscess in the depths of the incisional scar. The leaves of periosteum which have been outlined by these incisions are pushed aside with a raspatory and the deep periosteal investment of the rib is freed, using an elevator of the Doyen type. The rib is then cut close to the edge of the transverse incision through the periosteum at each end of the denuded segment which is to be removed. The incision is completed by cutting through the deep periosteal layer and the underlying pleura.

Special Considerations. Because such an incision is usually used for the drainage of empyema or a lung abscess, an opening through the pleura wider than that provided by a simple linear incision is required. This is obtained by excising semicircular portions of periosteum and pleura from each edge of the original incision through these membranes so as to secure a round or oval opening. In some cases, especially for the unroofing and packing of a lung abscess, it is necessary to enlarge the entire wound by the resection of a segment of one of the adjacent ribs and the wide excision of the subjacent periosteum and pleura. In this event portions of the intervening intercostal muscles and sections of the corresponding intercostal nerve and vessels must be removed. In every case, after resecting the rib segment it is advisable to excise a section of the corresponding intercostal nerve to minimize the pain from the pressure of the rubber drainage tube, and of the intercostal vessels to avoid the danger of secondary hemorrhage resulting from pressure necrosis.

Whenever an incision through the thoracic wall is to be used for prolonged drainage of an abscess or empyema, it should be made larger than would seem at first to be necessary because of the striking tendency of the incision to contract as the result of the healing of the tissues at its edges. In general, the greatest difficulty encountered in the after-care in such cases is the tendency of the wound to close prematurely.

MAJOR THORACOTOMY INCISIONS

The purpose for which a major thoracotomy is used demands the procurement of a wide exposure of the region within the chest which is to be the site of the surgical procedure. The choice of the position and direction of the incision in relation to the chest wall depends upon the location of the lesion and the locale of the greatest expected technical difficulty. In the case of an inflammatory process in the periphery of a lobe of the lung, the incision should be relatively high or low depending upon whether the process lies in the apical region of the upper lobe or in the basal segments of the lower lobe, with corresponding variations for localization of the lesion in segments between these extremes. If, on the other hand, the greatest difficulty is likely to be experienced at the hilus of the lung, the incision must be placed so as to secure the best exposure of that region, disregarding to some extent the possibility of difficulties at the periphery. Also in the case of operations within the mediastinum, the position of the incision across the chest should depend upon the level at which the lesion lies.

Furthermore, in placing the incision, it is important to consider the physical build of the patient. In those with a long narrow chest it is of greater importance to have the incision high or low in relation to the long axis of the thorax, depending upon the location of the lesion, than in a patient whose chest is short. In the patient whose chest is long, the incision should be unusually oblique, whereas in the patient with a short, broad chest it should have a more transverse inclination. These variations are necessary because of the characteristic differences in the obliquity of the ribs in the two types of body build.

A further consideration of importance, especially in young women, is the avoidance of disfigurement. Thus incisions which are carried transversely across the upper portion of the chest above the breast should be avoided. This is easily accomplished, even if a high exposure is required, by making the anterior portion of the incision below the breast or in the submammary fold and retracting the breast and pectoral muscle upward. Likewise, if it is necessary to operate upon the sternum or to enter the mediastinum anteriorly, a much better appearance is obtained by using a straight midline incision over the sternum than by elevating curved or U-shaped lateral flaps. If the elevation of a flap is necessary, the curved incision should be made in a transverse direction. If possible one should also avoid upward extensions of the posterior end of a thoracotomy incision too close to the shoulder because of the unsightliness of the scar in that region. In no case, however, should such cosmetic considerations be allowed to take precedence over the importance of obtaining a satisfactory exposure of the field of operation within the thoracic cavity.

Relative Merits of the Intercostal and Rib Resection Technics. There has been considerable discussion concerning the relative merits of the intercostal incisions versus those which involve the resection of a long segment of rib. The principles which apply to the use of these two types of incision can be reduced to simple terms.

An incision made through an intercostal space has the advantage that it can be made and closed rapidly. This is an important consideration in children because they do not tolerate long thoracic operations quite as well as adults. In children, also, the use of the intercostal incision eliminates the possibility that removing a rib might bring about structural abnormalities of the chest resulting from alterations in development, although this danger has been overemphasized in the past. In adults beyond the age of 30 years, and especially in elderly patients, the use of an intercostal incision is likely to be complicated by annoying fractures of the adjacent ribs as a result of the use of the rib spreader, no matter how carefully it may be applied. In this group, therefore, the rib resection technic is to be preferred because of the greater ease of obtaining an adequate exposure without the necessity for dividing the adjacent ribs. As a general rule it is best to confine the use of the intercostal type of incision to operations upon children of all ages and upon adults not more than 30 years of age, depending upon the apparent relative rigidity of the chest wall.

There is some reason for the belief that patients who have had an intercostal incision experience a shorter period of postoperative intercostal neuralgia than those who have been operated upon by the rib resection technic. This possibility, however, depends upon certain technical aspects such as the use of nonabsorbable pericostal sutures for closure and the avoidance of cutting the adjacent ribs to improve the exposure. Persistent, long-lasting pain is unusual, however, in either case.

TECHNIC OF MAJOR THORACOTOMY

Standard Thoracotomy Incision. Major thoracotomy incisions of several types are used according to the indications of the case and the preference of

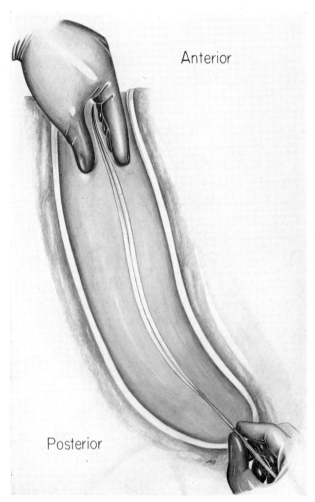

Anterior

Posterior

Fig. 42. Standard thoracotomy incision. First step: Incision through the skin.

the individual surgeon. There are few intrathoracic operations, however, which cannot be performed with maximum ease through a long incision extending from close to the nipple line in front almost to the region of the vertebral column behind (Fig. 29). This incision has such a wide field of usefulness that it may be called the *standard thoracotomy incision*. It is sometimes spoken of as *posterolateral*. This term is misleading because if it is to be completely successful, the incision must extend anteriorly as well. Through such an incision adequate exposure can be obtained for all operations upon the lung and for the majority of operations on the structures within the mediastinum.

The deep portion of the incision is made either through an intercostal space or through the bed of a rib, depending upon the age of the patient, the amount of exposure required, and to some extent upon the purpose of the operation and the personal preference of the surgeon. No matter whether

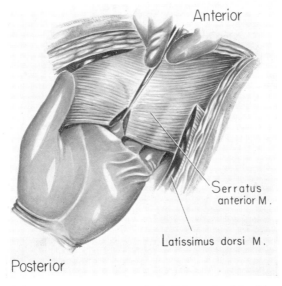

Anterior

Serratus anterior M.

Latissimus dorsi M.

Posterior

Fig. 43. Standard thoracotomy incision. Method of decreasing blood loss during the transection of the muscles by making pressure with the fingers from beneath while the muscle is being cut across.

a rib is resected or not, the incision through the soft parts is essentially the same (Fig. 42). After the skin and fat have been incised, a towel is attached to each skin edge by means of towel clips made especially for the purpose or a continuous suture of silk. The division of the muscle layers is begun by cutting across the latissimus dorsi muscle. In order to minimize the amount of blood lost as a result of cutting across the many vessels which must be severed during the transection of this and the other large shoulder girdle muscles, it is helpful to insert the fingers of one hand beneath the muscle. As the muscle is cut across, upward pressure is exerted by the fingers. This stops the bleeding from the vessels until hemostatic forceps can be applied. This maneuver is of great importance when making the incision for an operation in cases of coarctation of the aorta where the collateral vessels in the chest wall are enormously enlarged. By its use much loss of blood is prevented (Fig. 43). As the posterior portion of the incision is deepened, it is usually necessary to divide the lateral fibers of the trapezius muscle and sometimes of the rhomboid muscles, especially when the incision is being made relatively high (at or above the level of the seventh

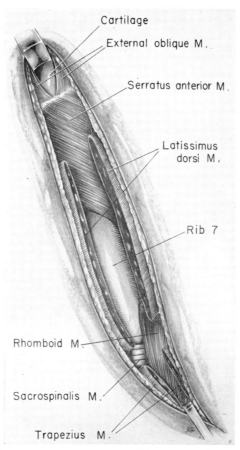

Cartilage

External oblique M.

Serratus anterior M.

Latissimus dorsi M.

Rib 7

Rhomboid M.

Sacrospinalis M.

Trapezius M.

Fig. 44. Standard thoracotomy incision. View of the incision after division of the latissimus dorsi muscle and partial division of the lower portion of the trapezius muscle; rib partially exposed.

rib). In low incisions these two muscles are not encountered unless the trapezius happens to be unusually wide. All of the muscles just mentioned have no costal attachments, so that the level at which they are divided need not be exact. On the other hand, before the muscles of the anterior thoracic wall are cut, a definite choice of rib or interspace must be made because of their insertion into the ribs. This can be predetermined by palpation through the skin before the incision is made, counting the ribs upward from the twelfth. The choice of rib may also be made by counting downward from the first rib, using direct palpation with the fingers inserted beneath the scapula after the latissimus dorsi muscle has been severed (Fig. 44).

If the incision is to be intercostal, it is carried forward through the serratus anterior and obliquus abdominalis externus muscles at a point where their fibers which insert into the ribs can be avoided. If a rib is to be resected, the incision is made through the interdigitations of these muscles and their rib insertions. From this step on, certain differences make it important to give separate consideration to the two methods of opening the rib cage.

INTERCOSTAL METHOD. A short preliminary incision is made with a scalpel through the intercostal muscles midway between the adjacent ribs at any suitable point. The pleura is opened and the lung is allowed to fall away from the thoracic wall. The remainder of the incision can be completed with either the knife or the scissors. If the lung is adherent to the parietal pleura, the knife is the more convenient. As the incision is lengthened, several small branches of the intercostal arteries which cross the intercostal space between the muscle layers will be encountered. These are found, one not far from the sternum, one close to the costochondral junction, several in the lateral aspect of the intercostal space, and another posterior to the angle of the rib. As the posterior extension of the incision approaches the region of the necks of the ribs, it should be made close to the superior margin of the inferior rib so as to avoid the intercostal vessels of the rib above as they cross the intercostal space to reach its lower margin.

If an adequate exposure is to be obtained through the intercostal space, the incision must extend from beyond the costochondral junction anteriorly to the region of the neck of the rib posteriorly. If a shorter opening is made it is almost always necessary to divide one or both of the adjacent ribs. This is usually done posteriorly. This manipulation should be avoided, however, because of the possibility of increasing the severity of the postoperative pain as a result of traumatizing one or both of the corresponding intercostal nerves.

RIB RESECTION METHOD. The rib periosteum is incised from the costochondral junction in front to the neck of the rib posteriorly. The periosteum is freed from the rib with a raspatory such as that developed by Alexander, Lewis or Matson. Because of the direction of the insertion of the fibers of the intercostal muscles, the freeing of the attachments to the edges of the rib is best accomplished by passing the instrument from back to front along the superior margin and from front to back along the inferior margin. The T-shaped end of the Alexander rib periosteal elevator, which is especially constructed for this manipulation, accomplishes the purpose admirably. The corresponding end of the Lewis elevator is equally useful. The deep surface of the rib is freed from its periosteum with an elevator of the Doyen type. These manipulations are illustrated in Figure 45. The rib is then cut

through the neck posteriorly and in front through the cartilage just anterior
to the costochondral junction. The reason for cutting through the cartilage
is to avoid both the inconvenience of tearing a glove on a spicule of bone
during the operation and the danger of traumatizing the reexpanded lung

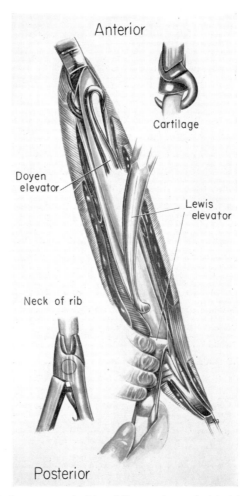

Fig. 45. Standard thoracotomy incision (rib resection technic). Muscles are completely
divided. Three phases of the elevation of the periosteum are shown, using the Lewis elevator
to strip the outer aspect of the rib and to free the edges, and the Doyen elevator to free the
inner surface of the rib. Inserts show the technic of transection of the neck of the rib posteriorly and the cartilage anteriorly.

after the chest wall has been closed. After the rib has been resected, the
pleural cavity is opened through a short incision made with a scalpel and
the entire length of the rib periosteum and underlying pleura is incised with
the knife or scissors (Fig. 46).

If the underlying lung is adherent, straight hemostatic forceps should be attached at intervals along each pleural edge for retraction by an assistant. If the surgeon then makes counterpressure against the lung so as to place the adhesions on the stretch, their division is made easier. The knife or scissors may be used, but if curved scissors are employed, the points should be directed away from the surface of the lung.

In order to secure a sufficient exposure of the interior of the thorax it is necessary to spread the wound edges with a mechanical rib retractor of some

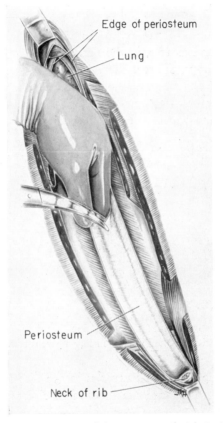

Edge of periosteum

Lung

Periosteum

Neck of rib

Fig. 46. Standard thoracotomy incision (rib resection technic). Incision of the periosteum and parietal pleura. The fingers of the surgeon's left hand are inserted to hold the lung away from the points of the scissors.

type. By far the best instrument available at the present time for this purpose is that designed by Finochietto (Fig. 37). It is available in adult and child sizes. This instrument is strong yet simple in construction and does not shift its position once it has been placed in the wound. For infants and very young children, one of the small sizes of the Tuffier rib retractor (or the Rienhoff modification) should be used. The spreading of the incision should be accomplished gradually, especially in elderly patients, in order to minimize the possibility of fracturing the adjacent ribs.

Enlargement of the Incision. If the exposure obtained through a standard thoracotomy incision is inadequate, the wound can be enlarged in one of two ways. The first method is by dividing one or more ribs posteriorly (Fig. 47). When this is necessary, it is wise to excise a 1 cm. segment of the neck of the rib in order to prevent friction between the two cut ends during the early postoperative period. It is likewise expedient to ligate and divide the intercostal vessels and to interrupt the nerve so as to avoid the results of trauma to these structures by the motion of the severed end of the rib. This applies particularly when more than one rib has to be cut. If it is necessary to secure better access to the region beneath the anterior end of the incision, as, for example, in the performance of a transthoracic gastrectomy or splenectomy, the second method of enlargement is used. This consists in cutting across the costochondral arch and incising the upper

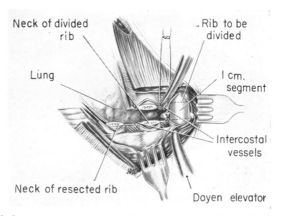

Fig. 47. Standard thoracotomy incision (rib resection technic). Method of enlarging the incision posteriorly by cutting adjacent ribs.

portion of the oblique abdominal muscles in the direction of the incision. It is rarely necessary to enlarge the incision in either direction when the rib resection technic has been used, provided an adequate segment has been removed.

Closure of the Incision. The closure of a standard thoracotomy incision is a relatively simple matter and does not require a deepening of the plane of anesthesia. In the case of an intercostal incision, the first layer consists of a row of pericostal sutures passed with a large curved needle through the intercostal spaces above and below the ribs which were separated. A rib approximator is then applied so as to hold the ribs as close together as they normally lie and the sutures are tied. Various especially developed instruments are available for this maneuver. None of these is necessary, however, if a Lambotte bone-holding forceps is at hand. The jaws of this instrument can be made to straddle the ribs and grasp them by their edges. The ratchet holds the ribs in the position desired and the sutures can then be tied (Fig. 48). If no instrument which is particularly adapted for the approximation of the ribs is available, the same result may be accomplished by using a tenaculum forceps, a towel clip or two small sharp rake retractors held across the wound by an assistant. If the rib approximation is difficult, especially in a heavy individual with a large chest, considerable assistance is gained by restoring the operating table to a level position, thus eliminating the lateral bend in the patient's thorax. In small children the ribs are best

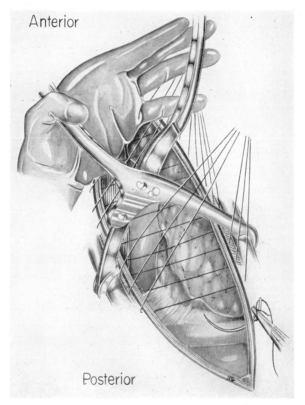

Fig. 48. Standard thoracotomy incision (rib resection technic). Closure of incision using Lambotte bone-holding forceps as a rib approximator. Sutures (all but the last) in place ready for tying.

approximated by the thumb and forefinger of the surgeon or his assistant. Pericostal sutures should be of chromicized catgut and not of wire, silk or other nonabsorbable material. In the closure of an incision made by the rib resection technic, the first layer consists of a row of silk sutures passed through the periosteum and subjacent pleura. After the sutures have been placed, the rib approximator is applied and the sutures are tied.

The remainder of the wound closure in both types of incision should be in layers. The divided edges of the muscles are approximated with two rows of sutures, one row placed in the deep fascial investment of each muscle and a second row used to bring together the superficial fascial investment. In the case of the latissimus dorsi muscle, which is thick in a well-developed patient, a third layer should be used in the center of the muscle edges to avoid leaving a dead space for the collection of serum. After the muscle approximation has been completed, the superficial fascial layer in the subcutaneous fat is sutured, and finally the skin. The choice of suture material, of course, rests with the surgeon. Interrupted silk sutures are highly satisfactory. If haste in closure is required because of the unsatisfactory condition of the patient, continuous chromic catgut sutures may be used after the first layer has been completed.

COMPLICATIONS AND SEQUELAE. FRACTURE OF RIBS. As a result of the forceful spreading of the edges of the wound, fractures of the ribs adjacent to the blades of the rib spreader may occur. This is true particularly in the case of intercostal incisions. Such fractures occur usually either at the point where the force of the blade of the instrument is applied or at some point posterior to the angle of the rib. In the first instance the fracture may be double, with a fragment of rib somewhat longer than the width of the retractor blade pushed aside and isolated from the remaining anterior and posterior segments. These fractures are usually irregular and leave jagged projections from the rib ends. In order to prevent injuries to the lung or intercostal vessels as well as to decrease the degree of postoperative pain, these jagged edges should be cut back with a costotome so as to produce smooth ends. The intercostal vessels should be inspected and tied if they have been injured, in order to prevent subsequent hemorrhage into the pleural cavity.

INJURY TO THE INTERCOSTAL NERVES. The avoidance of pain or paresthesia in the regions innervated by the intercostal nerve is an important consideration in the after-care of the patient. Long-lasting pain is an unusual occurrence after a thoracic incision if care is exerted to avoid injuring the nerve. Characteristically there is considerable acute pain which subsides within one or two weeks. After that there may be a period of gradually diminishing dull pain lasting from a few weeks to several months, or there may be an area of anesthesia or hypesthesia in the region of the anterior chest or upper abdominal wall supplied by the corresponding intercostal nerve, which is soon followed by hyperesthesia in the same area. This gives way in due course to a return of normal sensation.

Various methods of avoiding postoperative pain, including division or crushing of the nerve and the injection of long-lasting local anesthetic agents, have been advocated. These methods, however, are actually more likely to create greater discomfort after the anesthetic effect begins to wane, or when the proximal cut or crushed end begins to regenerate, than if the nerve is left undisturbed. The best results are obtained by avoiding the nerve in the placing of sutures and by using absorbable pericostal sutures for the closure of intercostal incisions.

In the case of low thoracic incisions, if there happens to be a permanent injury to the ninth or tenth intercostal nerves such as would result from crushing them with a hemostatic forceps, flaccidity and bulging of the musculature of the upper abdominal quadrant become annoying sequelae.

SPECIAL THORACIC INCISIONS

Under certain circumstances specialized thoracotomy incisions which do not have a wide application may be necessary. The specific indications for the use of these will be mentioned when the operations for which they are most appropriate are described.

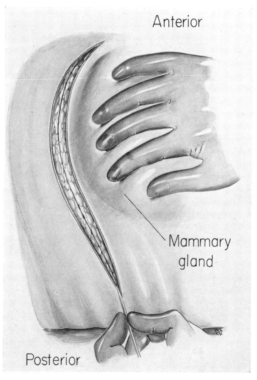

Fig. 49. Anterolateral intercostal incision. First step: Skin incision beneath the breast with lateral extension posteriorly.

Anterolateral Intercostal Incision. This incision is useful occasionally for the removal of anterior mediastinal tumors in certain cases when it appears that the standard thoracotomy incision might not be satisfactory. This situation is unusual. In the majority of such cases a better approach is by median sternotomy. Some surgeons employ it for pulmonary resections. From the purely technical aspect it is not so satisfactory for this purpose as the standard incision because it does not allow such ready access to the posterior aspect of the hilus of the lung or to adherent portions of the periphery of the lung in the costovertebral gutter. It is useful, however, in certain patients who have a large amount of secretion from the lung which is to be operated upon, because the dorsal recumbent position of the patient diminishes the possibility of aspiration of material into the opposite lung. The advantage in such cases arises, therefore, not from the technical superiority of the incision itself, but from the position of the patient during the progress of the

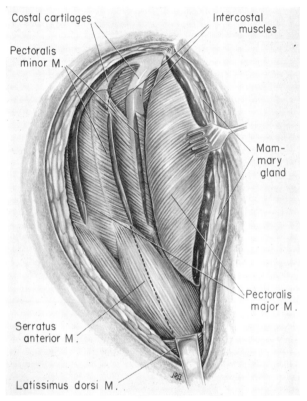

Fig. 50. Anterolateral intercostal incision. Pectoral muscles divided and retracted, revealing the ribs and intercostal muscles beneath.

operation. This purpose can be accomplished more successfully by placing the patient in the face-down position and by using a standard posterolateral thoracotomy.

TECHNIC. The patient is placed on his back. If it is likely that an unusually long posterior extension of the incision will be required, the shoulder and chest of the side to be operated upon is propped forward on low pillows or sandbags to allow greater access to the posterolateral region. The arm on the side of the operation is held in the position of abduction. This arm may then be used for the intravenous infusion. The skin incision begins close to the midline in front and extends beneath the breast to the region of the posterior axillary line (Fig. 49). The pectoralis major, the serratus anterior, and sometimes a portion of the latissimus dorsi muscle are divided, exposing the rib cage beneath (Fig. 50). A large retractor is used to reflect the soft parts, including the breast, so that any appropriate intercostal space can be entered. The fourth or fifth space is frequently chosen and entered by the technic described under the section dealing with the intercostal variation of the standard thoracotomy incision. Anteriorly care should be exerted to avoid injury to the internal mammary vessels. If they happen to be injured or if it seems to be necessary to divide the intercostal muscles all the way to the edge of the sternum, these vessels should be severed and both ends ligated.

It is not possible to obtain a wide exposure with this incision unless it is extended a long distance posteriorly, usually beyond the angles of the adjacent ribs, or unless the costal cartilages of these ribs are divided close to their sternal insertions. Even when the intercostal incision is long, it may be necessary to cut the cartilages. When this is done, the corresponding intercostal vessels and nerves must be ligated and divided in order to take full advantage of the amount of lateral retraction of the anterior portions of the ribs which is thus made possible.

The closure of the incision is made in the same manner as for any intercostal incision, using pericostal sutures of chromic catgut as the first layer. Abnormal mobility of the anterior ends of the divided ribs is prevented by using sutures of steel wire or heavy silk passed through the ends of the cartilages. This step should not be omitted. The usual layer by layer muscle approximation is made and separate layers of sutures are used for the superficial fascia and skin.

No special after-care is required.

Anterior Mediastinotomy (*Sternum-splitting Incision*). For direct access to the anterior mediastinum for the removal of the thymus gland, aberrant parathyroid or thyroid glands, or certain anterior mediastinal tumors, a midline incision through the center of the sternum is superior to all others.

TECHNIC. The incision through the skin begins with a short transverse extension across the base of the neck 1 or 2 cm. above the suprasternal notch. From the center of this cervical incision a long vertical extension is made straight down the midline over the sternum to the end of the gladiolus. After the protecting towels have been sutured to the skin edges, the wound is deepened through the fat and the superficial fascia to the periosteum of the sternum which is incised but not elevated from the surface of the bone. In the cervical portion of the incision a deep plane of dissection is exposed between the medial edges of the sternohyoid and sternothyroid muscles. By spreading the ends of a pair of curved scissors, with the tips of the blades directed against the deep surface of the manubrium, the anterior mediastinum is entered and, with the index finger of the left hand, the loose areolar attachments to the bone are pushed aside as far downward as can be reached. The midline cleavage of the sternum is begun at the suprasternal notch using either a sternum-cutting shears or the Lebsche sternum knife. The latter instrument has the advantage that it makes a neat clean cut with a minimum

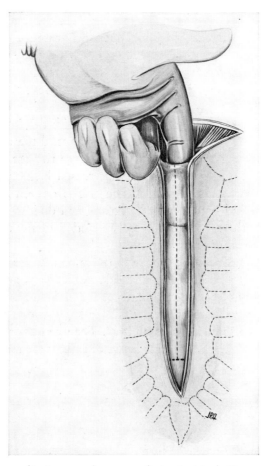

Fig. 51. Anterior mediastinotomy (sternum-splitting incision). First step: Skin and fascial incisions completed; index finger inserted behind the sternum from above to free the posterior attachments. Outline of sternum and rib cartilages shown in dotted lines.

of trauma. The knife is propelled from above downward by the tapping of a mallet directed against the surface which is provided for that purpose. The head of the mallet should be of nonmetallic material so as to avoid the possibility of striking sparks which might lead to explosion of the anesthetic gases. This is of especial importance when cyclopropane and oxygen are being used. It is rarely necessary to divide the entire sternum to secure adequate exposure of the anterior mediastinum. The vertical incision in the bone is carried to the level of the fourth or fifth intercostal space where a transverse cut is made across the gladiolar portion, using the sternum knife which is introduced beneath one edge of the bone, care being taken to avoid injury to the internal mammary vessels. The edge of the sternum should be freed of muscle and fascial attachments with the scissors before applying the knife to it (Figs. 51 and 52).

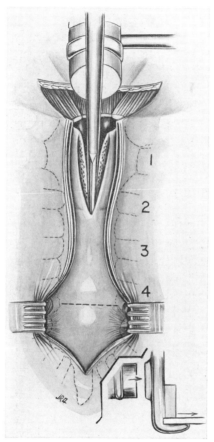

Fig. 52. Anterior mediastinotomy (sternum-splitting incision). Second step: Longitudinal cleavage of the sternum with the Lebsche sternum-cutting knife. Site of transverse section through the gladiolus shown as a broken line. Insert shows the direction of the impact of the mallet against the knife.

The cut edges of the bone tend to bleed freely. In some cases this bleeding is difficult to control. It is wise as a routine measure, therefore, to place strips of fibrin foam along each edge of the bone before the protecting pads of gauze are applied. The smallest Finochietto rib spreader or one of the Tuffier or Rienhoff retractors is used to force the edges of the sternum apart and the desired exposure of the anterior mediastinum is thereby obtained with ease.

5

The closure of a sternum-splitting incision is simple. No bone fixation sutures are required. After the retractor and gauze pads have been removed, the edges of the bone are inspected and if the fibrin foam strips have been displaced, they are readjusted or new ones are applied. A layer of interrupted medium heavy (00) silk sutures is then placed in the periosteum and tied. The fixation of the bone thus obtained is strengthened by the next layer which is used to approximate the deep fascia over the bone. The superficial fascia and skin constitute the remaining layers.

AFTER-CARE. A small gauze dressing is held firmly in place with adhesive plaster, preferably of the woven elastic type. If the closure of the wound has been made with care, there is relatively little tendency to abnormal motion of the divided bone and not much pain. In some cases, if the bone approximation has not been entirely successful, a tight swathe may be helpful during the first few days. The patient can be allowed out of bed as soon as he has recovered fully from the effects of the anesthetic, usually the first day after operation. By the time the sutures are removed on the ninth or tenth postoperative day, the anterior chest wall is firm and stable so that no further support of any kind is required. Ultimate healing is complete and no deformity of the chest wall ensues.

Anterior Incisions for Exposure of the Pericardium and Heart. Operations directed upon the heart or pericardium require a wide but localized exposure. Although the pericardial sac can be reached through an anterolateral intercostal incision with division of the cartilages, a somewhat wider anterior exposure is usually required than can be obtained by this means. Innumerable varieties of incision have been proposed. For practical purposes three modifications of the anterior approach to the pericardium are sufficient for the majority of cases (Fig. 53). The technic of each of these is as follows.

PERICARDIOSTOMY FOR DRAINAGE. To drain a purulent effusion in the pericardium a relatively simple procedure will suffice. A short incision is made along the course of the fifth costal cartilage on the left side extending from the edge of the sternum to the costochondral junction. The entire fifth cartilage is excised so as to avoid the probability of prolonged drainage from infection of any remnants which may not have been removed. The left pleural reflexion should be identified and if necessary pushed aside without opening it. The internal mammary vessels, which traverse the depths of the incision medially, should be ligated so as to avoid secondary hemorrhage. The anterior surface of the pericardium lies directly at the bottom of the incision and may be incised as widely as necessary (Fig. 53, *3*).

PERICARDIOTOMY FOR OPERATIONS ON THE HEART. To gain access to the heart for suture of lacerations or for extraction of intracardiac foreign bodies, a wider exposure of the pericardium is needed. The direction of the skin incision is immaterial as is also the method of dealing with the cartilages. The important consideration is the simplicity of the procedure, which must be carried out swiftly in many cases of cardiac injury. A useful method is as follows: A curved transverse incision is made over the left fourth intercostal space from the sternum to the region of the costochondral junctions. The incision is deepened by cutting directly through the pectoralis major muscle fibers which are retracted widely to expose the cartilages beneath. The fourth and fifth costal cartilages are excised. The left pleura is gently dissected away from the pericardium laterally. Medially, greater exposure

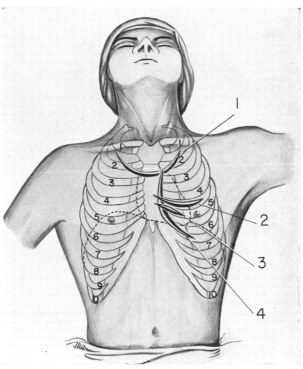

Fig. 53. Anterior thoracic incisions other than the sternum-splitting thoracotomy. *1,* Curved transverse incision for partial excision of the sternum. *2,* Pericardiotomy incision for operations upon the heart. *3,* Pericardiostomy incision for drainage of the pericardial sac. *4,* Classical incision for pericardiectomy.

is obtained by ligating and dividing the internal mammary vessels at the upper and lower limits of the operative field. The pericardium is opened transversely or obliquely, whichever seems to be most convenient. If a larger exposure is needed, the cartilages above or below can be divided close to their sternal articulations. If possible this maneuver should be avoided because of the need for fixing the cartilages to the sternum, which prolongs the time required for closure (Fig. 53, 2).

INCISION FOR PERICARDIECTOMY. The skin incision starts on the left side over the second costal cartilage near its articulation with the sternum and extends downwards along the left side of that bone, curving laterally along the course of the sixth costal cartilage to approximately the level of the costochondral junction of that rib. The deep fascia over the pectoralis major muscle is incised and the insertions of this muscle into the sternum and the rib cartilages are severed, making it possible to retract the muscle, the overlying breast and the skin. The third, fourth and fifth costal cartilages are removed with their perichondrium, cutting laterally at or behind the costochondral junction and medially through the sternal articulations. Comparable sections of the intercostal muscles, nerves and vessels are excised and the internal mammary vessels are tied and cut at both the upper and the lower limits of the area of denudation. The anterior surface of the pericardium is thus exposed (Fig. 53, 4).

If greater access to the region of the right ventricle is required, the exposure is widened by excising a portion of the left half of the body of the sternum, using a large bone-cutting shears or the sternum-cutting knife. The left lateral half of the sternum from the level of the third cartilage above to the lower limits of the incision below is removed as a piece roughly semicircular in shape.

Closure of the incision is made in three layers including the deep fascia over the pectoralis major muscle, the superficial fascia and the skin.

It should be mentioned that the sternum-splitting incision may also be used for the exposure of the pericardium. It provides particularly good access to the right side of the heart as well as the left. It has the further advantage that it leaves the patient with a stable chest wall.

AFTER-CARE. Because of the removal of cartilages and sometimes a portion of the sternum as well, a considerable degree of paradoxical motion of the chest wall occurs at the site of operation during the early convalescent period. This should be prevented by a tightly applied dressing. It is often helpful to apply a plaque of plaster bandage in the same manner as is employed after partial excision of the sternum (see Chap. 4). After eight to ten days no special support is necessary. The chest wall always remains flexible at the site of operation, however, and the motions of the heart beneath are readily seen.

CHAPTER 4

OPERATIONS ON THE THORACIC WALL

SUPERFICIAL STRUCTURES

Operations required in the treatment of lesions of the skin and subcutaneous tissues of the chest wall present no problems which demand special consideration in a work on thoracic surgery. Operations on the mammary gland are of great importance, but they have been so well dealt with in the various treatises on general surgery that they need not be included here.

THE STERNUM

Reference to Figure 2, Chapter 1, will serve to illustrate the muscle insertions of the sternum and its deep relations. The inner surface of the bone is covered by a tough fascial investment and in the lower portion by fibers of the transversus thoracis muscles. In attempting to free its mediastinal surface a deeper plane of dissection must be entered either inferiorly, under the xiphoid process, or superiorly, over the suprasternal notch starting in the cleavage plane beneath the sternothyroid muscles in the base of the neck. Through either approach the loose areolar tissues of the anterior mediastinum can be freely dissected away, thus pushing back the thymus gland, the innominate vessels and the pericardium which might otherwise be injured. The course of the internal mammary vessels which run beneath the deep endothoracic fascia on the undersurfaces of the costal cartilages and the intercostal muscles not far lateral to each sternal edge must be kept in mind.

Sternal Bone Marrow Biopsy

In the diagnosis of certain blood dyscrasias a bone marrow biopsy is sometimes required. This can be obtained from the sternum with relative ease. Using procaine hydrochloride (1 per cent) infiltration anesthesia, a short vertical or transverse incision is made over the gladiolar segment of the bone. The pectoral fascia and periosteum are incised and freed from a small surface over the outer cortex with a raspatory. A circular cranial trephine of small diameter is used to make an opening into the marrow cavity and pieces of marrow are removed with a bone curette (Fig. 54). The fragment of cortex is usually replaced at the completion of the biopsy, but this step may be omitted. The wound is closed with a layer of fine sutures and the skin edges are approximated with sutures of silk.

The only technical difficulty which may be encountered is the control of bleeding from the marrow. This can usually be overcome by stuffing the hole in the bone with fibrin foam soaked in thrombin solution.

No special after-care is required.

Excision of Sternum for Tumor

Because of the possibility of opening either pleural cavity during the operation, positive pressure inhalation anesthesia is necessary. The patient should lie on his back with the upper half of his body sloping slightly up-

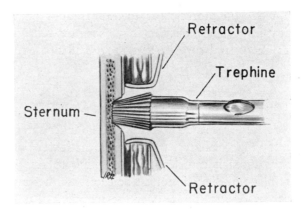

Fig. 54. Sternal biopsy. Use of trephine to remove a portion of the cortex of the sternum to obtain marrow for histologic studies.

ward. The head should be tilted slightly back. One arm should be fastened by his side. The other arm is held in the position of abduction on an arm board for the administration of the intravenous infusion.

Excision of the entire sternum without fixation of the rib ends by means of a bone graft or otherwise is usually followed by death from the effects of the uncontrollable paradoxical motion of the chest wall; this motion interferes with the respiratory function to an intolerable extent. Large segments of the sternum can be removed, however, if a portion is left behind to lend stability to the thorax. The usual indication for partial excision of the sternum is the removal of a neoplastic growth. These growths tend to involve either the gladiolus or the manubrium, without much tendency at first to overlap from one part to the other. The removal of the tumor-bearing segment can therefore usually be accomplished in such a way as to leave the other portion for strength.

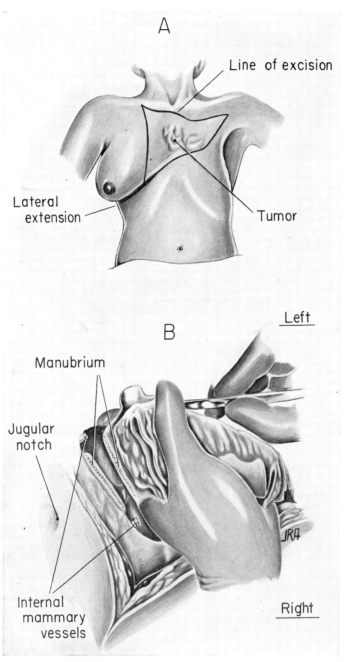

Fig. 55. Partial excision of the sternum. *A,* Outline of incision used to excise the recurrence of mammary carcinoma in the chest wall invading the sternum. Excision of previously grafted skin is a necessary part of the procedure to obtain edges of normal skin for approximation in that area at the completion of the operation. *Note:* The lateral extension of the incision was necessary to facilitate coverage of the defect using the right breast. *B,* Stage of the operation showing the manubrium and right second, third and fourth costal cartilages already divided. The division of the left cartilages is being accomplished with a knife. The incision across the gladiolar portion of the sternum remains to be done. Right and left internal mammary vessels are shown after division (lateral to the divided edge of manubrium).

83

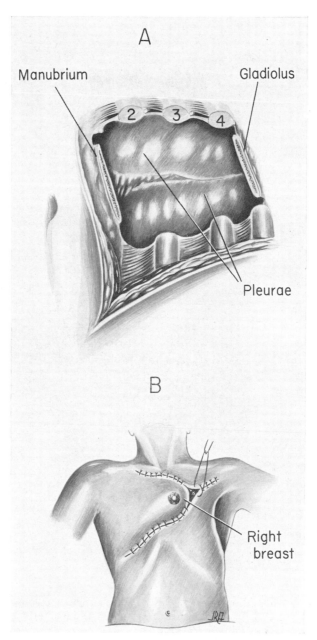

Fig. 56. Partial excision of the sternum. *A*, Operative field showing defect resulting from excision of the major portion of the manubrium and more than half of the gladiolus with sections of right and left second, third and fourth costal cartilages. A large area of the mediastinum lies exposed. *B*, Method of closure by swinging over a large flap consisting of the right breast and the underlying right pectoralis major muscle.

Technic of the Operation. EXCISION OF THE MANUBRIUM FOR MALIGNANT TUMOR. A transverse U-shaped incision is preferable to a vertical one in the midline to avoid the effect of the motion of the chest wall at the site of operation during the respiratory excursion. The curve should be downward and should pass over the normal portion of the gladiolus which is to be left behind (Fig. 53, 1). The flap consisting of skin, subcutaneous fat and fascia is reflected upward to the base of the neck. Because of the fact that the operation is almost always performed for the removal of a malignant tumor, a careful anatomic dissection cannot be made. Sections of the muscles, rib cartilages and often the inner ends of the clavicles must therefore be removed en bloc with the tumor.

The pectoralis major muscles and the lower ends of the sternocleidomastoid and sternohyoid and sternothyroid muscles must be cut an appreciable distance from their insertions into the bone. By blunt dissection through the base of the neck the inner surface of the bone is exposed, and the loose attachments of the tissues in the anterior mediastinum are freed by the finger passed beneath the manubrium from above the jugular notch. Disarticulation of the inner ends of the clavicles is permissible when the growth is a small one. This is done with a knife and scissors. However, in the majority of cases the inner ends of the clavicles must be removed with the tumor. This is accomplished with a Gigli saw. The costal cartilages on each side as far down as the point where the sternum is to be divided are then freed from the underlying pleura after incising the corresponding intercostal muscles. The internal mammary vessels are exposed beneath the inferior edge of the lowermost cartilage which is to be removed. At this level these vessels are divided between double ligatures. The costal cartilages are cut with a costotome, a knife or a pair of heavy scissors. After the lowermost pair of cartilages have been divided, the finger is inserted beneath the sternum below the level of the tumor, to be certain that nothing is adherent beneath, and the sternum is cut across at the appropriate level with a bone shears or a Gigli saw. The remaining rib cartilages are divided.

Before cutting the first rib cartilages all deep attachments which might make it possible to injure the innominate and jugular veins which lie so close beneath must be pushed away. If a finger is then inserted through the previously made dissection in the base of the neck so as to guide the points of the bone-cutting shears, the division of the first ribs can be accomplished safely. The upper portions of the internal mammary vessels are tied and cut, leaving the intervening segments attached to the specimen which is removed.

When an appreciable portion of the gladiolus is allowed to remain, no attempt to fix the divided rib ends by means of bone grafts or prosthetic appliances need be made. The ends of the clavicles are left to take care of themselves. In many cases it is possible to give strength to the closure of the wound by approximating as far as possible the cut edges of the pectoral muscles in the midline and also by suturing the cut ends of the sterno-cleidomastoid, sternothyroid and sternohyoid muscles to the upper portion of the sutured pectoral muscles. The superficial fascia and skin are closed as separate layers.

EXCISION OF THE GLADIOLUS. The same type of incision should be used as for the removal of the upper portion of the sternum. It should be placed somewhat lower or the direction of the curve can be made upward instead of downward, thus crossing the portion of sternum which is not to be removed. The principles of removal described previously are used. It is usually necessary to excise the xiphoid with the portion of gladiolus which is removed. The wound is closed in the same manner as for excision of the manubrium.

After-care. Whatever can be done to reduce the tendency of the chest wall to develop paradoxical respiratory motions in the region where a portion of bone has been removed will tend to make the early convalescent period safer and more comfortable for the patient. If no rigid protection of the weakened chest wall is provided, coughing is difficult, bronchial secretions may accumulate and pulmonary atelectasis or pneumonia may develop. Much relief is provided by the application of a rigid plaque made of plaster bandage to the anterior aspect of the chest. This is held in place by means of flexible adhesive bandage to the surrounding skin around its edges. This apparatus allows freer respiratory motions of the chest as a whole than would a circular bandage. After the expiration of ten to twelve days, external protection is no longer necessary because of the stiffening of the tissues which have been used to close the bony defect.

The ultimate functional result after the operation is amazingly satisfactory. The tendency to paradoxical motion almost disappears because of the formation of a tough layer of scar tissue over the defect. In cases where the upper half of the sternum has been excised, with disarticulation or partial excision of the clavicles, a more obvious deformity is noticed because of the abnormal mobility of the remaining portions of the clavicles. The abnormal motions of the clavicles consist in medial approximation of the ends when the shoulders are moved forward, and up and down motions of these ends when the arms are moved about. On the other hand, no serious impairment of arm or shoulder girdle function is ever experienced. Patients are able to lift heavy weights, row a boat or swing an axe, and perform almost all arm and shoulder motions.

An occasional source of local discomfort centering about the cut ends of the clavicles is the result of the development of a spicule of bone which grows upward from the divided end in a hornlike projection. This occurrence can be avoided by careful treatment of the end of the bone, with removal of all fragments of periosteum from which such an exostosis might arise.

Correction of Pectus Excavatum

In order to appreciate fully the importance of some of the steps for its correction, an understanding of the structural changes which are characteristic of pectus excavatum is necessary. The etiology of this condition is

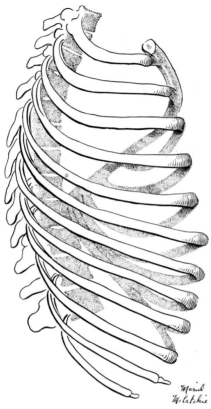

Fig. 57. Pectus excavatum. Diagram of rib cage to show the extent of depression of the gladioloxiphoid junction in a severe deformity.

unknown. It has been suggested that there is an unusually tight substernal fascia or a very short diaphragmatic attachment to the lower end of the sternum which pulls it in during inspiration. It is true that in this condition the deepest point at the bottom of the funnel tends to sink inward when the patient inspires, but whether it is pulled in by a strong attachment beneath or pushed inwards by the deeply incurved costal cartilages is not clear.

Certain anatomic changes are constant. The deepest point is always at the junction of the xiphoid with the gladiolus. The manubrium rarely takes part in the deformity, but the beginning of the inward inclination of the involved portion of the bone is often at or just below the manubriogladiolar junction. Those costal cartilages which articulate with the depressed portion of the sternum seem to be unusually long, and there is a peculiar distortion of their articulations with the sternum characterized by marked hypertrophy of their deep surfaces. These joints when viewed from the mediastinal side appear to be partially subluxated (Fig. 60). In cases in which the deformity is most pronounced, the lower end of the sternum pushes into the mediastinum as though it were a wedge which had been driven in, and ultimately lies against the anterior surfaces of the vertebral bodies at that level, almost cleaving the mediastinum into two lateral halves. The heart is

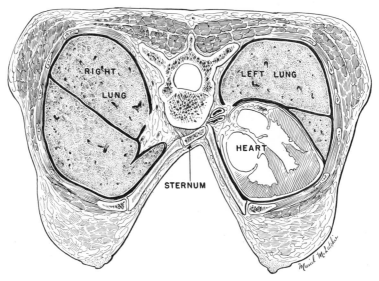

Fig. 58. Pectus excavatum. Diagram of a cross section of the body at the greatest depth of the depression. Note the striking deviation of the heart into the left hemithorax, the apex resting against the ribs in the anterior axillary line.

thereby pushed far to the left, sometimes as far as the left anterolateral aspect of the chest wall (Figs. 57 and 58).

Technic of Operation. None of the numerous methods of correcting a funnel chest deformity has proved satisfactory except that proposed by A. Lincoln Brown. A modification of that procedure is described here. The cases should be considered according to the age of the patient and the severity of the deformity. One of two procedures may then be chosen as the occasion demands.

MINOR PROCEDURE. In infants 2 years of age or younger, a limited operation directed toward the division of a tight substernal fascial or muscular attachment is worthy of trial if the deformity is not very deep and is sharply localized at the gladioloxiphoid junction. With the child lying on his back, under intratracheal general anesthesia, a short vertical or transverse incision is made over the region of the joint between the xiphoid and the gladiolus.

The attachments of the linea alba and rectus abdominis muscles are freed from the xiphoid which is grasped with a tenaculum and held up so that the lower portion of the anterior mediastinum can be entered by blunt dissection with the scissors and finger. A tight band of fascia or diaphragmatic muscle is sought for and divided if found. This should eliminate the excessive pull upon the lower portion of the sternum.

The wound is closed in layers consisting of the fascial edges of the linea alba, the subcutaneous fascia and the skin. The success of this relatively simple procedure depends upon the finding of a substernal band of tissue for division and upon the fact that the bone is unusually flexible in infants and has not yet become firmly fixed in the abnormal position. The number of cases in which this operation is completely satisfactory is small.

MAJOR PROCEDURE. In children beyond infancy and in adults a more radical operation is required because the bone has already assumed a permanently abnormal shape and the articulations of the costal cartilages with the sternum are held rigidly at an abnormal angle of partial subluxation. Success in producing a permanent correction of the deformity in such patients requires (1) the elimination of the abnormal downward inclination of the sternum, (2) the straightening of the attachments of the cartilages to the side of the sternum and (3) the correction of the abnormal inward curvature of the ribs which forms the side of the funnel.

To accomplish the first requirement a transverse wedge-shaped osteotomy must be made at the point in the sternum where the abnormal inward sloping begins. The second requirement depends upon the excision of the misshapen articulations and the reattachment of the freshened ends of cartilage to the bone. The third requirement is expedited by performing small transverse osteotomies on the outer cortex of each involved rib.

General anesthesia is used with an intratracheal tube for positive pressure to control the expansion of the lungs if either pleural space should be opened. The position of the patient on the operating table is the same as for any operation on the sternum (see *Excision of Sternum for Tumors*). A long, vertical, midline incision is made from the level of the manubrium superiorly to a point approximately equidistant between the xiphoid and the umbilicus inferiorly. The wound edges are protected with towels held in place by continuous sutures of silk. The incision is deepened to the bone in the thoracic portion and to the linea alba in the abdominal extension. The fascial insertions of the pectoralis major muscles into the sternum are cut so as to retract the medial edges of these muscles laterally. In order to gain exposure to the cartilages it is necessary to divide the attachments of these muscles to the medial ends of the cartilages. When this is done, the anterior perforating branches of the intercostal vessels must be divided and tied. At the lower end of the incision the linea alba is incised, exposing but not opening the peritoneum, and the insertions of the rectus abdominis muscles into the medial ends of the lower costal cartilages are divided. The skin, fat and muscles are then retracted laterally, exposing the sternum and the costal cartilages from the manubriogladiolar junction to the costal margins (Fig. 59).

The xiphoid is grasped with a tenaculum and with scissors dissection the anterior mediastinum is entered. A sweep of the finger serves to free the pericardium from the sternum. Working from below upward, the costal cartilages are cut across in turn as far as the point where the inward

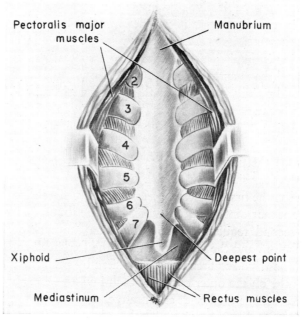

Fig. 59. Pectus excavatum. Operative technic, Step 1: The exposure of the sternum is produced by freeing the sternal attachments of the pectoralis major and rectus abdominis muscles.

inclination in the sternum begins. By this maneuver the depressed portion of the bone is freed, but its angular shape is not changed. By means of two transverse cuts across the bone at the point where the inward slant of the depressed segment starts, a narrow wedge–shaped section is removed from the anterior cortex of the sternum (Fig. 60). A small rotary saw can be used for this purpose, or a small hand saw such as is used for the amputation of small bones may be employed. After this small fragment has been removed, the depressed portion of bone can be swung outward to assume a normal position in relation with the remainder of the sternum. This position is maintained by means of two or three stainless steel wire sutures (22 gauge) passed through small drill holes in the anterior bony cortex.

The excessive inward curvature of the rib cartilages is corrected by cutting a small wedge from the anterior surface of each cartilage or from the bone itself lateral to the costochondral junction, whichever point happens to be at the maximum curve of the rib. Strong silk (No. 0 Deknatel) sutures (or wire if desired) are used to hold the cartilages in their corrected position. The abnormal articular surfaces on the sides of the sternum are trimmed with a knife. The cartilages are then shortened by excising the exact length of the articular end necessary to make an accurate fit between them and the

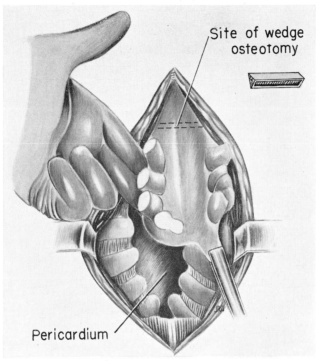

Site of wedge osteotomy

Pericardium

Fig. 60. Pectus excavatum. Operative technic: Sternum freed after cutting the cartilages. Note (1) the distorted partially subluxated costosternal articulations. These ends of cartilage are to be removed and the edges of the sternum smoothed as a preliminary to reapplication of the costal cartilages. Note also (2) the location and relative size of the wedge osteotomy at the level where the inward deviation commences (usually at the manubriogladiolar junction).

sternum in their newly assumed positions. In severe cases as much as 2 cm. of cartilage must be removed. In less marked deformities not more than 0.5 cm. need be trimmed away. After this trimming of cartilages and sternal articulations has been completed, the newly created surfaces of sternum and cartilage must fit flat against each other in each case. The cartilages are fastened to the sternum with strong silk or wire sutures passed through the entire thickness of bone and cartilage. At the lower end the xiphoid is removed and the sternum is trimmed in a V-shaped manner so as to fit the newly trimmed lowermost costal cartilages. All of these sutures are tied (Fig. 61).

The correction of the deformity is now obvious, but the stability of the anterior chest wall depends upon the strength of the sutures which must maintain the new position until healing is well advanced. It is wise in many cases, therefore, to lend assistance by providing traction on the sternum. This is accomplished by means of a steel wire passed beneath the central portion of the gladiolus, each end of which is brought up through the muscle, fat and skin by means of a large needle. After the correction of the deformity has been accomplished, the pectoral fascia is sutured with inter-

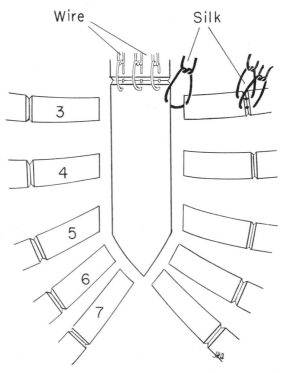

Fig. 61. Pectus excavatum. Diagram of the sternum and cartilages after trimming and performance of wedge osteotomies on both sternum and ribs to correct the deformity. Note: Sutures of the sternum are wire; sutures of the rib cartilages are heavy silk (Deknatel).

rupted silk sutures to the periosteum of the sternum, and in the lower portion of the wound the fascia of the linea alba is approximated. The subcutaneous and skin layers are then closed with interrupted fine sutures.

After a small gauze dressing has been placed over the skin incision, a light plaque of plaster in which a heavy wire loop is incorporated is molded over the anterior surface of the thorax, and when this is dry the two ends of steel wire are suspended from the heavy wire loop in the plaster. Enough tension is used to keep the sternum up in its new position so as to prevent sagging until the healing process has begun. In some patients, especially in children, the wire can be omitted.

After-care. The patient may be allowed out of bed early in the convalescent period with the traction apparatus in position. The wire support may be removed after ten to fourteen days. From then on, and from the beginning in those who have not been supplied with external support, the patient must be encouraged to maintain a proper erect position at all times. Partial recurrences of the deformity which have been reported after the operation have been the result of the failure of the patient to cooperate in the maintenance of correct posture during the first few months. This applies particularly, of course, to young children.

RIBS AND COSTAL CARTILAGES

Excision of Costal Cartilage for Tuberculous Chondritis with Cold Abscess of the Chest Wall

If tuberculous abscesses of the thoracic wall do not arise primarily in the breast or in axillary lymph nodes, they are usually secondary to infections involving the costal cartilages. Whether or not the chondritis is secondary to tuberculous lymphadenitis of the anterior mediastinum, it is necessary to find and excise all diseased cartilage in order to cure the condition.

An incision is made through normal skin in the vicinity of the cold abscess which is entered directly and emptied of its purulent contents. One or more deep sinus openings can always be found leading off from the bottom of the abscess cavity. These sinuses are explored with a probe and laid open down to the point where they communicate with the diseased portions of the underlying cartilages. The pleura beneath the cartilage is pushed away with a blunt instrument such as a Matson periosteal elevator, and the infected cartilage is excised with its perichondrium. A careful search must be made for ramifications of the sinus tracts which might lead to other foci of diseased cartilage which must also be removed. After all the diseased cartilage has been excised, the pus and debris of tissue should be thoroughly wiped away and the incision closed tightly in layers consisting of muscle, fascia, fat and skin. It is important not to insert a drain because of the danger of introducing infection from the exterior.

After-care. Primary healing occurs promptly. The prophylactic use of penicillin and streptomycin is a valuable adjuvant. Recurrence of the abscess is unusual if all diseased cartilage has been removed, provided that contamination with pyogenic bacteria can be avoided.

Excision of Rib for Neoplastic Tumors

Excision of segments of rib is rarely practiced for metastatic tumors unless there is reason to believe that one may be dealing with a single metastasis which may, therefore, be removed successfully. Such a rare occurrence may be observed in the case of carcinoma of the thyroid or in renal cell carcinoma of the kidney (hypernephroma), but not often in the case of other malignant tumors.

The great majority of rib tumors are primary and are usually malignant. The most frequent type is the chondrosarcoma. As with malignant tumors everywhere in the body, the best chance of cure depends on the performance of a wide excision of the tumor with a large margin of adjacent normal tissue in all directions. Chondrosarcoma of the rib is notorious for its tendency to recur in the portions of the rib which are left behind after local excision of a short segment of the rib. It is therefore necessary to remove the entire bony portion of the primarily diseased rib. This means that the anterior section should be through the costal cartilage and the posterior division through the neck as close as possible to the head of the rib. If feasible the head of the rib should be disarticulated from the spine.

Although radical surgical excision offers the best prognosis in the majority of cases, it has been found that in the exceptional instance of a sarcoma of the Ewing's tumor type, high voltage roentgen-ray treatment has given better results than surgery.

Technic of Operation. General inhalation anesthesia with positive pressure is necessary. A standard thoracotomy incision made with the patient lying on the opposite side is used in the majority of cases. If the growth is not adherent to the overlying skin, a long linear incision is made over the tumor in the direction of the rib. If there is suspicion that the skin may be adherent, a long ellipse should be outlined by two incisions and the segment of skin thus circumscribed should be left attached to the mass of tissue which is to be removed. The wound is deepened through the muscles away from any point of possible infiltration by the tumor. If the muscle is apparently involved, a section must be left attached and removed with the growth. The rib is exposed both anterior and posterior to the growth, and the intercostal muscles and pleura are incised not far from the tumor so as to palpate the inner surface of the chest wall in the tumor-bearing area. If the underlying lung is adherent, a portion of it may have to be excised. The examining finger will tell the surgeon if such is the case and also serve to detect any extension of growth to the adjacent ribs on the pleural surfaces (Fig. 62). If inspection and palpation indicate that one or more of the adjacent ribs are involved or if the growth is so close to these ribs that not a sufficiently large margin of intercostal muscle can be obtained, sections of these ribs must be removed in continuity with the tumor-bearing mass. The rib which is the site of the tumor must be excised as nearly as possible in its entirety by dividing the cartilage in front and cutting through the rib neck behind. The usual rib-cutting instruments are used. The resection of the rib or ribs, however, must be done extraperiosteally so as to remove the periosteum and the adjacent endothoracic fascia and pleura as well. This maneuver, of course, necessitates the ligation and division of the inter-

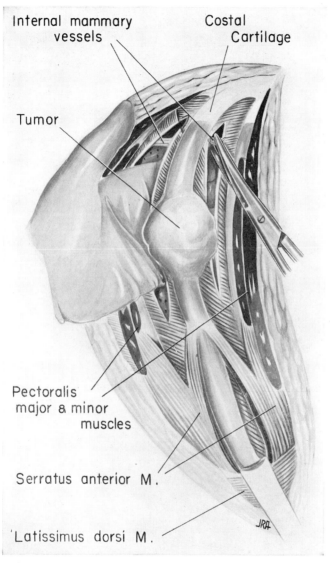

Internal mammary vessels

Costal Cartilage

Tumor

Pectoralis major & minor muscles

Serratus anterior M.

Latissimus dorsi M.

JRA

Fig. 62. Technic of extraperiosteal excision of a rib for primary malignant tumor; left side. Note (1) the exposure obtained by means of an anterolateral submammary incision, and (2) the surgeon's left hand inserted through a tentative short intercostal incision to determine the inner extent and relations of the tumor for decision as to amount of chest wall to be removed.

costal vessels both anteriorly and posteriorly. Thus a large bloc of tissue including in many cases portions of skin, muscle, segments of adjacent ribs, intercostal muscles, vessels, nerves, endothoracic fascia, pleura, and sometimes portions of lung is excised en masse (Fig. 63). If the lung is invaded, the adherent portion may be isolated by means of straight clamps applied in such a direction as to make it possible to excise a wedge of the involved pulmonary tissue along with the growth. The remaining defect in the lung

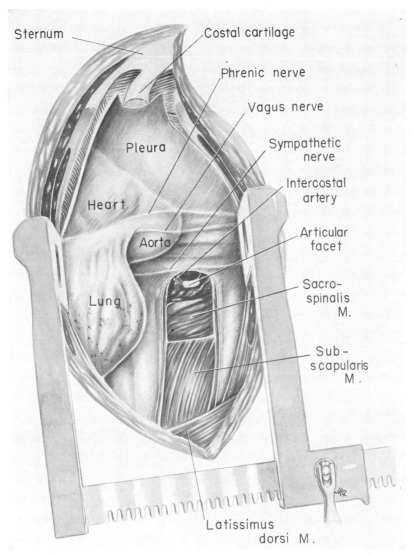

Fig. 63. Technic of excision of rib for primary malignant tumor. Same case as Figure 62, showing the appearance of the chest after the entire rib has been removed by section of the cartilage anteriorly and by disarticulation from the spine posteriorly.

is closed either with interrupted mattress sutures placed close together so as to control hemorrhage and to prevent leakage of air from small bronchi and the alveolar surfaces, or with a continuous suture of fine catgut on an atraumatic needle.

Even when only one rib has been resected, closure of the pleural cavity is impossible except by roofing over the defect with muscle, fat and skin. A careful layer by layer approximation of the fascia, muscle, fat and skin, however, produces an ample closure. In cases where large portions of the thoracic wall, including muscle and skin, have been removed, it is necessary to construct flaps of skin or skin and underlying muscle from an adjacent area such as the abdominal wall or some portion of the back. Such flaps can be sutured in place over the defect so as to close the pleural cavity. The region from which they come is closed either by undercutting and sliding of the remaining skin and fascial edges or by means of primary Thiersch grafts taken from the thigh. In some cases a combination of both methods may be used.

After-care. Excessive paradoxical motion of the chest wall at the site of excision should be minimized by the application of a tight bandage. Large effusions of serosanguineous fluid often develop in these cases because of the presence of large denuded surfaces. Thoracentesis should be resorted to if the accumulation of fluid becomes large.

Excision of Ribs for Pulmonary Collapse

Extrapleural Thoracoplasty. This operation is used primarily for the collapse therapy of pulmonary tuberculosis. It is occasionally employed also after total pneumonectomy in order to overcome the tendency of the mediastinum to shift too far to the operated side. So much has been written regarding the subject of thoracoplasty that there is need of simplification of the subject. One hears of posterior operations, anterolateral operations, revision thoracoplasties, thoracoplasties performed through muscle-splitting incisions, and others. The existence of such modifications of the procedure arises from the desire of the surgeon to avoid a primary radical operation for cosmetic reasons or otherwise, or the failure to realize that once a thoroughly comprehensive procedure has been performed, no further operation short of lobectomy or pneumonectomy can be expected to improve the clinical result. In the vast majority of cases, therefore, a standard thoracoplasty operation is all that is required. No modifications of the extrapleural procedure will be described.

The principle of the operation is to induce a collapse of the underlying lung by the intraperiosteal resection of several ribs, the number depending on the extent of the diseased area. The regeneration of bone from the periosteum of the resected ribs then maintains the collapsed condition of the lung. Because of the characteristic distribution of the disease, which tends to involve chiefly the upper portions of the upper lobe and the superior segment of the lower lobe, the maximum degree of collapse must be secured in the upper half of the chest. In general it is necessary to resect the entire length of the upper three ribs, which should be divided through the cartilage in front and the neck behind. Because the neck of the first rib lies actually above the apex of the lung, the posterior division of this rib need not be so far back as the others.

Because of their downward inclination the anterior ends of the ribs below the third lie below the level of the portion of the lung which is to be collapsed; therefore, beginning with the fourth, the anterior division of each of the succeeding lower ribs is made further back toward the midaxillary line and, if the seventh or eighth is resected, actually posterior to that line. Thus shorter and shorter segments of the lower ribs are resected, but the division of each rib posteriorly should be through the neck. The average thoracoplasty involves the resection of segments of from five to seven ribs.

In order to improve the efficacy of the collapse, two additional maneuvers are of value. In order to secure the maximum degree of collapse of the portion of the lung which lies in the paravertebral gutter, the tip of the transverse process of each vertebra should be removed as the neck of the rib is cut close to its head. This tends to diminish the depth of the posterior groove along the bodies of the vertebrae. In certain cases, furthermore, the extent of collapse of the apical portion of the upper lobe can be increased by freeing the extrapleural attachments of the superior, medial and posterior surfaces of the dome of the pleura so as to allow the pulmonary apex to sink downward in the direction of the hilus. This so-called apicolysis is valuable only in cases where the apical pulmonary tissues are flexible. In rigid fibrotic disease, even though the apex may be dissected free, very little improvement in the degree of the collapse results.

When more than three or four ribs must be resected, the operation should be performed in two or more stages, depending upon the extent of the disease and the condition of the patient. The majority of patients are able to withstand the performance of a seven rib thoracoplasty in two stages with the removal of the first three ribs at the first and portions of the next four ribs at the second stage.

Technic of Standard Thoracoplasty. Local anesthesia with procaine hydrochloride solution (1 per cent) injected into the intercostal nerves and infiltrated in the region of the operation can be used, especially for the second or third stages of the procedure. The chief advantage of the use of local anesthesia is the fact that the cough reflex is maintained so that secretions may be raised from the trachea and bronchi. On the other hand, when used for a first stage it is difficult to obtain good anesthesia of the upper end of the incision, and during the resection of the first rib there is likely to be considerable pain which is difficult to control. Many patients complain also of fatigue and discomfort resulting from lying in one position on the operating table for a prolonged period of time. Inhalation anesthesia is therefore preferable in the majority of cases. An intratracheal tube is desirable because of the possibility of opening the pleura but is not absolutely necessary. Furthermore, the presence of such a tube within the larynx and trachea might, theoretically at least, be objectionable because of the possibility of inciting a flare-up of preexistent subacute or quiescent foci of tuberculosis.

A standard lateral position is used, but the uppermost arm should be placed at the patient's side instead of being held forward over his face. This position of the arm makes easy the retraction of the scapula which then rolls off of the chest after the shoulder girdle muscles have been divided. If the arm is held forward in the usual position, it acts as a prop to wedge the scapula against the chest wall, and retraction is difficult.

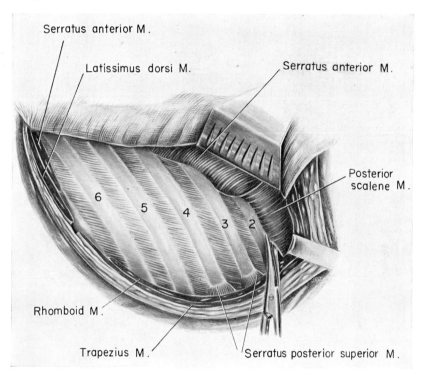

Fig. 64. Extrapleural thoracoplasty. First stage: Exposure is obtained through a standard incision curving beneath the scapula and dividing the latissimus dorsi and portions of the serratus anterior, rhomboid and trapezius muscles.

FIRST STAGE. The incision starts at the midaxillary line slightly below the level of the angle of the scapula and extends posteriorly, curving slightly upward to a point midway between the angle of the scapula and the spine whence it proceeds straight up almost to the top of the shoulder. In order to obtain a wide enough exposure to the upper ribs, especially the first, the scapula must be liberated so that it can be retracted several inches away from the rib cage. To accomplish this it is necessary not only to cut completely across the body of the latissimus dorsi muscle, but also to divide portions of the body of the serratus anterior muscle anteriorly and of the trapezius and rhomboid muscles posteriorly and superiorly. The division of the latter muscles must be carried upward to the level of the superior margin of the scapula. A wide Davidson retractor, held by an assistant, is useful to keep the scapula away from the chest wall while the ribs are being resected (Fig. 64).

In order to gain access to the anterior portions of the ribs, the costal insertions of the serratus anterior and pectoralis major muscles are cut extraperiosteally. In the upper portion of the chest the costal insertions of the scalenus muscles are divided, also extraperiosteally, so as to expose the entire length of the first and second ribs. Posteriorly the insertions of the serratus posterior superior muscle must be divided, and also the tendinous insertions of the erector spinae muscle, so as to expose the necks of the ribs. In the usual first stage operation the upper three ribs are resected. In order to make the approach to the second and first ribs easier, the third rib is resected first. The periosteum is incised with a knife and freed from the rib in the usual manner. The inner surface of the rib anteriorly and the intercostal muscle insertions beyond the costochondral junction may present some difficulty. The best procedure is to free the periosteum and perichondrium along the inner surface of the anterior aspect of the rib with the Matson elevator, pushing the periosteum and pleura away as far forward as possible. The intercostal muscle insertions are then cut almost as far forward as the internal mammary vessels with a long pair of curved scissors. The posterior end of the rib must be freed as far around as the head. This can be done on the inner surface by blunt dissection with the finger or with the Matson elevator. The outer surface of the neck of the rib, of course, articulates with the transverse process of the corresponding vertebra. A short segment of the process should be removed. To accomplish this the tendinous and ligamentous attachments to the process are divided with a heavy pair of blunt scissors. With a large bone-cutting shears the neck of the rib and the transverse process are cut across simultaneously, leaving the tip of the process attached by its articular surface to the resected segment of rib. The remaining portion of the transverse process and the short proximal segment of rib should be smoothed off with a rongeur if any irregular spicules of bone are left behind. The anterior end of the rib is cut through the cartilage with a large bone shears or preferably with the Coryllos costotome which was made for that purpose (Fig. 65).

The second rib is then dealt with in the same manner as the third, removing the tip of the transverse process with the rib and cutting through the cartilage anteriorly. It should be kept in mind that the second rib, although much larger than the first, has some of the same physical characteristics as the first and can be mistaken for it. If this error is made, the first rib may then be left behind. This difficulty can be avoided if an adequate exposure is obtained, as described above. Furthermore, it should be possible to identify

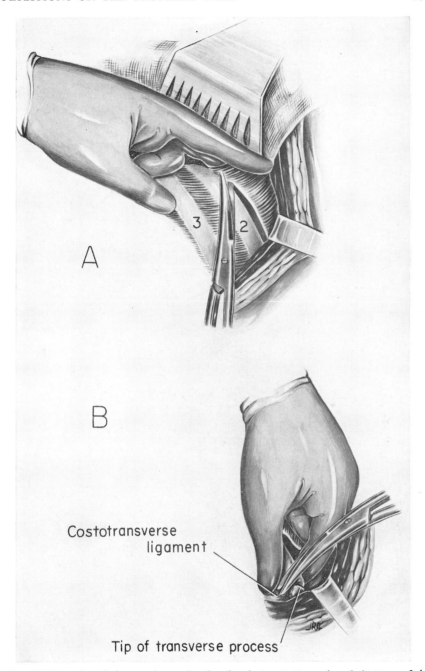

Costotransverse ligament

Tip of transverse process

Fig. 65. Extrapleural thoracoplasty: details of technic. *A,* Extrapleural division of the scalene muscle insertions, using scissors. The fingers are inserted beneath the muscle to insure against injury to the subclavian vessels. This is of paramount importance in the division of the first rib attachments. *B,* Preparation of the neck of the rib and end of the transverse process of the vertebra for simultaneous transection with large bone-cutting shears.

the second rib because it is larger than the first and does not present the nodule on its inner margin which is known as the scalene tubercle.

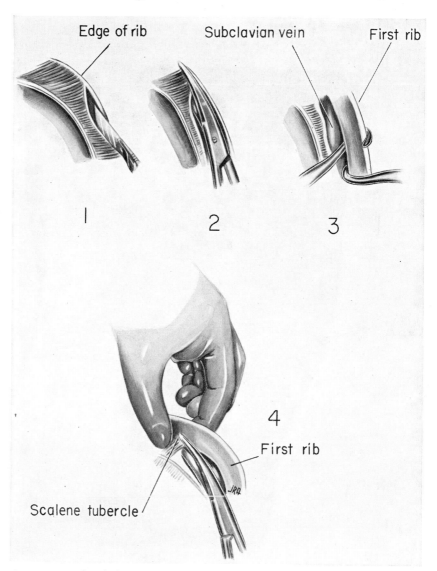

Fig. 66. Extrapleural thoracoplasty: Steps in the technic of freeing the first rib. *1,* Start of periosteal incision on the outer edge of the rib using a knife. *2,* Cutting intercostal muscle insertions at an unusually adherent point with scissors. *3,* Method of freeing the inner edge and superior surface of the rib so as to avoid injury to the subclavian vein; use of special first rib periosteal elevator. *4,* Section of the musculofascial attachment to the scalene tubercle with scissors.

The technic of resection of the first rib deserves special consideration (Fig. 66). This rib is short and rigid. Its surfaces are superior and inferior instead of lateral and medial as in the lower ribs. The division of the scalene attachments to the rib should be completed. These muscles must be cut extraperiosteally because if they are left attached to the rib periosteum, their upward retraction will cause the regenerated bone to lie high in the apex of the chest with the result that the lung can expand upward into a space which should have been obliterated. The purpose of the operation would thus be defeated. The inferior surface of the rib can be cleared of its periosteum with ease, using a Matson elevator. The intercostal muscle insertions along the outer margin of the rib are cut with a pair of curved scissors. The freeing of the superior surface and inner margin of the first rib is best done with a periosteal elevator, the end of which is curved in the direction of its long axis (Figs. 36 and 66). With this instrument passed under the inner margin of the rib, with its point directed toward the rib, the fascial attachments are freed. The tough attachments to the scalene tubercle should be cut with the scissors. In order to be certain that the subclavian vein, which lies against the first rib in this region, will not be injured, the index finger of the left hand should be used to push the vein away and direct the points of the scissors against the bone. The rib is cut posteriorly with the Sauerbruch first rib cutter, but no attempt need be made to remove any of the vertebral transverse process. The rib is then pulled outward away from the sub-clavian vein beneath, and the cartilage is cut as far forward as possible with a heavy scissors or a bone-cutting shears.

If the apex of the lung is rigid and indurated so that no greater degree of collapse could be expected, an apicolysis need not be performed. In all other cases, however, the few minutes required to complete this additional step are well spent. To accomplish this the intercostal nerves, vessels and muscle bundles must be divided posteriorly close to the spine. The extra-pleural fascial plane is then developed by blunt and sharp dissection with the scissors so that the attachments of the apical pleura to the sides of the vertebral bodies and the tissues of the mediastinum are freed. The apex of the lung can then be made to sink down behind the level of the fourth rib posteriorly (Fig. 67). The wound is closed in layers without drainage.

SECOND STAGE. At the second stage of a multiple stage thoracoplasty, from two to four additional ribs are resected. The number of ribs depends upon the predetermined decision of the surgeon based upon the preopera-tive roentgen-ray examination and upon the condition of the patient. If the lesion is small enough to require merely a five rib thoracoplasty, the second stage in the average case will involve only the resection of segments of the fourth and fifth ribs. On the other hand, even in cases where because of the size or location of the diseased area a seven or eight rib procedure is required, the patient's condition may be such that not more than two or three ribs should be removed at the second stage. In that case a third stage is necessary to obtain the degree of collapse which the disease requires.

The second stage is performed through the same incision as was used for the first. It is not necessary, however, to reopen the upper 2 or 3 inches of the incision. The latissimus dorsi and serratus anterior muscles are divided if possible at the point where they were cut before. It may be necessary also, if it is unusually wide, to redivide a small portion of the lateral margin of the trapezius muscle. As the scapula is retracted, the lower portion of the extrapleural space which was created at the first stage is often entered and

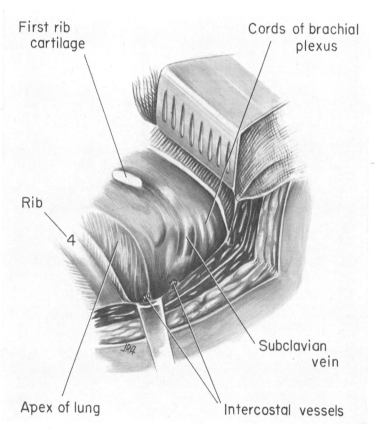

First rib
cartilage

Cords of brachial
plexus

Rib

4

Subclavian
vein

Apex of lung

Intercostal vessels

Fig. 67. Extrapleural thoracoplasty: First stage. The field of operation after removal of the first three ribs and the performance of an apicolysis. Note the dropping of the pulmonary apex from its normal location to the level of the fourth rib.

the serous fluid which is usually found there is evacuated. The attachments of the serratus anterior muscle to the ribs which are to be resected are severed extraperiosteally. The periosteum is elevated from the rib next below the last rib resected at the first operation. This is usually the fourth. The freeing of the rib and transverse process posteriorly is identical in extent with that used in the resection of the third and second ribs. However, anteriorly the periosteum is reflected to the point where the rib is to be cut, not quite to the costochondral junction. Therefore, the resected portion of the fourth rib includes the neck with the tip of the transverse process of the fourth thoracic vertebra attached, but not the entire length of the bony portion anteriorly. The exact point of division in front depends, of course, upon the amount of the lung which is to be collapsed. A shorter segment of the fifth rib is removed in the same manner. The anterior division of this rib is usually at the midaxillary line.

In some cases the removal of sections of the upper five ribs will produce a sufficient extent of collapse of the underlying lung. In others, however, it is necessary to resect a section of the sixth rib or, in some cases of more extensive disease, the seventh and sometimes even the eighth as well. If inspection of the preoperative roentgen-ray films indicates that a six rib thoracoplasty would be adequate to produce the degree of collapse which is required, particular attention must be given to the postoperative function of the scapula. In such cases the tip of the scapula almost invariably becomes caught momentarily on the edge of the seventh rib as the patient moves his arm, if nothing is done to prevent it. This causes a most annoying discomfort or a considerable amount of functional impairment of the shoulder girdle motions.

This sequela of a six rib thoracoplasty may be prevented in one of three different ways. By far the simplest and best method is to resect a portion of the seventh rib in all cases when at least a six rib collapse is required. The eighth rib is low enough so that it does not interfere with the scapular motions, and the resection of a short segment of one additional rib, the seventh, adds very little to the duration or severity of the operation. The other two methods need only be mentioned. One is to develop an extrapleural space between the seventh and eighth ribs and the lung in the region where the tip of the scapula lies. The tip of the scapula is then pushed into this artificially created space in the hope that it will remain there. The other method is to excise a short length of the tip of the scapula so as to shorten it and thus make it impossible for it to reach the seventh rib. This method involves an undesirable amount of trauma resulting from the severance of the attachments of the muscles to that portion.

After resection of the ribs has been completed, the wound is sutured in layers in the usual manner.

THIRD STAGE. In the present day few patients are observed who require a collapse so extensive as to make it necessary to carry out the procedure in three stages. Occasionally even when the disease is less extensive, the frail condition of the patient may make it necessary to proceed with caution, with the removal of fewer ribs at the first and second stages. When this is necessary, a third stage must inevitably follow to complete the surgical program. In the majority of cases, however, the third stage is performed because of the extent of the disease.

A second incision is usually required to obtain easy access to the ribs which are to be removed at the third stage. This incision starts anteriorly approximately at the midaxillary line at a point about 3 inches below the incision used for the first and second stages, and extends parallel to the first incision until the region of the angles of the ribs is reached, where it curves upward to meet the upward curve of the first incision. The muscles are divided and the ribs exposed for resection in the same manner as for the upper two stages. It is not necessary to retract the scapula because of the low location of the operative field. Only relatively short segments of the lower ribs need be resected in the average case. The closure of the incision is made in the usual manner.

After-care, Prevention of Complications and Unfavorable Sequelae. The alarming degree of shock which at one time complicated the early recovery period in many cases of thoracoplasty was the result of the failure to recognize the fact that in almost every case a considerable degree of blood loss occurs. The amount varies, depending upon the factors which have to do with the control of hemostasis, the size and build of the patient and the stage of the procedure. The blood loss is likely to be largest at the first stage because of the great vascularity of the large amount of tissue which must be divided. The present-day practice of administering blood intravenously during the progress of the operation has corrected this situation so that shock no longer occurs. Furthermore, the replacement by transfusion of the blood lost during the operation prevents the anemia which might otherwise make it necessary to prolong the interval between the stages of the operation.

The use of antibiotics to safeguard the early recovery period need only be mentioned at this point. Streptomycin is undoubtedly valuable in certain cases to minimize the tendency to reactivation of quiescent foci of disease or even to prevent the occasional spread of the process. Penicillin may be helpful to reduce the incidence of nonspecific pneumonia and wound infection resulting from the occasional contamination with pyogenic organisms.

Much may be accomplished during the early phase of convalescence to diminish the disfigurement and functional disturbances which are to some extent the more or less inevitable sequelae of the operation, especially when a large number of ribs have been resected. Here again the superior results of the present day arise from the abandonment of some of the older concepts. For example, hardly any improvement in the eventual degree of collapse accrues from the application of external pressure in the form of specially padded bandages, chest swathes or braces. The routine use of a flat cloth bag filled with lead shot is likewise of little value except to make it easier for the patient to cough during the first few days after the operation, when the abnormal mobility of the chest wall may make the act of coughing painful or may diminish the ability of the patient to raise secretions from the lung. Furthermore, if the arm is kept bound to the patient's side for even a few days a very prolonged and disabling degree of stiffness of the shoulder can hardly be avoided.

The best results are obtained by using a minimum of restraint. The wound is covered with a small dressing held in place with woven adhesive strapping. A chest swathe is not used. The patient is encouraged to move freely in bed and to use his arm in all motions as soon as he is able to do so comfortably. It is necessary to give some patients special encouragement to do this early. If coughing and raising sputum are too painful, the support of a shot bag lying on the chest may be helpful during the first few days, but its use is rarely required. Sitting upright in bed should be encouraged, and later postural exercises to overcome the instinctive tendency to favor the operated side should be practiced. The patient should be allowed to get out of bed for short periods of time each day between the stages so as to help him assume a better posture and to prevent excessive weakness which may result from insufficient utilization of muscles. By following these precautions exceptional degrees of scoliosis and long-lasting stiffness of the arm may be avoided.

It should be kept in mind that in the majority of cases at least two and sometimes three stages are required to complete what is in fact one surgical procedure. The interval of time which should be allowed to elapse between the various stages must depend upon the favorable concatenation of several circumstances. In the first place, the incisional wound must be well healed and free from evidences of infection no matter how superficial it may appear to be. The hemoglobin level of the blood must be within a normal range. The well-being of the patient should be at a satisfactory level and in particular there should be no evidence, either clinical or roentgenological, of a spread or reactivation of the disease. The usual safe interval is about two to three weeks. In some cases a week or more of additional time may be necessary, but if there is evidence of reactivation or spread or if for any other reason after any of the stages of the operation the patient becomes too ill to proceed, it is imperative to postpone the next stage indefinitely.

When it becomes necessary to wait three or more months between the stages of the operation, a complication arises from the fact that the regeneration of bone from the periosteum of the previously resected ribs tends to fix that part of the chest wall in a position which prevents the most effective degree of collapse. It is necessary in such a case to repeat at least a part of the previous stage by removing much of the regenerated bone along with the resection of additional ribs which the subsequent stage requires. If this is not done, the ultimate collapse of the lung cannot be so complete and effective as it is in cases where the stages can be performed in the normal sequence after the usual intervals of time.

Intrapleural (Schede) Thoracoplasty

In certain cases of chronic empyema where an extrapleural thoracoplasty would fail to close the cavity, it becomes necessary to perform a type of operation which involves not only the resection of the overlying ribs but also the removal of the thickened parietal pleura and intercostal muscle bundles, nerves and vessels. This procedure is used almost exclusively in cases of tuberculous empyema in which the diseased condition of the underlying lung makes it inadvisable to attempt to obliterate the cavity by pulmonary decortication and expansion of the lung. In many such cases there is a complicating bronchopleural fistula, with a mixed infection of the pleural cavity consisting of various contaminating pyogenic organisms superimposed upon the primary tuberculous involvement. In this situation preliminary external drainage of the pleural cavity by rib resection is necessary before proceeding with the thoracoplasty.

The principle underlying the use of intrapleural (Schede) thoracoplasty in the treatment of a chronic empyema cavity is to eliminate the cavity by excising its outer wall. This unroofing allows the soft parts of the thorax in the corresponding area to fall in against the lung where they then adhere. The ultimate closure of the wound is by granulation and epithelization of the surface by proliferation from the adjacent skin edges. In order to encourage the healing and to prevent the development of persistent sinuses which communicate with the deep recesses of the wound, it is essential to unroof the cavity widely so that no shelving edges remain around the periphery. The length of ribs which should be resected must therefore be greater than the diameter of the cavity at the level where each resected rib crosses it. The excision of the overlying pleura must also be carried beyond the actual periphery of the cavity, leaving only the pulmonary surface behind.

The longitudinal extent of many of these chronic empyema cavities is frequently almost equivalent to that of the chest wall itself. It is necessary, therefore, in a majority of cases to resect a large number of ribs, often from the second above to the tenth below. Such a radical procedure can be performed in one stage only in patients whose general condition is good. Many patients on whom the operation must be performed, however, are in relatively poor physical condition because of the debilitating effects of prolonged sepsis, chronic protein loss from drainage of pus, and sometimes amyloid disease involving the liver and kidneys. In addition there is always the possible effect, either actual or imminent, of activity within the collapsed lung. These considerations make it important in some cases to divide the operation into stages. The physiologic disturbance which would ordinarily be expected as a result of the elimination of the rigidity of much of the thoracic wall is not a very important factor because of the relative fixation of the underlying lung and mediastinum. It is usually possible, therefore, when a one-stage operation seems too radical, to perform the procedure in two stages, with the resection of from four to six ribs at a time.

Patients are often seen who have had a previous attempt at closure of a chronic empyema cavity by means of an extrapleural thoracoplasty. Such attempts are almost universally attended by failure. The most that is ever accomplished, with rare exceptions, is to change the shape of the cavity by flattening it and to reduce to some extent its cubic capacity. The altered cavity remains, however, and in the majority of such cases final resort must

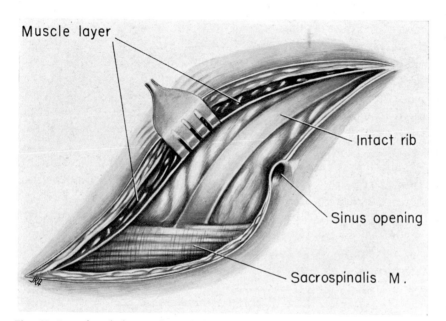

Fig. 68. Intrapleural thoracoplasty (Schede): Preliminary incision passing through the sinus opening and exposing the intact rib below the last resected rib in a case of chronic empyema with bronchopulmonary fistula previously treated unsuccessfully by extrapleural thoracoplasty.

be made to intrapleural thoracoplasty in order to bring about a complete cure of the condition.

Technic. Because the wound is to be packed open with gauze until it closes by granulation, only one incision is used no matter how many stages may be necessary to complete the operation. In the average case the incision begins anteriorly at approximately the anterior axillary line and extends backward along the course of the rib which lies over the lowermost extent of the cavity, usually the ninth or tenth. On reaching the region of the angle of the underlying rib it is curved upward and extended parallel with the spine as far as the upper limits of the cavity. When a drainage sinus exists, the incision is placed so that the sinus tract may be excised (Fig. 68). However, if the sinus is in an unusual location and is inaccessible for excision in this way, it may be ignored or excised locally if desired. The resection of ribs is begun over the lower end of the cavity and long segments of the lower five or more are resected (see above). The condition of the patient should then be assessed by the anesthetist and the surgeon before proceeding with any further resections of rib unless a two stage operation has already been decided upon. In a few cases the entire unroofing can be done at once, but in others it will be obvious that the operation should be interrupted at that point and completed at a later stage. After all of the ribs which are to be removed at any given procedure have been resected, the corresponding portion of the cavity is uncovered by excising the thickened parietal pleura over it. This of course involves the resection of long sections of the corresponding intercostal nerves, vessels and muscles. The vessels are ligated at the anterior and posterior margins of the denuded portion of the cavity, using suture ligatures of chromic catgut (0). The overlying muscles are allowed to fall into the floor of the cavity against the visceral pleura to whatever extent they will and the remainder of the wound is packed with long strips of folded gauze.

When the operation is performed in two stages, a careful evaluation of the patient's condition is made before deciding on the proper time to proceed with the second stage. This may be two or three weeks or it may be a matter of several months. The gauze packing (which of course has been renewed from time to time during the interval) is removed and the wound is enlarged upward as far as necessary. This in many cases involves cutting the lower portions of the trapezius and rhomboid muscles in order to gain access to the ribs beneath the scapula. The resection of the ribs and the excision of pleura, nerves, vessels and intercostal muscles is carried out in the same manner as in the first stage.

At the completion of the operation, whether in one or two stages, the muscle, fat and skin layers of the upper third or more of the wound can be sutured so as to reduce the extent of the wound which must heal by granulation. The remainder of the wound is then packed with gauze.

In those cases which are complicated by the fact that an extrapleural thoracoplasty has been done at some previous time, the performance of a Schede operation is unusually difficult. A neat resection of the regenerated ribs cannot be made. It is usually best in such cases to resect the one or two untouched (normal) ribs which lie below the last resected rib of the previous operation, and at the same time to enter the cavity, removing some of the overlying parietal pleura. The remainder of the roof of the cavity, including the parietal pleura, intercostal muscles, nerves and vessels as well as the regenerated ribs and their periosteum, is then cut as one layer around the periphery of the cavity with heavy, double action bone-cutting shears used like scissors (Fig. 69). As this is done, the portion of chest wall which is

being excised should be grasped with a tenaculum or heavy clamp and retracted outward so that the proximal cut ends of the intercostal arteries can
be secured with hemostatic forceps. Because these arteries lie embedded in
chronic inflammatory tissue behind the thickened parietal pleura, the only
type of hemostat which can be used with much success for this purpose is
that of the Ochsner or Kocher type, with teeth at the ends of the jaws.
If this precaution is not taken, much unnecessary blood loss will occur as

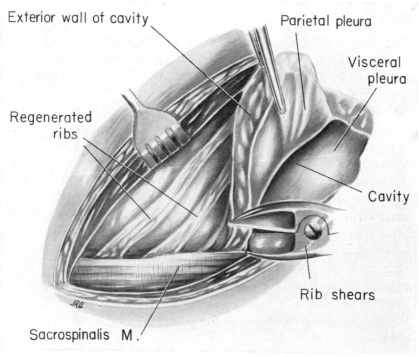

Fig. 69. Intrapleural thoracoplasty (Schede): Same case as in Figure 67. Method of excising
the rigid portion of chest wall with bone-cutting shears, including parietal pleura, periosteum, intercostal muscles, nerves and vessels, and the regenerated ribs over the cavity as a
single plaque.

the unroofing is carried out. The operation is completed in one or two
stages as described above.

After-care. Treatment for shock is rarely required because of the fact that
ample blood replacement is made by transfusion during the progress of the
operation. The blood loss, especially in patients who have had a previous
extrapleural thoracoplasty, is often so massive and so rapid in occurrence
that it is necessary to start a second transfusion in another vein during the
course of the procedure. Such double transfusions administered through
different veins simultaneously are sometimes barely sufficient to compensate for the excessive hemorrhage which may occur. The administration

of blood must be continued after the patient is returned to his bed until an amount equivalent to the amount lost has been given.

Except for the necessity of changing the gauze packing every few days, the care of the patient differs in no important respect from that of those treated by extrapleural thoracoplasty.

The ultimate closure of the wound is slow, often requiring six or more months for its completion, but permanent healing is the rule in the vast majority of cases and the results of the operation are highly satisfactory.

Resection of a Rib With Additional Procedures for Inducing Pulmonary Collapse

Extrapleural Pneumothorax. In certain cases where the obliteration of the pleural space by the adhesion of the lung to the parietal pleura makes it impossible to induce artificial pneumothorax to obtain collapse of the lung, an extrapleural space for the introduction of air may be created artificially by surgical means. This space may be made as large as desired, but it must be maintained by the repeated introduction of air at frequent intervals. There is no uniformity of opinion regarding the indications for the use of this procedure. Certain surgeons use it freely, others not at all. It has had a wide vogue in Europe, especially in France. There are few cases, however, where an intrapleural pneumothorax is not superior in every respect.

Technic. A short incision (5 to 6 inches) is made between the scapula and the spine. The fibers of the trapezius and rhomboid muscles are divided, exposing the ribs beneath. Deep blunt rake retractors are used to increase the exposure and a 3 to 4 inch segment of the third or fourth rib is resected after reflecting its periosteum by the usual technic. An incision is made into the extrapleural fascial plane through the deep rib periosteal layer. With blunt dissection the parietal pleura is then freed from the rib cage over the entire apical portion of the lung, which falls away from the chest wall so as to produce a collapse of the liberated portion. The dissection may be carried downward as far as the sixth or seventh rib posteriorly and anteriorly to any desired level, usually the fourth or fifth costal cartilage. A certain amount of extrapleural freeing of the mediastinal pleura may be accomplished in many cases so as to increase the collapse of the apex of the lung if it is not too rigid because of fibrosis.

During the dissection care must be exerted to avoid injury to the intercostal vessels, especially posteriorly where they are most exposed. Small branches of these vessels may require division and ligation. If the main vessels are torn or cut, they can usually be secured only by means of suture ligatures or dura clips. A further important consideration is to avoid breaking into a superficial cavity within the lung. The control of the mixed bacterial infection which results from such an accident is exceedingly difficult. A fatal outcome from chronic sepsis of the thoracic wall may result.

After the amount of space required to produce a sufficient collapse of the lung has been developed, the wound is closed in layers placed in the rib periosteum, muscles, superficial fascia and skin.

AFTER-CARE. Because of its rapid absorption from the extrapleural space, it is necessary to refill the cavity with air every few days during the first few weeks after the operation. Later the interval may be lengthened as the rate of absorption decreases. In all cases, however, there is a gradual tendency for the lung to creep out along the edges of the cavity so as to reduce its size by the slow process of adhesion around the periphery. In this way the ultimate degree of collapse may not be so large as the size and location of the underlying lesion require. Recourse in such cases must be made to the performance of an extrapleural thoracoplasty over the region which was freed originally at the first operation.

The late occurrence of infection in the extrapleural space, usually from erosion through the thin wall of a superficial pulmonary cavity, is not a subject for discussion in this work and need only be mentioned.

Paraffin Plombage. In certain cases of extensive disease where artificial pneumothorax is unsuccessful and for some reason thoracoplasty or extrapleural pneumothorax may be contraindicated, it may be desirable to bring about a focal collapse in a localized area of the lung. This can be done by producing a circumscribed extrapleural space between the ribs and the parietal pleura in the region of the pulmonary lesion. The resultant focal collapse of the lung is then increased in degree and rendered more permanent by filling the newly created space with some substance which can be molded easily to fit its size and shape. Paraffin which has a melting point a few degrees above body temperature serves the purpose well.

The use of paraffin plombage is usually confined to the production of a localized collapse and compression of a pulmonary cavity which is in a location unfavorable for collapse therapy by other means. One of the most frequent indications is bilateral cavitary disease where a thoracoplasty or artificial pneumothorax has been used on one side, making it unwise to induce a large collapse on the second side.

TECHNIC. An accurate preliminary localization of the pulmonary cavity which is to be the subject of collapse must be made by roentgen ray studies. A short incision (5 to 6 inches) is made over the rib which lies directly over the cavity. Through this a 3 to 4 inch segment of rib is resected subperiosteally. The deep periosteal layer is incised, but the pleura is avoided. The parietal pleura is dissected free from the surrounding portion of the chest wall over an area which is considerably wider in diameter than the diameter of the underlying cavity in the lung. Caution must be exerted to prevent perforation of the cavity during the performance of the dissection. A sufficient quantity of paraffin is softened by immersion in a heated water bath to the point where it can be molded between the fingers. The entire extra-pleural space which has just been created is then filled tightly with the paraffin. It is necessary to introduce more of the substance than might at first seem to be necessary because the success of the operation depends to a large extent upon the local compression produced over the pulmonary cavity. After its introduction has been completed, the mass of paraffin should have a dome-shaped contour equivalent to that of a hemisphere whose diameter is that of the extrapleural space in which it lies. Its con-vexity is, of course, against the lung.

The wound is closed in layers consisting of the rib periosteum, the muscles, the superficial fascia and the skin.

AFTER-CARE. No particular immediate after-care is required and the operation need make only a temporary interruption (not more than a few days) in the general treatment program of the patient. Patients who have been treated by paraffin plombage, however, should be kept under careful scrutiny because of the danger of erosion of the thin layer of pulmonary tissue over the apex of the pulmonary cavity. This would lead to a serious mixed organism infection of the extrapleural space. If this complication should occur, the wound must be reopened, the paraffin removed com-pletely, and wide open drainage of the space provided by gauze packing or the introduction of rubber tube drains.

Subsequent slipping of the paraffin from its original ideal position has been described, but does not occur if material of the correct melting point (higher than body temperature) is used.

There is some difference of opinion regarding the duration of time during which the paraffin should be allowed to remain in position. There is reason to believe that it can be left in place indefinitely without causing harm. On the other hand, if the underlying pulmonary cavity is large and does not tend to close, the longer the paraffin is left in place, the greater the proba-bility of erosion through the cavity. This accident rarely occurs within one to two years after the operation. Furthermore, if the cavity is to close, it will probably have done so by the expiration of that time. It is possible, therefore, in the majority of cases, to remove the foreign body after one to two years. Because of the density of the shadow produced by the paraffin mass on the roentgen ray film, however, it is difficult to determine what the condition of the cavity may be. In practice the decision as to when to remove the substance must be made on a purely arbitrary basis.

For the removal of the paraffin the previous incision is used. The extra-pleural space in which the material lies is found and the entire mass is lifted out. This is accomplished with ease because the paraffin does not become adherent to the surrounding tissues. Some attempt should be made before closing the incision to obliterate the extrapleural space which remains. This may be done by filling it with a large flap of muscle developed from the adjacent latissimus dorsi or trapezius muscles or by resection of long segments of all the ribs which form the outer surface of the space. It is not possible by either method to prevent a partial reexpansion of the lung into the space which is left. The muscle flap method is the less effective of the two because of the well-known tendency of such flaps to undergo atrophy. The localized thoracoplasty produced by rib resection is therefore the method of choice in the average case.

Operations Made Necessary by Trauma to the Chest Wall

Superficial Lacerations. Lacerations of the skin and other soft parts of the thoracic wall, unless complicated by fractures of the ribs or evidences of injury to intrathoracic organs, do not require special consideration. The principles of débridement and closure of wounds of the soft parts anywhere in the body apply equally well in those of the chest.

Sucking Wounds of the Chest Wall. Much has been written on the treatment of sucking wounds of the chest wall, which are those which penetrate the pleural cavity and tend to produce a tension pneumothorax. Prompt closure of the opening with an occlusive airtight dressing followed by aspiration of a large volume of the air which has entered the pleural cavity is the emergency treatment required. Often the life of the patient may be saved by this means. The definitive treatment of such a wound involves of course not only the débridement and closure of the soft part portion, but also the initiation of whatever measures may be required to correct the effects of injuries to the intercostal vessels, splintering of the ribs, or lacerations of the lung or injuries to any other intrathoracic structures. The necessity for observing the general principles of the treatment of shock, for replacement of extravasated blood by transfusion, for procurement of adequate intratracheal anesthesia, and for insistence upon proper conditions for the performance of a major thoracotomy is self-evident. The exact procedure, of course, depends entirely upon the nature and extent of the internal injuries. Only injuries to the chest wall are considered here.

Fractures of the Ribs. Fractures of the ribs rarely require surgical intervention, but there are three circumstances when a thoracotomy may be indicated. These occur usually in injuries of great severity produced by direct violence to the chest wall and are as follows:

1. In cases in which the fractured ends of the rib are unusually jagged, often with long splinters which have been driven inward towards the lung, it may be necessary to expose the region of the fracture and to resect the fragmented segment of bone. This prevents continued injury to the lung beneath with the resulting escape of air from the alveoli. Intratracheal inhalation anesthesia is necessary to control the expansion of the lung. An incision of sufficient length is made through the skin and muscles. The region of the fracture is exposed and the periosteum is elevated from the normal

portions of rib at each end of the broken segment. The rib is then cut squarely across and the broken fragments are removed. A search should be made at the same time for evidences of injury to the intercostal vessels, which should be tied if need be. The pleura should be opened widely enough to discover the nature and extent of the pulmonary injury or the presence of injury to vessels other than the intercostals. If intrathoracic injuries requiring surgical intervention are found, the wound should be enlarged by whatever method seems best and the necessary procedure carried out.

2. In certain cases of severely fractured ribs, there is a recurring hemothorax. Although this condition may be the result of injury to other vessels, in the overwhelming majority of instances it is the result of laceration of the intercostal artery and vein. In such a case it is necessary to make an incision and to deal with the vessels and jagged ends as described above.

3. A third indication for active intervention in cases of rib fracture occurs when a large number of ribs have been broken, both front and back. This condition, popularly referred to as "stove-in chest," allows the occurrence of marked paradoxical motion of the chest wall on the injured side. This abnormal motion, together with the intense pain produced during respiration and especially during attempts to cough, often interferes to an alarming degree with the effective exchange of air within the respiratory passages. As a result the raising of secretions is interfered with and the oxygenation of the blood is seriously impaired. In such cases open exposure and fixation of the fractured rib ends by wire sutures is a life-saving measure.

TECHNIC. Intratracheal anesthesia is administered. An incision similar to that used for a thoracoplasty is employed. The division of the muscles is made extensive enough to permit a wide exposure of the posterior portions of the ribs. The ends of the ribs at the site of fracture are trimmed with a costotome or rongeur so that no jagged points remain. With a small bone drill a hole is made through each end of the broken bone. This is repeated with every fractured rib and a piece of stainless steel wire (22 gauge) is passed through the holes in each rib. The wire is drawn tight and the ends are twisted so as to hold the two ends of each fractured rib in firm apposition. It is not necessary in the average case to fix the broken ribs anteriorly if a firm posterior fixation is accomplished.

AFTER-CARE. The improvement in the condition of the patient which results from this operation is usually very striking. The severity of the pain is greatly diminished. Breathing is more comfortable and the expectoration of secretions is more effective. The discomfort of the incision is inconsequential when compared with the pain experienced before the operation. Healing of the wound presents no special problems. Furthermore, the ultimate healing of the fractured ribs is hastened and a considerable degree of distortion of the bones is prevented because of the fact that the broken rib ends are brought together posteriorly.

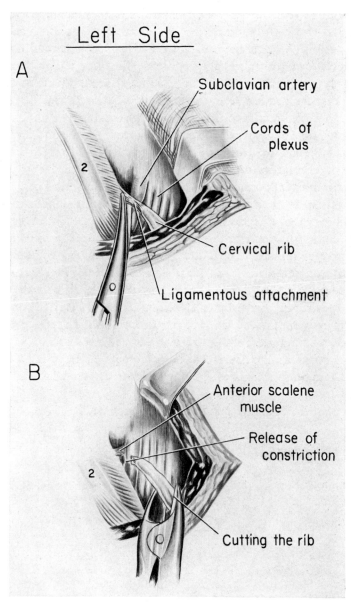

Fig. 70. Thoracic approach for the removal of cervical rib. *A*, Exposure obtained showing cervical rib and ligamentous attachment to the first thoracic rib at the scalene tubercle with marked constriction of the subclavian artery and the lower trunk of the brachial plexus. *B*, Release of the constriction after cutting the ligamentous attachment showing the insertion of a portion of the anterior scalene muscle on the scalene tubercle. The excision of the rib is portrayed.

Excision of Cervical Rib by the Thoracic Approach

Under certain circumstances the technical difficulties attendant upon the removal of a cervical rib and release of a tight anterior scalene attachment result in postoperative sequelae which may be prolonged and disturbing. Furthermore, it is sometimes difficult to make the operation sufficiently thorough to bring about the desired relief of symptoms. A new approach to the region involved has been shown to simplify the procedure and make it possible to avoid trauma to the trunks of the brachial plexus. This operation consists in the exposure of the cervical rib and scalene attachment from below, using an incision similar to that employed in the performance of the first stage of a thoracoplasty.

The incision extends from the level of the superior border of the scapula down between the medial border of that bone and the spine, curving forward a short distance beneath the angle of the scapula. The rib cage is exposed by cutting portions of the trapezius, rhomboid, latissimus dorsi and anterior serratus muscles. The scapula is retracted and the middle scalene muscle is freed from the first and second ribs. The exposure obtained in this manner reveals the cervical rib and tight anterior scalene attachment without touching the trunks of the brachial plexus or the subclavian artery (Fig. 70, A). The release of the constriction of these structures is readily accomplished by cutting the muscle attachment with scissors and excising the rib with a bone-cutting forceps. A long segment of rib can be removed without causing any trauma to the important structures which lie above it (Fig. 70, B).

The incision is closed in layers in the usual manner.

CHAPTER 5

OPERATIONS CONCERNING THE PLEURAL CAVITY

There is no entirely logical manner in which to classify the procedures which concern primarily the pleural cavity. Some of these, such as the aspiration of fluid or the introduction of air into the pleural space, can hardly be considered surgical. Certain others, on the other hand, require the application of great technical skill and the exercise of mature surgical judgment. Emphasis will be placed upon the more strictly surgical procedures.

THE MANAGEMENT OF ACCUMULATIONS OF FLUID IN THE PLEURAL CAVITY

Thoracentesis

The withdrawal of fluid from the pleural cavity by aspiration with a needle and syringe may be used either to obtain specimens for diagnostic purposes or as a method of treatment to remove accumulations of thin pus or to relieve respiratory embarrassment produced by large extravasations of fluid of any type. An airtight syringe and a needle of sufficient caliber to allow the passage of fluid through it are sufficient for diagnostic thoracentesis. The needle should be long enough to penetrate the structures of the chest wall. The length required varies, depending upon the physical build and age of the patient.

An accurate determination of the location of the fluid is made by physical examination and roentgen ray visualization so as to choose the best site for the needle puncture. In dealing with large accumulations of fluid which rest upon the diaphragm, it should be borne in mind that on the right side the diaphragm rises higher than on the left, so that if the needle is inserted at too low a level, the liver may be punctured and nothing but blood will be obtained. In general, the eighth or ninth intercostal space in the postero-lateral aspect of the chest is satisfactory in the case of a massive effusion. When the fluid is loculated or confined to a small localized area, the inter-costal space which lies directly over the point where the fluid accumulation makes its largest contact with the chest wall must be chosen. The location of this point, of course, varies depending upon the individual case.

A separate small syringe with a needle of fine bore is used for the infiltration of procaine hydrochloride solution. An intradermal wheal is made at the site chosen for the aspiration. The anesthetic solution is then introduced into the subcutaneous fat and muscles, including a generous amount in the intercostal muscle layer so as to perfuse the intercostal nerve. The point for the injection of the intercostal space can be determined by inserting the needle deeply until the pleura is felt. The touching of the pleura usually causes the patient to feel a transitory painful sensation. If the needle has gone deeper, slight negative pressure produced by pulling on the plunger of the syringe will cause a small gush of fluid. The needle is then withdrawn while suction is being exerted with the syringe until fluid cannot be obtained. At that point several cubic centimeters of anesthetic solution should be injected. The subsequent manipulation of the aspirating needle through the region where the injection was made is then quite painless.

After the desired amount of material has been aspirated into the barrel of the syringe, the needle is withdrawn. In theory an effort should be made throughout the procedure to avoid accidentally disconnecting the aspirating needle from the syringe until its withdrawal from the chest, to avoid the entrance of air into the pleural cavity. In practice, however, the introduction of small amounts of air is of little importance. In certain cases where the pleura is acutely inflamed, it is wise to introduce 100 or 200 cc. of air to avoid the friction of lung against the hypersensitive parietal pleura whenever the major portion of a fluid accumulation has been withdrawn.

It sometimes happens that the fluid obtained at thoracentesis, though not bloody of itself, is suffused with blood which results from the trauma of the procedure. The blood under such circumstances comes from the intercostal veins of the chest wall, from the lung, or from the liver when the needle is inserted at too low a level. This occurrence must be recognized so as to avoid errors of interpretation of the characteristics of the fluid.

Operative Treatment of Acute Empyema

Aspiration and Introduction of Antibiotics. Aspiration followed by the instillation of a solution containing penicillin or streptomycin, or a combination of these antibiotics, has become an established method of treatment, especially when the purulent fluid is thin. The technic of this manipulation is essentially the same as that described under the section dealing with diagnostic thoracentesis. However, the removal of large quantities of fluid is greatly facilitated by modifying the apparatus so as to include a two-way stopcock valve which is connected with the needle and the syringe by pieces of rubber tubing of suitable size. The stopcock is arranged so that suction applied by withdrawing the plunger of the syringe will cause the fluid to enter the syringe without the access of air into the apparatus. After the barrel of the syringe is full, the stopcock valve is turned and the fluid is evacuated from the syringe through a side nozzle with a rubber tube attachment to direct it into a collecting basin. This process is then repeated until all of the fluid has been withdrawn. The aspirating needle can, if desired, be attached directly to the stopcock, but the interposition of a short length of tubing between the valve and the needle makes the procedure easier because it eliminates the effect of transmission to the chest wall itself of forces created in the manipulation of the valve.

The dosage of antibiotic solution and the interval between treatments depend upon the indications in each individual case and are not matters for discussion here.

Closed Thoracotomy. In certain cases of empyema where for some reason it is impracticable to rely upon repeated thoracentesis with a needle, continuous aspiration by means of a catheter introduced through an intercostal space is advantageous. The purpose of this method is to provide drainage which will avoid the ingress of air to the pleural cavity at a time when the lung might collapse because of its failure to become adherent to the chest wall. Its use in the management of empyema is therefore confined to those cases where the fluid is thin with a low fibrin content, as in streptococcal infections.

TECHNIC. Because many patients on whom this operation is to be performed are desperately ill or are suffering from serious embarrassment of the respiratory function due to the magnitude of the effusion or the effects of the coexistent pneumonic infiltration, the operation must often be performed without moving the patient from his bed. The majority of such patients are unable to lie flat and can rarely be placed upon the opposite side. The operation must therefore often be performed with the patient in the sitting position or reclining at an angle and leaning slightly toward the opposite side. As in all procedures which involve puncturing the thoracic wall, the dangers of cerebral air embolism caused by the ingress of air to the intercostal veins which communicate with the vertebral veins must be kept in mind. The theoretically ideal position with the head slightly lower than the chest cannot be assumed by these patients, however, and the risk of air embolism must be accepted. Fortunately its occurrence is very infrequent.

The intercostal space which lies over the lowermost portion of the extravasation is identified and the exact site for drainage is determined. At this point the structures of the chest wall are anesthetized by local infiltration of procaine hydrochloride solution (1 per cent) in the same manner as for the performance of a thoracentesis. An aspirating needle attached to a syringe is introduced to verify the presence of pus. If pus is found, a 1 cm. incision is made in the skin. Through this a trocar and cannula are introduced and thrust directly through the intercostal space into the pleural cavity (Fig. 71, *A*). A rubber catheter is selected to fit exactly the internal diameter of the cannula and the correct length of the catheter which should lie within the chest is determined and a small scratch made upon it at the point which should lie at the skin level. This catheter, with the free end closed by a hemostatic forceps, is then pushed into the chest through the cannula immediately after the trocar is withdrawn. In this manner the entrance of more than a negligible quantity of air into the chest is avoided. While this maneuver is being carried out, the cannula is withdrawn by sliding it out along the catheter, which is held securely to prevent its escape. When the cannula reaches the outer end of the catheter, an occluding hemostat is placed between it and the patient and the terminal hemostat is removed

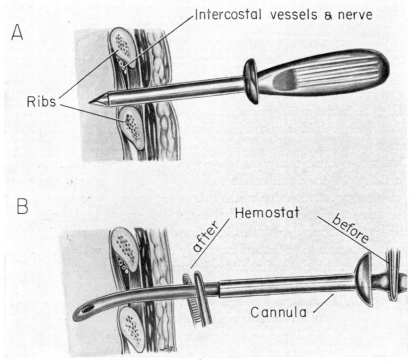

Fig. 71. Technic of closed thoracotomy. *A*, Trocar and cannula inserted correctly through an intercostal space, avoiding the vessels and nerve along the inferior margin of the upper-most rib. *B*, Method of preventing ingress of air while the catheter is being inserted. First hemostat on the end of the catheter is removed and a second hemostat is put on near the patient as the cannula is removed.

so as to allow it to be passed off the free end of the tube (Fig. 71, *B*). A single silk suture is used to tighten the skin edges around the catheter, and the free ends of this strand are tied securely around the catheter at the point where the mark upon it lies. This suture prevents the subsequent accidental withdrawal of the catheter from the chest. A long connecting tube of rubber is fastened to the free end of the catheter by means of a connecting link of glass tubing.

Provision for continuous drainage without the entrance of air into the pleural cavity may be made by introducing the end of the rubber connecting tube under an accumulation of water in a bottle which rests upon the floor at the bedside. If continuous aspiration of the fluid is desired, the tube may be connected to a bottle on which slight negative pressure is made by means of continuous suction with an interposed safety valve to control the pressure relations (see Chap. 3).

Following the operation special precautions must be observed to make certain that the drainage system remains airtight. The importance of this matter must be explained to the nurses or attendants. As the evacuation of the pus approaches completion, the previously compressed lung expands to the point at which it begins to make contact with the chest wall, where after a few days it will usually become adherent. In the meantime the pus usually becomes thickened and full of fibrin so that ultimately (seven to ten days) it is too viscid to pass readily through the catheter. By this time the lung will have become adherent and it is then safe to shift to open drainage. For this purpose, except in young children, it is usually necessary to resect a rib in order to provide an adequate opening.

Open Thoracotomy for Drainage of Empyema. When the pus is thick and full of fibrin, as in a pneumococcus infection, the lung is likely to be adherent. In such cases and in all cases of encapsulated empyema which require drainage, an open thoracotomy for the insertion of one or more large drainage tubes is necessary.

Local infiltration of the structures of the chest wall using procaine hydrochloride solution (1 per cent) is the anesthesia of choice for the drainage of empyema by open thoracotomy. In addition to the infiltration of the tissues which are to be incised, it is necessary to produce an anesthetic bloc of the intercostal nerves corresponding to the ribs above and below the rib which is to be resected. This is done because of the tendency of some of their fibers to overlap.

The position of the patient on the operating table should follow the principles outlined in the section on trocar thoracotomy.

TECHNIC. The technic of rib resection for minor thoracotomy as described in Chapter 3 is applied in the treatment of empyema. After the incision has been made and a suitable dependent point opened, a drain must be inserted in order to keep the wound open long enough to allow obliteration of the cavity. If the empyema cavity is unusually large, two tubes of rubber, each with a diameter of ½ to ⅝ inch, should be inserted. One of these tubes can be eliminated after three or four weeks of drainage and the other maintained. In many cases a single large tube is sufficient. The tube should be long enough to extend a short distance within the pleural cavity but not too deeply. Lateral holes can be cut near the end of the tube if desired. This may improve the efficiency of the drainage to some extent, but after several weeks a new tube which does not have side holes should be substituted for the original tube. If this is not done, the granulation tissue from the drainage sinus will grow through the lateral openings and cause it to become obstructed.

A suture of catgut passed through one side of the tube is used to fasten it to the fascia of one of the muscle edges. This avoids suturing to the skin edges which is unnecessarily painful. Ultimate fixation of the tube with adhesive tape passed through a safety pin attached to the tube is resorted to after the catgut suture becomes loosened.

AFTER-CARE. The after-care of patients whose empyema is treated by open thoracotomy involves merely the frequent changes of dressing and the use of precautions such as adhesive strapping to the skin to prevent escape of the drainage tube. Great care must be exerted also that a tube or a portion of drain be not lost within the empyema cavity; whoever changes the dressing must each time observe that the drain or drains are in place. The presence of a foreign body of this sort within the pleural cavity is a ready source of failure of the cavity to close properly.

By far the most important consideration in the management of these cases is to leave the tube in place long enough. If the drain is removed prematurely, the chest wall sinus will close over in a few days and a localized accumulation of pus will be left still undrained. Subsequent surgery to re-establish adequate drainage is required in such cases. The decision as to when to remove the tube cannot be made arbitrarily on the basis of the expiration of a certain period of time after the operation. The proper time for the removal of the tube may be determined in either of two ways. One method is to wait until the cavity is so reduced in size that it amounts to hardly more than the volume of space required to accommodate the tube itself. This can be determined by palpation, using a small probe. The other method is to make periodic measurements of the amount of sterile saline solution which the cavity will hold and remove the drain when the volume of the space is reduced to no greater than 5 or 10 cc.

Irrigation of adequately drained empyema cavities is rarely necessary except when there may be accumulations of fibrin or necrotic tissue from a focus of gangrene in the lung. In all other cases it is preferable not to resort to irrigation.

Chronic Empyema

A rare but unfortunate sequela of cases of acute empyema treated by thoracotomy is the failure of the cavity to become obliterated. This leads to a state of chronicity which makes it necessary to maintain a drainage tube indefinitely or subject the patient to further surgery. The most frequent causes are premature removal of the original drain, the presence of a foreign body such as a portion of drainage material or a fragment of sequestrated bone from a rib end, the presence of a bronchopleural fistula or the exist-tence of certain types of infection, notably tuberculosis and actinomycosis. Intelligent treatment requires a consideration of these possibilities in each case.

Operations for the Treatment of Chronic Empyema. The surgical management of cases of chronic empyema must of course depend upon the etiology. Wide open drainage of the cavity must be established as a preliminary measure. At that time foreign bodies should be searched for and a generous biopsy should be obtained from the chronically thickened pleura. If tuberculosis or actinomycosis is present, the histologic examination of the tissues will usually confirm the diagnosis. After the above causes of chronicity have been excluded, there remain two methods of surgical treatment which may be applied according to the indications in each case. These are (1) thoracoplasty, to obliterate the cavity by collapsing the overlying portion of the chest wall, or (2) decortication of the lung, to eliminate the cavity by allowing the reexpanded lung to fill it. Of these the latter is superior because it avoids disfigurement and permits an almost complete return of respiratory function.

THORACOPLASTY FOR THE CLOSURE OF CHRONIC EMPYEMA CAVITIES. The method of closure of a chronic empyema cavity by thoracoplasty is confined nowadays almost exclusively to the cases of empyema which occasionally follow as a complication of total pneumonectomy, and to the cases in which the lung beneath the cavity is too extensively diseased to make it safe to bring about its expansion or to make it worth while from a functional standpoint. This holds true particularly in pulmonary tuberculosis.

TECHNIC. The operative technic which should be employed in these cases has been described in the section dealing with thoracoplasty (Chap. 4). The Schede technic is the method which is most likely to be completely successful.

DECORTICATION OF THE LUNG. The elimination of a chronic empyema cavity by releasing the partially collapsed lung which lies beneath it is the method of choice for the reasons already cited. Its use is most applicable in the cases of chronic nontuberculous infection. In certain unusually favorable cases of chronic tuberculous empyema, however, the method may also be used, but the amount of disease in the underlying lung must be small and the stage of activity quiescent or apparently arrested. Otherwise a reactivation of the process is almost inevitable.

In all cases of chronic empyema the lung beneath the pleural cavity is covered by a membrane of fibrous tissue which forms over the visceral pleura and by contraction becomes ultimately stretched as tightly as a drumhead over the lung. This membrane is distinct from the visceral pleura. The operation of decortication involves the removal of this layer of tissue.

TECHNIC. A standard thoracotomy incision is made. In order to gain an adequate exposure it is usually necessary to resect a rib. The empyema cavity is entered and cleansed by irrigation with sterile saline solution or by wiping with gauze. The layer of tough fibrous tissue which lies tightly stretched over the lung is incised with a knife at any convenient point. This incision must be deep enough to reach the visceral pleura (Fig. 72, *A*). Between this pleura and the overlying fibrous layer there is usually enough loose areolar tissue to make it relatively easy to develop a satisfactory plane of cleavage. The tough membrane can thus be dissected away from the visceral pleura with the scissors and sometimes even with the fingers. Only in fairly recent cases is much sharp dissection necessary. As the constricting

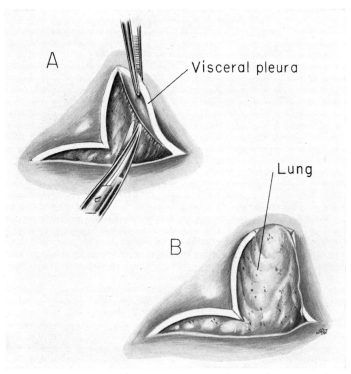

Fig. 72. Decortication of the lung. *A,* Incision through the thickened pleural membrane started and removal of membrane begun by dissection with the scissors. *B,* Bulging of the lung through the area of partial decortication noticed as the freeing progresses.

pleural membrane is removed, the liberated lung beneath begins to expand immediately in response to the positive pressure in the anesthesia system (Fig. 72, *B*).

It is sometimes easiest to find the correct plane of cleavage, however, by making the initial incision through the fibrous membrane at some point near its attachment to the thoracic wall where the fixation to the underlying lung is usually not so intimate (Fig. 73). Starting at the initial incision the entire layer is peeled from the lung and any adhesion of the margins of the lung to the mediastinal surface, the pericardium or the bodies of the vertebrae is divided. In the majority of cases the lung is found to be not atelectatic but merely compressed and reduced in volume. Its complete expansion is brought about by increasing the pressure within the anesthesia system. The lung in this way is made to assume its normal relation to the chest wall and the negative pressure which results from an airtight closure of the wound serves to keep it expanded.

In some cases the interior of the chest wall is lined by an unusually thick layer of fibrous tissue covering the parietal pleura. Excision of this layer as an adjunct to the pulmonary decortication improves the functional result by permitting better expansion of the thorax on the operated side.

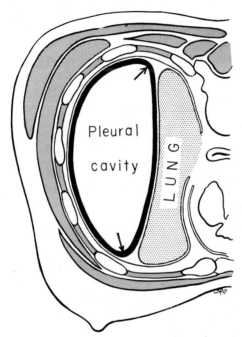

Fig. 73. Decortication of the lung. Diagram: Arrows indicate the areas where it is easiest to start the subcortical dissection in order to avoid trauma to the underlying lung.

Closed catheter drainage of the pleural cavity may be necessary if there is enough oozing from raw surfaces to cause the accumulation of a large extravasation of serosanguineous fluid in the pleural space, or if there has been damage to the pulmonary tissue which might give rise to a leakage of air.

OPERATIONS USED FOR THE RELIEF OF HEMOTHORAX (TRAUMATIC)

The management of hemothorax should include both measures necessary to stop the bleeding and evacuation of blood to avoid the crippling fibro-thorax which results from failure to remove it.

Thoracentesis. As soon as the condition of the patient permits, the extravasated blood should be removed from the pleural cavity by thoracentesis. In some cases the enormous volume of blood in the chest interferes mechanically with the respiratory function to an alarming extent, making prompt aspiration imperative even though the loss of blood from the circulation has been replaced by transfusions. The technic of this procedure has been described (section on *Thoracentesis for Acute Empyema*).

Exploratory Thoracotomy. If the bleeding does not cease and the hemothorax recurs after one aspiration, a prompt resort must be made to open thoracotomy. A standard thoracotomy incision is used. After the blood has been evacuated, a careful search is made for the source of the bleeding which is often one of the intercostal vessels at the site of the injury. Bleeding from a major pulmonary vessel or from the heart or great vessels of the mediastinum is usually so excessive that death occurs before an exploration can be performed. Bleeding from lacerations of the lung parenchyma, on the other hand, frequently stops of its own accord. As soon as the bleeding vessel has been secured by ligature and any injury to other structures dealt with according to the indications found, the lung is thoroughly expanded and the chest wall closed in the usual manner after thorough evacuation of any residual blood or clots. Drainage is not required in the usual case.

After-care. The after-care is essentially the same as that required in any case of thoracotomy. Adequate blood replacement must be made by multiple transfusions.

When the presence of blood in the pleural cavity has been unrecognized or ignored, coagulation occurs after several days and ultimately fibrous tissue organization of the clot results. This in turn leads to the development of a tight membrane over the collapsed lung and also to the fixation of the chest wall because of the formation of a layer of tough, inflexible tissue on the parietal wall. Considerable impairment of the respiratory function is the inevitable result of the influence of these two factors. Such cases of neglected hemothorax require treatment by decortication of the lung and often of the parietal pleura as well. The technic which must be employed is identical with that described in the section dealing with decortication of the lung for chronic empyema.

THE MANAGEMENT OF ACCUMULATIONS OF AIR IN THE PLEURAL CAVITY

Operations for Tension Pneumothorax. THORACENTESIS. A single aspiration of air from the pleural space may be curative in some cases of tension pneumothorax, providing the source of the leak is small and prompt sealing over of the opening occurs. The technic used for the aspiration of fluid may be used. Because of the tendency of air to occupy the portion of the pleural cavity which is uppermost, the most convenient site for the needle puncture is the second intercostal space in the midclavicular line when the patient lies in the dorsal recumbent position with the headrest elevated. This site makes it possible to avoid injury to the internal mammary vessels. If the apparatus used for the induction of artificial pneumothorax is available, the removal of air can be much more easily effected by its use. A sufficient quantity of air should be withdrawn to relieve the distress of the patient.

CONTINUOUS ASPIRATION. In cases where the leakage of air continues after a single aspiration has been carried out, the recurrence of respiratory distress makes it apparent that continuous aspiration is necessary. This may be accomplished either with a needle or with a rubber catheter introduced through an intercostal space and connected with a water seal by means of a length of rubber tubing. The second intercostal space in the midclavicular line is usually the best site for the introduction of the needle or catheter. If a needle is used, it should be passed through a cork or a piece of rubber sponge, leaving just enough of its length to penetrate the pleural cavity when the cork or rubber is held tightly against the skin of the chest wall by adhesive strapping. This method of fastening the needle insures continued operation of the apparatus by avoiding shifting of its position. It also makes it possible to avoid having the needle protrude too far within the chest cavity, thus reducing the possibility of injury to the expanding lung.

If a trocar and cannula of small diameter are available, a small rubber catheter can be introduced by the method described in the section on empyema drainage. The use of a catheter has the obvious advantage that there is no danger of traumatizing the surface of the lung.

In either case, the needle or catheter is attached by means of a suitable adapter to a rubber tube, the opposite end of which is put beneath a volume of water in a large bottle beneath the patient's bed. The development of positive pressure from a continuous leakage of air within the pleural cavity is thereby avoided by the automatic simultaneous escape of air through the water. As the leak seals over, the normal intrathoracic negative pressure is restored because of the fact that air cannot gain access to the pleural space from the outside. Continuous suction at not over 8 to 10 cm. of water negative pressure may be substituted for the water seal if desired.

In the average case of spontaneous pneumothorax reexpansion of the lung occurs within a few days and the apparatus can usually be removed soon thereafter. It is wise to try the effect of occluding the tube during a twenty-four hour period before its removal to be sure that a recurrence of the leak will not make it necessary to reintroduce it subsequently.

SUTURE OF THE LUNG. Under certain circumstances when the tension pneumothorax is the result of the rupture of an emphysematous bleb of the lung, it may be advisable, in order to shorten the period of disability, to perform an open thoracotomy to stop the continued or recurrent leakage of air. The technic of this procedure is described in Chapter 6, which deals with the operations performed on the lung.

Operations Concerning the Utilization of Artificial Pneumothorax. The artificial or instrumental introduction of air within the pleural cavity is used either as a method of diagnosis or as treatment.

DIAGNOSTIC ARTIFICIAL PNEUMOTHORAX. Artificial pneumothorax is occasionally induced as a method of diagnosis in order to improve the visualization of the inner surface of the thoracic wall or more often to determine whether certain peripheral shadows are caused by a mass within the lung or by one in the chest wall itself. The interposition of air between the chest wall and the lung makes such a differentiation possible. This method is rarely used nowadays because of the wider application of exploratory thoracotomy. Air is sometimes introduced into the pleural cavity as a preliminary measure to facilitate the performance of a diagnostic thoracoscopy.

THERAPEUTIC ARTIFICIAL PNEUMOTHORAX. As a method of treatment artificial pneumothorax is used occasionally to overcome the pain of acute pleurisy by preventing the lung from rubbing against the parietal pleura. Its widest application, however, is in the collapse therapy of pulmonary tuberculosis. The indications for its adoption and the details of its use are not the subject of this book. It is not ordinarily regarded as a surgical procedure. A brief description of the technic follows:

The patient is made to lie upon the opposite side resting on a pillow so as to arch upward the side to be treated. Local infiltration anesthesia of procaine hydrochloride solution (1 per cent) is used. The most convenient site for the needle puncture is usually the sixth intercostal space in the midaxillary line. For the initial injection of air it is necessary to take special precautions to avoid injury to the surface of the lung. This makes it wise to use one of the especially constructed pneumothorax needles which has a short bevel and an obturator which insures against plugging the needle tip with tissue or blood. The needle is inserted slowly through the anesthetized area until the pleural space is entered. This event can usually be determined by the sudden release of the sense of resistance which is imparted to the fingers of the operator by the tissues of the thoracic wall. When it seems that the space has been found, the obturator is withdrawn and the needle is connected with the pneumothorax apparatus for the determination of the pressure. If a negative pressure reading in the vicinity of −7 to −12 is obtained, the space has been entered and the introduction of air may be started. If only a slightly negative pressure reading is obtained, it may mean that the needle has entered the lung. A positive pressure may be the result of the penetration of a pulmonary vessel. The amount of air to be injected and the frequency of subsequent injections need not be discussed here.

COMPLICATIONS AND SEQUELAE. A rare but alarming complication of the introduction of air into the pleural cavity is the so-called "pleural shock" which is now known to be the result of the injection of air into the blood circulation, with ensuing cerebral air embolism. This occurrence is probably caused by the entrance of air into a pulmonary vein. However, the injection of air into a vein in the chest wall may produce the same result by way of the collateral communications of the intercostal veins with the vertebral veins which anastomose with the cerebral venous system, thus by-passing the pulmonary circuit. Syncope, fall in peripheral blood pressure, pallor and convulsions announce the occurrence of this accident. These attacks may be fatal, but recovery frequently occurs unless the amount of air injected before the difficulty is recognized has been large.

SURGICAL TREATMENT OF COMPLICATIONS. Although the introduction and maintenance of artificial pneumothorax for the collapse therapy of pulmonary tuberculosis is not usually regarded as a surgical procedure, some of its complications and sequelae may demand surgical treatment. This is particularly true of chronic empyema which may occur spontaneously or result from injudicious management such as increasing the pressure within the cavity to the point where adhesions may be torn. The most frequent requirement for surgical intervention, however, is the persistence of adhesions between the lung and the chest wall which interfere too greatly with the collapse of the lung. In such cases, in order to convert a partially successful collapse into one which has therapeutic value, it is necessary to divide the adhesions which hold the lung out. Two methods for the accomplishment of this result are available.

CLOSED PNEUMONOLYSIS. For the division of attenuated single adhesions or of thinned-out, fanlike adhesive bands, cutting with an electrically actuated cautery under thoracoscopic visualization is satisfactory. There are several excellent instruments available for this purpose. A simple and effective apparatus is the Coryllos thoracoscope which is a modification of an earlier instrument developed by Jacobaeus. This consists of a light carrier through which a thoracoscope is introduced, the two acting as one instrument after they have been articulated, and an electric cautery which is introduced separately at another point. Various accessory instruments such as biopsy punch forceps, long needles for anesthetizing painful adhesions, and aspirating tubes are available.

After the general location, direction, size and shape of the adhesions have been determined, the most advantageous site for the introduction of the thoracoscope is chosen. This is usually at some point in the midaxillary line, often over the sixth or seventh intercostal space. The chest wall at the point where the cannula is to be inserted is anesthetized with procaine hydrochloride after the manner described previously (see section on trocar thoracotomy). A short incision (1 cm.) is made through the skin and the trocar and cannula are introduced into the pleural space. The trocar is withdrawn and the light carrier is inserted through the cannula. The thoracoscope is then put in place within the tubular portion of the light carrier and the latter is connected by means of a light wire cord with the proper socket in the rheostat box. The switch is turned on and the interior of the pleural cavity is inspected. The inner lens of the thoracoscope may become fogged with moisture from the air within the pleural cavity if the thoracoscope is much colder than body temperature. This occurrence can be prevented by holding the end in hot sterile saline solution for a few moments to warm it. The end must be wiped dry before reinserting the instrument.

The number, location and characteristics of the adhesions which are to be divided are studied carefully. Some may be too broad for division, others

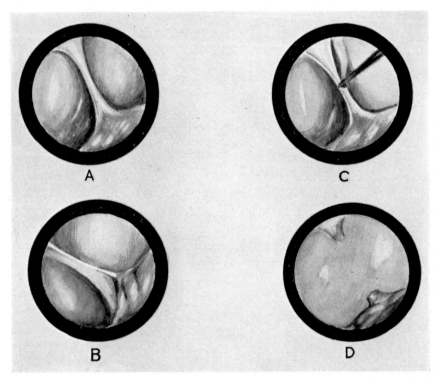

Fig. 74. Closed pneumonolysis. *A* and *B,* Views of adhesion obtained through the thoracoscope; *C,* division of the adhesion with electrocautery, showing optimum site for transection in the majority of cases; *D,* adhesion divided.

may be too short or attached too intimately to some vital structure like the superior vena cava or the vessels which cross the dome of the pleura to reach the neck or arm. If adhesions are found which lend themselves to safe division, the next step is to decide at what point it would be best to intro-duce the cautery. A survey of the interior of the chest wall will usually make it possible to choose an intercostal space which lies most nearly oppo-site the adhesions which are to be cut. This is usually rather high in the region of the anterior axillary line or in the second or third intercostal space anteriorly. The intercostal space chosen as a result of inspection within the chest is identified externally by making pressure with a finger over various interspaces until the correct one is seen to bulge with each impulse transmitted from the pressure of the finger outside. The second cannula is then inserted through the intercostal space thus chosen, after local anesthetization. The cautery tip is introduced a short distance into the chest through the second cannula. The operator, by looking through the thoracoscope, then sights the cautery as it enters the pleural cavity. From that time on the manipulation and direction of the cautery must be carried out with one hand under direct vision through the thoracoscope which is operated with the other. The cautery is moved slowly to the first adhesion and after its tip has been applied at the point where the adhesion is to be divided, the current is turned on and the cutting of the adhesion is completed under vision (Fig. 74, C).

If more than one adhesion exists, the cautery is allowed to cool after turning off the current and then carefully moved to the next adhesion. One advantage of the Coryllos instrument is the fact that both the cautery and the thoracoscope can be introduced through the same size cannula. If the division of a given adhesion, therefore, proves to be difficult from one angle, an entirely different approach can be obtained merely by interchanging the two instruments without shifting the cannulas.

Certain rules of procedure regarding the safe division of adhesions should be mentioned. The cutting of the adhesions should be done slowly with the heat in the cautery tip adjusted to the point where considerable coagulation of the tissues takes place as the division proceeds. If the instrument is allowed to be too hot, the cutting effect is augmented at the expense of the coagulating effect and bleeding may occur. In general, the least vascular point at which to cut an adhesion is midway between the lung and the chest wall. Very long and thin adhesions should be cut in this way. However, if the adhesion is large around, even though it may be long, there is danger that lung tissue may be tented up a considerable distance within it. Such adhesions, therefore, should be divided close to the chest wall to avoid entering a focus of tuberculosis. When it is necessary to cut an adhesion almost at its attachment to the parietal pleura, the danger of hemorrhage must be kept in mind and the cutting must be made slow so as to allow time for thorough coagulation. Under such circumstances the procedure is usually very painful because of the sensitiveness of the parietal pleura. It is wise, therefore, in such a case to withdraw the cautery from the chest and to insert the especially made long needle through the cautery cannula for the injection of procaine hydrochloride solution into the tissues beneath the parietal attachment of the adhesion. This will render the completion of the operation painless. Adhesions which seem to be attached to the pleura overlying the superior vena cava or the vessels at the dome of the pleural cavity had better be left untouched if they are so short that their division might endanger these structures. Also, in the case of adhesions whose parietal base covers a large area, it is wise to be content with partial division because of the dangers of hemorrhage and injury to the lung. A second operation several months later will often permit the completion of the division of such an adhesive area without danger to the lung beneath. In the same way, if certain adhesions seem to be so short that their division might carry the cautery too close to the lung for safety, it is wise to terminate the operation and wait for the time when they may have become sufficiently elongated to make the operation safe.

Failure to exercise the necessary precautions against the development of hemorrhage from inadequate coagulation or the injury of the lung by cutting too close to it may lead to very serious consequences. Hemothorax of alarming extent may occur. It must be treated as described above (section on hemothorax), sometimes by open thoracotomy for ligation of the bleeding vessel. Damage to the lung may lead to the development of tuberculous empyema which, if it does not cause the death of the patient, may require the application of major surgical procedures to overcome its effects. Closed pneumonolysis should therefore be regarded as a surgical procedure requiring great skill and experience for its successful application.

OPEN PNEUMONOLYSIS. An open thoracotomy for the division of adhesions between the lung and the chest wall is occasionally used. In the majority of cases, if the adhesions are too broad or too widespread for the successful lysis of the lung by the closed method, it is usually preferable to abandon the use of artificial pneumothorax in favor of thoracoplasty as a method of obtaining collapse of the lung. On the other hand, if there is any particular reason for avoiding thoracoplasty, an open thoracotomy for the purpose of liberating the lung can be accomplished without great risk to the patient. It is possible that the use of streptomycin as an adjuvant prophylactic measure during the phase of surgical treatment may lead to a wider use of this operation.

Intratracheal inhalation anesthesia is used. A standard thoracotomy incision is made. With the rib spreader in position the adhesions are easily surveyed and in the majority of instances their division can be carried out safely by sharp dissection, using a knife or scissors. Vascular areas are treated by ligation of the bleeding points with suture ligatures. In certain cases, the fixation of the lung to the parietal pleura over a focus of chronic tuberculosis is so intimate and so firm that it is impossible to secure a cleavage plane between these structures. It is possible in such cases to free the lung without breaking into the diseased area by entering the extrapleural fascial plane where the dissection can usually be carried out easily. In this way a small plaque of the parietal pleura is left attached to the lung over the adherent area which had to be freed. This method is useful chiefly for the freeing of relatively small areas having a diameter of a few centimeters only. The need for using it for large areas would mean that the case is probably unsuitable for treatment by artificial pneumothorax and that a thoracoplasty should be resorted to.

If in any case where an open thoracotomy is performed for the division of adhesions it is decided that the operation is injudicious and that a thoracoplasty would be preferable, the opening through the rib cage can be closed and a first stage thoracoplasty operation done at the same time. This, of course, presupposes that the condition of the patient is satisfactory and that not too much operating time has been consumed before the decision to alter the procedure has been made.

CHAPTER 6

OPERATIONS ON THE LUNG

DRAINAGE OF LUNG ABSCESS

Because of the great reduction in the mortality of the operation in recent years there is now a growing tendency to use primary lobectomy in the treatment of lung abscesses which do not respond favorably to medical management. The superiority of this procedure over drainage alone is emphasized by the avoidance of certain complications such as hemorrhage from the lungs, spreading pulmonary sepsis, metastatic brain abscess and the persistence of a chronic state after the acute infection has subsided. Thus by lobectomy the period of disability is shortened and the overall mortality is diminished. On the other hand, there are still cases which demand surgical drainage either because of the advanced age or the poor condition of the patient or the extent and activity of the local septic process. The criteria for drainage, the proper time for its performance and other clinical considerations relative to management of the disease are not discussed here.

Technic. LOCALIZATION OF THE ABSCESS. It is well known that all putrid abscesses of the lung are located peripherally in relation to the hilus. They arise in one bronchopulmonary segment, although occasionally more than one segment may be involved. In a relatively short time after the onset of the disease, the inflammatory process reaches the visceral pleura. As the abscess develops, the cavity which forms can be reached by a direct approach to the pleural surface of the exact pulmonary segment in which it lies. This does not imply, however, that access to every lung abscess is easily obtained. If it should happen to involve the apical segment of the upper lobe, or if it presents along the mediastinal surface of the lung, the approach for drainage may be exceedingly difficult. In such cases it is usually preferable to decide in favor of primary lobectomy rather than to attempt to drain a relatively inaccessible area. Accurate localization of the cavity can be made almost invariably by means of anteroposterior and lateral roentgen ray films. A careful comparison of the relations of the diseased area within the lung to the overlying ribs as visualized in these two projections provides the only

136

information necessary to make it possible to determine the best situation for a direct approach to the cavity.

Unless the amount of cough and expectoration make it impossible, the patient should lie upon the unaffected side with his head slightly lower than his chest to minimize the danger of cerebral air embolism. For anesthesia local infiltration and regional block of the intercostal nerves with procaine hydrochloride (1 per cent) is satisfactory. Inhalation anesthesia is to be avoided except in patients treated by lobectomy because of the possibility of disseminating the septic material from the diseased area throughout the bronchial tree. Very young children who are unable to cooperate may be given intravenous pentothal to produce somnolence before the injection of procaine hydrochloride solution is begun. This practice is unwise, however, under any other circumstances because of the danger of abolishing the reflexes in the upper respiratory tract.

With accurate knowledge of the exact location of the abscess the incision can be made directly over the diseased area and therefore, with few exceptions, in the direction of the long axis of the rib. In two types of case a different incision may be preferable. In the case of an abscess located in the apical segment of the upper lobe and presenting posteriorly at the top of the chest the incision should be vertical, midway between the spine and the medial border of the scapula. To gain sufficient access to such a cavity it is necessary to resect short segments of the three or more ribs which overlie it, and also to excise sections of the corresponding intercostal muscles, nerves and vessels. The other variation from the usual type of incision is required with an abscess in the lateral portions of the posterior or anterior segments of the upper lobe presenting high in the axillary region. In this situation an inverted U-shaped incision gives the best access to the rib or ribs which must be resected in order to gain adequate exposure to the cavity (Fig. 40).

No matter what segment may be involved, if the incision is placed correctly there is scarcely ever any necessity for performing the operation in two stages because the lung is practically always adherent at the point where the abscess approaches the surface. If, on the other hand, the incision is not accurately placed and therefore only near but not actually over the diseased area, it is wise to pack gauze against the pleura to stimulate adherence between the lung and the chest wall. The opening of the cavity is then postponed until another day.

INCISION OF CAVITY. A useful rule of procedure is as follows: The rib is exposed through the incision of the soft parts and the periosteum is reflected from it in the usual manner, taking care to cut the periosteum transversely at each point where the rib is to be divided. A 3 to 4 inch section of rib is denuded, but before it is resected the surgeon should inspect and palpate the pleura beneath. By this means it is usually possible to determine whether or not the lung is adherent at that point. If the pleura is thin and transparent and the lung can be seen moving beneath it, the chances are either that the abscess has not yet become sufficiently adherent or, more often, that the incision has not been made directly over the place where the abscess has pointed on the surface of the lung. In either case it is best to postpone opening the cavity until the development of adhesions between the lung and the parietal pleura. The rib is therefore not resected at this stage, but gauze is packed tightly between it and the periosteum and the pleura beneath. If the rib is resected at the first stage, the gauze packing may not be tight enough to be effective for the production of adhesions. The outer portion of the wound is then packed lightly with dry gauze and the skin is approximated loosely with interrupted silk sutures. The drainage of the abscess is deferred in such a case for several days. Two or three days usually suffice for the production of firm adhesions of the lung, but if the patient is very ill and badly in need of the relief which can only be obtained by providing egress for the pus, it is best to accept a possible risk that the adhesions are inadequate and proceed after the expiration of twenty-four hours only.

It should be mentioned in this connection that formerly a second reason for the drainage of a lung abscess in two stages was to diminish the danger of developing cellulitis of the thoracic wall, which may occur if the freshly incised tissues are bathed immediately in pus full of virulent bacteria. The danger of this complication, however, is practically eliminated by the use of penicillin and streptomycin. If these agents, especially penicillin, are not available, this possibility should be kept in mind.

If in a one-stage procedure or at the second operation in a two-stage procedure it is obvious that the lung is adherent, an aspirating needle with a syringe attached is used to make certain of the presence of the cavity beneath the site chosen for drainage. If the cavity has not been evacuated through a bronchus, pus will be obtained; however, even if such a cavity is completely or partially empty, its presence is determined by the free escape of air into the barrel of the syringe. The previously denuded segment of rib is then removed. With the exact location of the abscess cavity known, and often with the aspirating needle still in place as a guide, an incision is made through the deep periosteum, parietal pleura and thin peripheral shell of lung. It matters little what cutting instrument is used for this purpose. A knife serves perfectly well although custom has led to the use of the cautery in the hope of diminishing the tendency of the cut surfaces of the lung to bleed. The electrosurgical cautery with both cutting and coagulating currents is useful for this purpose. If, on the other hand, the chest wall incision has been accurately placed over the abscess, the tissues which must be divided are relatively avascular and coagulation of vessels is not necessary.

It is important to unroof the cavity widely by excising a circular portion of the tissues, including the visceral and parietal pleurae and the periosteum of the resected rib. If the abscess is unusually large, it may be necessary to resect sections of two adjacent ribs instead of one in order to open it widely enough. If this is done, sections of the intervening intercostal muscle bundle and the corresponding intercostal nerve and vessels must be excised along with the pleura and periosteum of each rib. After a wide opening has been made, the unroofed abscess cavity and the chest wall incision which lies in continuity with it are packed with dry gauze. It is important to pack the superficial portion widely, and in order to avoid the tendency of all such openings to close prematurely no sutures should be put in the ends of the incision.

After-care. The after-care of a patient with a lung abscess involves daily renewal of outer dressings and the changing of the gauze pack at intervals of several days. The original packing usually becomes soaked with pus and sufficiently loosened to allow its removal in four to six days after operation. After the abscess cavity has made considerable progress toward closure and the outer portion of the wound has begun to close in, it is possible to shift from gauze packs to a soft rubber tube which can be removed when the cavity is practically obliterated, leaving only the chest wall sinus. This will usually close promptly once the drain has been omitted. Several weeks or even months are necessary to allow sufficient time for healing. However, it should be kept in mind that complete and permanent healing of the average lung abscess treated by drainage alone occurs in not more than one third of the cases even though the external opening may ultimately heal over. In the remaining cases of those who survive it is necessary to perform a lobectomy to effect a definitive cure.

EXTIRPATION OF PARTS OR ALL OF THE LUNG

General Principles

Anesthesia. As for all intrathoracic operations which are performed through an open thoracotomy incision, those upon the lung require positive pressure inhalation anesthesia. Ether mixed with oxygen remains the safest agent in the majority of cases (see Chap. 2).

Position of the Patient. The position of the patient on the operating table depends to some extent upon the nature and location of the condition which prompts the performance of the operation, but principally upon the preference of the surgeon. There are no cases which cannot be handled satisfactorily in the lateral thoracotomy position (Chap. 2).

Incision. In the majority of cases the standard thoracotomy incision may be used. It should be long and placed in such a manner as to provide the best access to the region where the greatest technical difficulty is to be expected. In general, a high rib or intercostal space such as the fourth or fifth should be used when peripheral adhesions are to be expected over the apex of the lung. Likewise, a lower rib or interspace such as the seventh or eighth may be necessary for a densely adherent lower lobe. In all other cases, especially when technical difficulties are anticipated in the region of the hilus of the lung, the sixth or seventh ribs or interspaces give the best exposure (Chap. 3, *Thoracic Incisions*).

Division of Adhesions. In many patients who require a pulmonary operation, the lung is discovered to be adherent to the parietal wall, the diaphragm or the mediastinal surface. The adhesions may be of long standing and therefore relatively avascular, or they may be recent and inflammatory, with great vascularity and suffused with edema fluid. They may be localized and filmy or widespread and dense. In some cases of chronic pulmonary sepsis, especially those with a history of complicating empyema in the past, the lung may be so intimately adherent that no plane of cleavage can possibly be recognized.

In general, the adhesions of *tuberculosis* tend to be most prevalent and most dense over the apex and along the posterior surface of the upper lobe and superior segment of the lower lobe. Those of *chronic bronchiectasis* are likely to be most pronounced over the basal segments of the lower lobe, the lingular segment of the left upper lobe, and the middle lobe on the right. In *lung abscess* the adhesions are usually localized over the region of the abscess itself and are likely to be exceedingly vascular even after the acute process seems to have subsided. Inflammatory adhesions of the inferior surface of the lower lobe to the diaphragm are always unusually vascular and are more dense near the margin of the lobe than over the central portion. Peripheral adhesions of an inflammatory nature, except in certain cases of tuberculosis of the upper lobe, are rarely as dense or as frequent on the mediastinal surface of the lung as they are elsewhere.

The division of inflammatory adhesions between the lung and the parietal pleura or diaphragm must usually be accomplished by sharp dissection with scissors or knife (Fig. 75). In the separation of adherent surfaces which are distant from the wound edges the illumination provided by the usual operating room lights may be inadequate. In such a situation great benefit results from the use of a small light which can be sterilized and held inside the chest cavity, often actually beneath the adhesion itself. When this is done, the transillumination provided is an important factor in avoiding injury both to the lung itself, because of failure to recognize its relation to the adhesion, and to important structures at the dome of the pleural cavity or on the mediastinal surface (Fig. 76).

In certain cases of inflammatory fixation of the lung to the pleura where it is impossible to find an intrapleural plane of cleavage, it is necessary to enter the retropleural fascial plane of the chest wall and remove a section

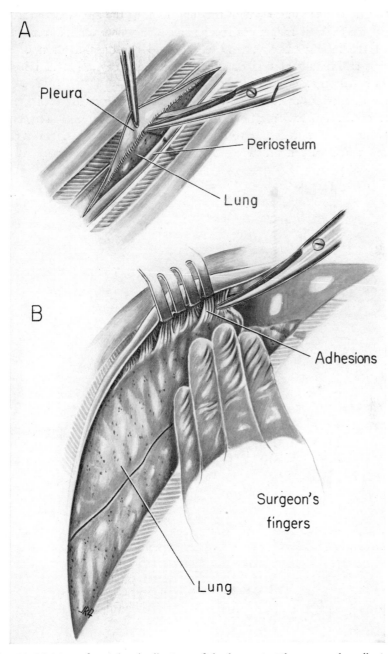

Fig. 75. Division of peripheral adhesions of the lung. *A*, Filmy avascular adhesions resulting from long past pleural inflammation. These are easily separated, partly by sharp
and partly by blunt dissection. *B*, Dense fibrous vascular adhesions of recent or subacute
inflammatory process. These require cutting with knife or scissors. Ligation of vessels is
frequently necessary.

7

of the parietal pleura along with the lung itself in the area where the dense fixation exists. This maneuver is advantageous whenever inadvertent cutting of the lung parenchyma might lead to the dissemination of septic material, as in lung abscess or tuberculosis with cavitation and in some cases of carcinoma.

Pleural adhesions are often so vascular that considerable bleeding results from their severance. Sometimes this bleeding tends to stop of itself, but not infrequently active measures must be instituted. Simple ligation or the placement of suture ligatures of silk usually suffices. Occasionally in inac-

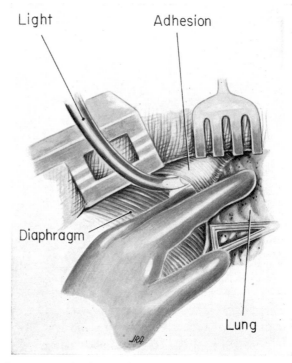

Fig. 76. Transillumination of a dense inflammatory adhesion to determine the proper area for division.

cessible regions, such as the dome of the pleural cavity, the application of metal dura clips to small bleeding points is helpful. In certain cases the oozing of blood takes place over a broader surface. In such a situation one can try the effect of suturing a piece of muscle over the area or, better still, the application of oxidized cellulose gauze or fibrin foam plaques soaked in thrombin solution. In a few instances, however, widespread oozing continues in spite of every effort to stop it. Prolongation of the operation beyond a reasonable length of time in an attempt to prevent such bleeding, however, is unwise. It is far better in such a case to close the wound, terminate the administration of the anesthetic, and rely upon copious transfusions to maintain an adequate volume of circulating blood until the oozing tendency ceases over the course of a few hours postoperatively. The assumption is made, of course, that all patients who are subjected to a major thoracic operation will have had adequate preoperative studies of their blood so that any correctable abnormalities such as alterations of prothrombin level can be treated before the operation is undertaken.

Dissection of Fissures. It is a rare lung, especially on the right side, whose interlobar fissures are anatomically complete from the surface all the way into the hilus. The most frequent locations for incompleteness of the fissures are on the right side between the upper and middle lobes and on both sides between the superior segment of the lower lobe, especially over its posterior extent, and the contiguous surface of the upper lobe. Abnormalities of the fissures elsewhere are much less frequent. In addition to the underlying anatomic fusion between the lobes in certain cases, the superimposed amalgamation of adjacent free surfaces which results from inflammatory processes within the lung may make separation still more difficult.

In general, the separation of inflammatory adhesions between the lobes of a lung presents little difficulty except in very recent acute cases or in certain cases of lung abscess which may be complicated by the spread of the infection across the septum into the adjoining lobe. The separation of the adhesions is effected by cutting with the knife or scissors, often with the guidance of transillumination. While dissection within the fissure is being carried out, it is important to have the anesthetist keep the lung expanded; otherwise the flaccidity of the collapsed lung may make it more difficult to follow the interlobar cleavage plane.

Once the inflammatory adhesions have been divided, it becomes necessary, in a lung upon which a lobectomy is to be performed, to complete the fissure if it is congenitally partially absent. Proximity to the region of anatomic incompleteness of the fissure can always be recognized by the presence of small vessels, both arterial and venous, which cross from one lobe to the other directly beneath the visceral pleural reflection at the bottom of the incomplete fissure. Some of these are branches of the bronchial vessels. They must be divided and ligated. From this level to the depths of the hilus, the separation between the lobes must be made artificially through lung parenchyma. A detailed knowledge of the course and distribution of the pulmonary vessels within the hilus of the lung is necessary to avoid injury to them. However, unless a large vessel is divided, little active bleeding is encountered if the distance to be traversed is short and if the dissection is kept within the proper intersegmental plane between major pulmonary vessels (see Chap. 1).

If, as so often happens in the case of the fissure between the upper and middle lobes of the right lung, there is a long section of lung to be cut, it is helpful to apply long straight Ochsner or Kocher hemostatic forceps in pairs and to cut the lung between them with a knife. When this method is used, it is necessary also to identify the important pulmonary arteries and veins as well as the bronchi of the lobes which are being separated so that the clamps can be applied to a relatively free area. Several pairs of clamps may have to be applied before the limits of the fissure are reached (Fig. 85). After the division has been accomplished, the cut edge of the lobe which is to be left behind is closed by means of a continuous suture of fine chromicized catgut attached to an atraumatic needle. This suture is started beyond the end of the clamp nearest the hilus, avoiding the artery, vein and bronchus which are always found there. It is then passed back and forth through the lung beneath the clamps. As the limit of the jaws of each clamp is reached, the clamp is removed until all have been removed in turn. The suture is then continued over and over the cut edge of the lung back as far as its starting point, where the two portions are tied together. This provides effective control of any tendency to bleed and prevents leakage of air from small bronchi which may have been severed (Fig. 80, B).

Dissection of Structures of Hilus of Lung. The manner of dissecting the structures of the hilus of the lung depends to a large extent upon the type of operation to be performed and even more upon the nature of the pathologic process. In carcinoma obviously a wide excision of hilar lymph nodes and a high proximal division of the bronchus are essential. In inflammatory lesions other considerations such as the enlargement and adherence of the peribronchial lymph nodes may have an influence upon the ultimate technic employed. In general, however, these differences are unimportant in relation to the broad principles which are to be employed.

In any case, wherever possible it is wise to reflect the pleura away from the posterior surface of the hilus so that this flap can be utilized to cover the bronchial stump. If the patient manifests a tendency to cough during these first manipulations around the hilus, local infiltration of 1 per cent procaine hydrochloride solution into the perihilar tissues will often be effective in controlling the reflex stimulation. This avoids the necessity for deepening the plane of anesthesia.

One of the greatest technical improvements in pulmonary surgery has been the abandonment of the tourniquet method of lobectomy or pneumonectomy in favor of individual ligation of the pulmonary vessels, separate ligature of the bronchial arteries, and careful closure and covering of the bronchial stump. Except in certain cases in which it may be important to avoid aspiration of pus or secretions from a diseased lung by placing a clamp on the bronchus at the earliest possible moment, it is convenient to deal with the pulmonary vessels first. It is unnecessary to mention that an accurate knowledge of the hilus of the lung is essential. Ideally the pulmonary artery should be secured first. This demands separate ligation and division of the various lobar or segmental branches in cases of segmental excision or lobectomy, or of the entire artery proximal to its branches in the case of a pneumonectomy. In some cases, however, it may be expedient to ligate and divide the vein first in order to gain better access to the artery. The necessity for this maneuver, of course, depends upon the topographical anatomy of the hilar structures in the particular lobe or lung which is being removed, upon variations which are sometimes encountered in the normal anatomic arrangement of these hilar structures, and often upon the pathologic conditions in and about the hilus itself.

In every instance it is necessary to clear the pulmonary vessels of the tissues which envelop them. In doing this accurate hemostasis is essential to avoid obscuring the field of dissection by extravasations of blood. After the reflection of the pleura, the surrounding fibrous tissues in which numerous small systemic arteries and veins are encountered must be dissected off. These small vessels must be divided and tied, usually with suture ligatures. In the performance of a lobectomy, portions of lung tissue in the hilus may have to be cut across in order to gain access to the pulmonary vessels. Furthermore, there are always numerous lymph nodes which lie in the perivascular fibrous tissues. These must be dissected away from the vessels. In the removal of lymph nodes with the lung it will be noticed that each node has a small artery and vein which must be ligated.

Ligation and Division of Pulmonary Vessels. The details of technic of the ligation and division of the pulmonary vessels will depend upon the preference of the surgeon. It should be mentioned, however, that these vessels are relatively thin-walled and more fragile than those of comparable size in the systemic circulation. In order to avoid tearing them it is best whenever possible not to apply hemostatic forceps. A method of accomplishing this is to pass a ligature of heavy silk around each vessel after it has been isolated by careful dissection. A curved clamp such as the cystic duct forceps of the Lowsley or Moynihan type is a useful instrument for this purpose (Fig. 77, *A*). The vessel which is to be divided is then tied firmly. While the first knot is being set, all traction which is being exerted upon the lung must be relaxed so that the vessel will not be tied on the stretch. If this precaution is not observed, the ligature may be so loose that it will slip off after the vessel has been cut. Certain vessels may be long enough to permit the placing of a second ligature distal to the first before cutting the vessel between them. In the majority of cases, however, it is best to apply a hemostatic forceps at the farthest possible distal point. The vessel is then cut between the clamp and the proximal ligature. The distal portion is then tied so that the clamp can be removed. In the case of the pulmonary veins and the smaller branches of the pulmonary artery, a single proximal ligature applied in the manner described is sufficient.

When one of the large branches or the main trunk of the pulmonary artery proximal to its branches is tied, special precautions to avoid slipping of the ligature should be used. This is important especially if the vessel is so short that the cuff on the proximal end is small after division. A proximal ligature is placed and tied and a distal hemostatic forceps is applied after the manner described previously. The artery is then cut half way across with the scissors (Fig. 77, B). At this point a hemostatic forceps is applied to the incompletely severed vessel distal to the ligature. The division of the vessel is then completed (Fig. 77, C). The advantage of this technic is the fact that in case the ligature should slip, the proximal end of the artery cannot escape completely from the surgeon's grasp before a second tie can be applied. It is wise also to apply a transfixion ligature behind the forceps distal to the

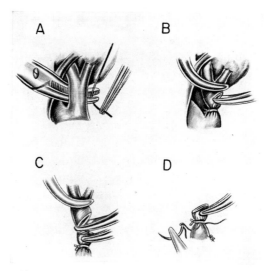

Fig. 77. Technic of ligation of a major pulmonary artery. *A*, Passing a ligature around the vessel after it has been isolated by dissection. *B*, Proximal ligature tied. A hemostatic forceps has been applied to the vessel at a point distal to the site of division and the artery has been cut half through in preparation for *C*, the application of a hemostatic forceps distal to the ligature but proximal to the site of division. The vessel is then completely severed, but the proximal end is held by the hemostat for *D*, the insertion and tying of a second ligature passed through the stump of the vessel with a needle.

proximal tie (Fig. 77, *D*). If the main trunk of the artery is long, as for example in the average case on the left side, a single ligature is sufficient if the cuff of the vessel which remains after division is large and if the vessel is not tied under tension.

Division of Bronchus. Once the pulmonary vessels have been ligated and cut, there remains merely the problem of dealing with the bronchus of the lobe or lung which is being excised. In preparation for the actual division of the bronchus at the level which has been chosen, the peribronchial lymph nodes must be dissected away and the bronchial arteries divided. Only in cases of carcinoma is it necessary to make an attempt to remove a large number of the hilar lymph nodes. The bronchial arteries approach the hilus of the lung from behind and send branches which ultimately surround the bronchi in a loose network of vessels so that in cutting across any of the larger bronchi, branches will be encountered at several points. These tend to group themselves so that the largest vessels lie on the posterior, anterior and inferior surfaces of the respective bronchi. Small vessels are often encountered on the superior surface as well. In each case, therefore, several ligatures are usually necessary to secure all the branches of the bronchial artery. Because the healing of the bronchial stump takes place at its end, it is of great importance to sever the bronchial arteries at a point only slightly proximal to the level at which the bronchus is to be cut across. This precaution insures the preservation of an adequate blood supply to the tissues and tends to minimize the occurrence of necrosis which would inevitably lead to delayed healing. The importance of maintaining the nutrition of the bronchial tissues in the prevention of bronchial fistula formation cannot be overemphasized. Hemostasis is secured by means of suture ligatures of silk.

No matter whether a lobectomy or a pneumonectomy is being performed, the level at which the bronchus is to be cut should be selected so as to leave the shortest possible stump. This diminishes the possibility of the accumulation of secretions in the stump. The technic for division, closure and covering the bronchus is as follows: A heavy clamp such as a curved kidney pedicle clamp is placed across the bronchus at a point between the lung or lobe and the level selected for division. This serves as a handle to manipulate the lung and also prevents the escape of material from the diseased portion of the lung into the tracheobronchial tree. A suture of medium silk is placed in the superior or inferior margin of the bronchus and tied. This is given to an assistant to hold. With a knife which has a blade curved on the flat side (Beaver No. 14) the division of the bronchus is begun (Fig. 78, A). After cutting a short distance a suture is passed from edge to edge across the partially divided end. This is held tightly by the assistant so as to avoid the escape of the anesthetic gases which would lead to a reduction in pressure within the anesthesia system. The bronchus is then divided slightly further and a second suture is applied and held as before. This process is continued until the severance is complete and the lobe or lung is removed from the chest (Fig. 78, B). The sutures which are still held tightly, so as to occlude the cut end of the bronchus, are then tied in turn and cut, keeping the first as a guide for traction (Fig. 78, C). If a sufficient number of sutures has been used, the bronchial stump will now be airtight. If leakage is observed, one or more additional sutures will usually correct the difficulty. When the cartilage is unusually rigid, the airtight closure of the stump is made easier by cutting across the cartilage at each end. This eliminates the springlike tendency of the folded cartilage to force the bronchus open at each corner of the closure. The division and closure of the bronchus must be accomplished rapidly so as to safeguard the patient against the effects of diminished aeration of the remaining lung which results from escape of anesthetic gases through the severed end. The division of the bronchus and especially the placing of the sutures in the divided end is facilitated by starting at the margin which corresponds with the heel of the clamp. In this way the handle of the clamp can be more easily turned so as to be out of the way of the surgeon as he works on the bronchus itself (Fig. 78, *B*).

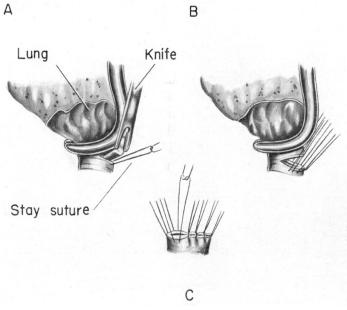

Fig. 78. Division of the bronchus and closure of the bronchial stump. *A,* Shows the stay suture ready for tying and the start of the division of the bronchus proximal to the clamp. *Note:* The knife has a blade curved on the flat side (Beaver type No. 14). *B,* The bronchus is partially severed; sutures have been placed through that portion which has already been cut; these are held taut by the assistant to prevent leakage. *C,* Division of the bronchus completed; all sutures in place and some of them already tied.

It is important not to place a clamp on the proximal portion of the bronchus because the resultant crushing of the tissues at the end of the stump would interfere greatly with the healing process.

No lobectomy or pneumonectomy is complete unless the closed bronchial stump is also covered. There is no doubt that this part of the operative technic is of equal importance with preservation of the blood supply and the avoidance of the crushing of the sutured end of the bronchus. Various methods have been described. In practice the success of this detail depends rather upon the ingenuity of the surgeon in using the structures which may be available in each individual case than upon the arbitrary adoption of any particular method. In a few instances, especially after a pneumonectomy, enough peribronchial areolar tissue is available to make it possible to bury the stump where it lies. This is done by approximating the mediastinal tissues over the stump by means of a series of sutures (Fig. 79, *A*). In certain cases of lobectomy or segmental excision the stump of the severed bronchus can be buried beneath the surface of an adjacent lobe or within the sub-

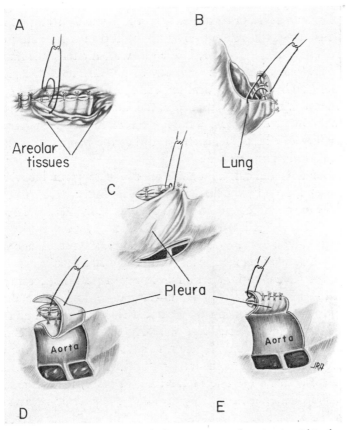

Fig. 79. Methods of covering the bronchial stump. *A*, By burying it within the peribronchial areolar tissue of the mediastinum; applicable almost exclusively in pneumonectomy. *B*, By infolding it within contiguous surfaces of the lung; applicable in segmental excision and some cases of lobectomy. *C*, By sliding an edge of pleura over it, sometimes with an additional relaxing incision as shown. *D*, By covering with a hinged flap of pleura sutured to both sides of the stump (almost a free graft). *E*, By covering with a hinged flap of pleura held with one row of sutures (when the attached edge of the flap is thoroughly secure).

stance of the remaining segments by suturing portions of pulmonary tissue over it (Fig. 79, *B*). In other cases a generous flap of mediastinal pleura can be preserved during the dissection of the hilus, usually from its posterior surface. This may be laid over the bronchial stump and sutured to its surface proximal to the end or to the surrounding areolar tissues. In some cases the flap, though available, is not large enough to be brought over without too much tension. In this event a linear relaxing incision is made several centimeters behind its edge. This will allow the pleura to be slid over the stump and sutured in place as described (Fig. 79, *C*). It is sometimes necessary to divide the areolar tissue attachments beneath the pleural flap to accomplish this. In other instances, however, it is necessary to construct a rectangular flap of sufficient size which is allowed to remain fixed at the edge nearest the bronchus so that it can be turned over the bronchial stump as if it were hinged. This flap is then sutured over the stump in the manner described previously, but it lies, of course, inside out with the serous surface against the bronchus. This difference in relation of the surface of the pleural flap to the bronchus is of no practical importance (Fig. 79, *E*). In certain instances when this method is employed, the attachment of the flap may be insecure and might come loose, leaving the stump inadequately covered. This possibility can be prevented by suturing the flap to each side of the stump as shown in Figure 79, *D*.

Sometimes it is difficult to obtain an adequate pleural cover for the bronchial stump even by the methods described. In these cases recourse may be had to the use of a free graft of pleura obtained from an undiseased portion of the lung which has just been removed. This can be sutured over the stump and usually makes a satisfactory protection against leakage.

Closure of Space Within the Pleural Cavity. The closure of the space which remains in the pleural cavity after a lobectomy or pneumonectomy depends upon shifting of the mediastinum, upward extension of the diaphragm, flattening of the chest wall on the operated side by approximation of the ribs and, in lobectomy cases, compensatory emphysematous enlargement of the remainder of the lung. There is in addition, of course, the organization of serosanguineous transudate by fibrous tissue. In pneumonectomy cases, because of the large size of the residual space, it is advantageous to favor the rise of the diaphragm by crushing the phrenic nerve before the chest incision is closed. In lobectomy cases the action of the diaphragm should be preserved to further the respiratory function of the remaining portion of the lung.

Drainage of Pleural Cavity. Drainage of the pleural cavity after lobectomy or pneumonectomy depends upon the nature of the case and upon the preference of the surgeon. The use of a drain placed on suction or water-seal collection is indicated whenever an unusually large amount of fluid might be anticipated, as in inflammatory diseases with very vascular adhesions, and when air leakage from the lung is anticipated, as in cases of segmental excision. In general it is wise to insert a drain after lobectomy to allow the remaining portion of the lung unimpeded access to the pleural space to insure its complete expansion. On the other hand, it is preferable to omit drainage after pneumonectomy because of the favorable effect of the effusion of fluid in preventing too sudden or too pronounced a shift of the mediastinum to the operated side; also, fluid aids in the ultimate obliteration of the pleural cavity.

Special Considerations Relative to the Type of Operative Procedure

Local Excision of a Portion of Lung (Wedge Excision). In certain cases of peripherally located benign primary tumors of the lung or in certain cases in which a metastatic tumor is presumed to be single and therefore amenable

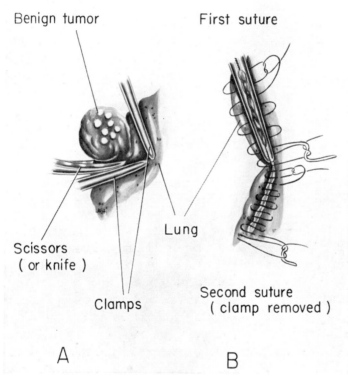

Fig. 80. Local excision of benign tumor. *A,* Method of wedge-shaped excision of involved area using clamps to secure the divided surfaces of the remainder of the lobe. *B,* closure by continuous suture: Upper portion shows start of suture by passing through and through beneath the jaws of the clamps; lower portion shows completion by passing the suture over and over back to the starting point where it is tied to the free end.

to surgical extirpation, the excision of a small, wedge-shaped section from the peripheral portion of a lobe is practicable. No effort is made to isolate and ligate separately the pulmonary vessels or to secure the bronchi individually. With the lung rendered partially atelectatic by reduction of the pressure within the anesthesia system, a wedge-shaped section of lung containing the lesion which is to be removed is blocked off by means of two series of straight hemostatic forceps applied in succession in the manner described previously for the separation of two lobes of the lung with an incomplete fissure between them. By cutting along the jaws of the clamps with a sharp knife the portion of lung thus outlined is excised (Fig. 80, *A*). The defect in the lung may be closed by either of two methods. The first method is to approximate the cut edges with mattress sutures passed beneath the clamps and placed in such a manner that they interlock one with the other. The sutures are held by an assistant until all are in place. After the clamps have been removed, they are tied. To complete the closure the cut edges of the lung, which are turned up one against the other by the mattress sutures, are sutured over with a continuous strand of very fine chromicized catgut on an atraumatic needle. Such a closure is airtight and hemostatic. The other method is to use a continuous suture of chromicized catgut passed back and forth beneath the clamps and then over and over to the starting point in the same manner as was described for the closure of a portion of the lung after the surgical separation of an incomplete fissure (Fig. 80, *B*). No drainage is required in either case.

Segmental Excision (Resection). The practice of excising a bronchopulmonary segment of a lobe of the lung as an anatomic unit is now well established. Its principal application is in the extirpation of pulmonary segments which are involved in localized bronchiectasis. The technical success of this procedure, however, depends upon the accurate isolation and separate division of the segmental branches of the pulmonary artery and vein and the corresponding bronchus of the segment which is to be removed. The older method of cutting blindly across the lung without knowledge of the location of these structures led to a high incidence of complications including hemorrhage, empyema, tension pneumothorax, spread of infection in the remainder of the lobe, and failure of the lobe to expand or to remain expanded after the operation was terminated. Accurate knowledge of the intricate anatomic relations of the pulmonary vessels and bronchi in the hilus and in the individual lobes and segments of the lung is essential. It must be kept in mind also that there are various anomalous arrangements of these structures which must be looked for. These usually fall into several more or less characteristic categories, but very rare and unusual anomalies may be found occasionally (Chap. 1).

Knowledge of the exact segment which is to be removed must be obtained during the preoperative investigation of the patient by study of roentgen ray films of the chest obtained after the intratracheal injection of iodized oil.

The dissection is begun in the hilus of the lung where the artery and vein of the diseased segment are identified, tied and cut. In some segments there may be more than one of these vessels, as for example in the superior segment of the lower lobe where there are often two independent arteries. Before any artery which is presumed to be the principal vessel supplying a given segment is divided, one should search for branches which may come from it to supply an adjacent normal segment. In some cases the segmental artery to the diseased segment comes from the main branch of another segment.

After the segmental vessels have been ligated and severed, the bronchus must be dealt with. Because of variations in the branches of the larger bronchi, it is not always possible to be exactly certain that the correct bronchus has been found. More often this difficulty is confined to determining whether a given bronchus is the chief segmental bronchus or one of its primary branches. The differentiation can be made, however, by temporarily occluding the bronchus with a clamp which is applied only tightly enough to close the lumen and then having the anesthetist inflate the lung. A study of the portion of lung which remains atelectatic will inform the operator as to whether or not the correct bronchus has been isolated. During its inflation the lung should be watched closely, because in certain patients the tendency of the segment whose bronchus has been occluded to become inflated through alveolar communications with adjacent segments is so great that in a short time the entire lobe may take on a uniform appearance. If this should happen, the anesthetist should be instructed to reduce the intrapulmonary pressure, whereupon the occluded segment can be distinguished from the remainder of the lobe because of the fact that air remains trapped within it while the portion with an open bronchus becomes deflated. Once the segmental bronchus has been correctly identified, it is clamped, cut proximal to the clamp and sutured in the manner previously described.

It remains then to cut across the parenchymal portion of the lung along the limits of the segment which is being excised. The determination of the peripheral extent of the segment is made in the manner just described for the selection of the correct bronchus. The division of the lung can be accomplished in one of two ways. The first is to apply a series of straight hemostatic forceps across the presumed limits of the segment to be removed (Fig. 85). The application of the clamps is usually begun at the periphery and carried to the hilar limits of the segment where the divided bronchus and vessels serve as a guide to avoid injury to the structures which serve the remaining segments. After the diseased portion of the lung has been removed, the cut edge of the remainder of the lobe is closed over in the manner described under separation of fissures and local excision of lung (Fig. 80, B).

The above technic has been supplanted by the more anatomic procedure which comprises the second method. The principle of this method is to bring about a separation without the use of clamps by blunt and sharp dissection as required, beginning at the hilar portion and working outward along the adjacent distended portion of the lobe which is being preserved (Fig. 81, B). If the proper plane of dissection is followed, there is relatively little bleeding because no large vessels are encountered unless the adjacent

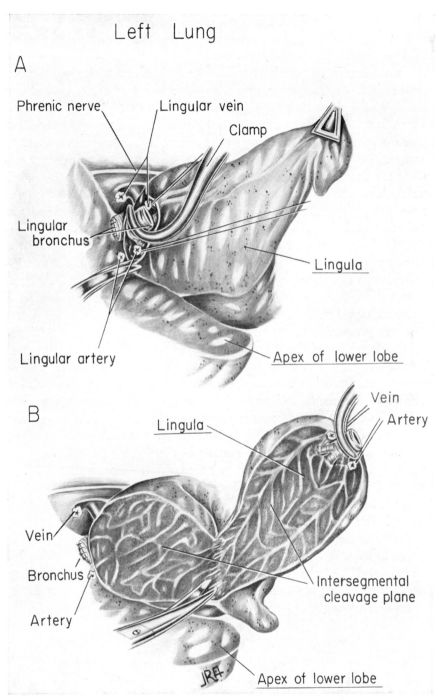

Fig. 81. Technic of segmental excision: Lingulectomy. *A*, First step: Ligation and division of segmental artery and vein; division and proximal closure of the segmental bronchus. *B*, Removal of the segment (lingula) by cutting with scissors along the intersegmental plane using the segmental vein as a guide.

segment is entered. What small vessels may bleed are clamped with hemostats and tied individually. Several small bronchi are usually cut during the procedure. These can be tied individually also. The advantage of this method is the fact that it is often possible to preserve more of the remaining portion of the lobe, but it has the disadvantage that there is a greater tendency to serosanguineous effusion postoperatively. There is also a greater tendency to develop pneumothorax and atelectasis of the remainder of the lung. The raw surface of lung which remains after the removal of a segment in this manner can be left as it is, accepting the greater probability of air leakage; otherwise it can be closed by means of a continuous fine catgut suture which approximates the edges of the lobe, thus pleuralizing the entire surface. A modification of this method is to preserve a long sheet of pleura from the surface of the segment which is being removed as the dissection is carried out. This sheet of pleura is then turned over the denuded area and held in place by sutures around the periphery. There is reason to believe that the incidence of complications is considerably reduced by closing the denuded surface of lung.

The final step in the technic of segmental excision is to cover the bronchial stump. In many cases, especially in lingulectomy, the stump can be buried within the lung at the base of the area of excision where a series of three or four sutures of fine silk can be made to approximate the edges of the remainder of the lobe over it (Fig. 79, B). In some cases this method of covering the stump is impossible or can be only partially accomplished. It is then necessary to use a flap of the pleura from the mediastinum for this purpose. When this maneuver is necessary, it is imperative to avoid drawing the flap too tightly over any of the pulmonary vessels of the remaining segments or an adjacent lobe.

Before the chest is closed, it is essential to observe the lung while it is being expanded by the anesthetist. In this way any errors of technic such as transfixion of an adjacent bronchus by sutures or the presence of a plug of mucus in the bronchus may be detected by the failure of the remainder of the lobe or a part of it to expand. When complete expansion has been obtained, the position assumed by the remainder of the lobe should be observed. In some cases this portion of the lung may rotate or fall into a position which might interfere with the free passage of air through its bronchus. This occurrence is most frequently observed in the case of the superior segment of the lower lobe after basal segmental excision when there is a complete fissure between the superior segment and the adjacent surface of the upper lobe. In this situation a few fine silk sutures placed in the edges along the fissure so as to hold the two lobes together will prevent atelectasis which might arise after the chest has been closed.

In all cases of segmental excision closed drainage should be provided for a period of at least forty-eight hours to provide egress for the fluid which often accumulates and to prevent the development of tension pneumothorax if there should be a small leak of air (see Chap. 2).

Lobectomy (Modern Technic). In general the technical difficulty of a lobectomy is greater than that of a pneumonectomy but not often so great as that of a segmental excision. The difference is chiefly on an anatomic basis. A thorough knowledge of the anatomy of the hilus of the lung and of all the common anomalies of the pulmonary vessels and the bronchi is necessary. The differences between the various lobes and the two lungs must be understood. For a review of these details reference should be made to the appropriate section in Chapter 1. In the case of the upper lobes there are several branches of the pulmonary artery. Some of these must be sought within the fissure. In the middle lobe there may be one or two arteries, both arising from within the fissure. In the lower lobes it is often possible to ligate the artery as a single structure, but on the right side the middle lobe artery (or one of two in some cases) may arise from the lower lobe artery below the origin of the artery to the superior segment. When this occurs, in order to preserve the blood supply of the middle lobe it is necessary to cut separately the superior segment branch and the main trunk of the lower lobe artery below the origin of the middle lobe branch. On the left side a similar situation may be encountered when the lingular artery arises from the lower lobe artery below the origin of the superior segment branch. Separate division of the lower lobe vessels is necessary when this anomaly is found. Anomalous distributions of the veins must be watched for also and dealt with in the appropriate manner.

Abnormalities of the primary branches of the bronchi also may require special attention in the performance of a lobectomy. In the right upper lobe little difficulty is usually encountered, but two infrequent anomalies must be kept in mind. One is the occasional occurrence of a tracheal bronchus which arises usually along the right side of the trachea and extends directly into the apical segment of the right upper lobe. Such an anomaly is a rare occurrence on the left side. The other is the separation of two of the primary upper lobe bronchial divisions by the passage of the azygos vein between them in the case of so-called "azygos lobe" of the lung.

Another more frequent difficulty which arises from variations of the bronchi in the right lung results from the unusually low origin of the middle lobe bronchus. In some cases this bronchus arises opposite the superior segment branch of the lower lobe bronchus. In a few it may be found at an even lower level. If a middle lobectomy is being done, this occurrence is of no importance; however, if the lower lobe is to be removed, the removal of the middle lobe as well may be necessary if it does not appear feasible to divide the superior and basal segmental bronchi independently in an attempt to leave the middle lobe bronchus intact.

On the left side variations of the bronchi are of less importance in the performance of a lobectomy, except in the rare case when the lingula bronchus arises from the lower lobe bronchus instead of the upper. The relation of this bronchus to the origin of the superior segment branch of the lower lobe bronchus may then make it necessary to divide the superior segmental branch and the main trunk of the lower lobe bronchus separately

Right Lung

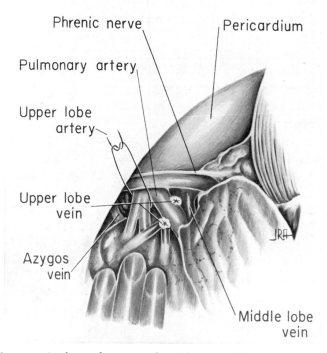

Fig. 82. First steps in the performance of a right upper lobectomy or right pneumonectomy. Anterior portion of superior pulmonary vein divided to give better access to the pulmonary artery. For lobectomy: ligature around the upper lobe artery to the apical and anterior segments; for pneumonectomy: additional ligature to be placed around the artery below this branch. Anterior aspect of the hilus.

as on the right side. Occasionally it may be necessary to remove the lingula to surmount the difficulty.

Aside from the technical difficulties which arise from anomalies of the origin and relations of the pulmonary vessels and the bronchi, and those which result from incompleteness of the fissures, there are few other matters of technic which are peculiar to the performance of a lobectomy as compared to pneumonectomy. The covering of the bronchial stump, however, is sometimes more of a problem. It is almost always necessary to turn up a rectangular flap of pleura to cover a lobar bronchus. This is especially so in the case of the upper lobe. Furthermore, if the stump of the bronchus is short, as it should be, it is sometimes difficult to place sutures in the side of the bronchus to hold the flap in place without interfering with the pulmonary vessels of the lobe which is not removed. Advantage should be taken of any hilar lymph nodes which may be present for the placing of sutures to hold the flap. The flap can also be sutured in some cases to that portion of the remaining lobe which lies close to the stump which is being covered. As in the case of segmental excision, in suturing a pleural flap over a lobar bronchus one should avoid drawing it tightly across a pulmonary vessel of the remaining lobe because of the danger of interference with the circulation.

Pneumonectomy (Modern Technic). From the technical point of view the performance of a pneumonectomy is relatively more simple than a lobectomy. However, conditions secondary to the pathologic process which may be present at the hilus may make the operation exceedingly difficult. Certain details of technic which have a particular importance should be mentioned. The method of ligating the pulmonary artery may vary depending upon which lung is being removed. On the right side, because the main trunk of the artery is short, it is often wise to tie the first upper lobe branch independently. The remainder of the vessel can then be secured with another ligature, but it will be found usually that this portion can be reached best after the superior pulmonary vein has been tied and cut. This step allows an unobstructed view of the artery (Fig. 82). It is then only necessary to exert precautions against tearing the vessel while the dissection between the artery and the bronchus is being completed. On the left side, because the main trunk is usually relatively longer than on the right, it is almost always possible to ligate and divide the main trunk of the pulmonary artery proximal to any of its branches.

Except for the presence of anomalies in arrangement of their branches, the pulmonary veins do not present any particular problem in the performance of a pneumonectomy. With the exception of the branches which traverse the hilar portion of the lung and are reached from within the fissures, these veins are more readily accessible than the arteries because they are more superficial. They are often covered merely by pleura and a thin film of areolar tissue. The inferior pulmonary vein lies at the upper limit of the pulmonary ligament. Its exact location can be determined, as this ligament is being divided from below upwards, by the presence of a small artery which runs in the perihilar areolar tissues along its inferior aspect. There is also a lymph node which lies below the vein at the upper limits of the pulmonary ligament.

The division and closure of the bronchial stump are performed in the same manner as in lobectomy. However, it is important to keep in mind that the main bronchus is large and that the loss of pressure in the intratracheal anesthesia system is rapid if much anesthetic gas is allowed to escape. The closure of the bronchial stump should therefore be accomplished as rapidly as possible by the method already described. Covering the stump is

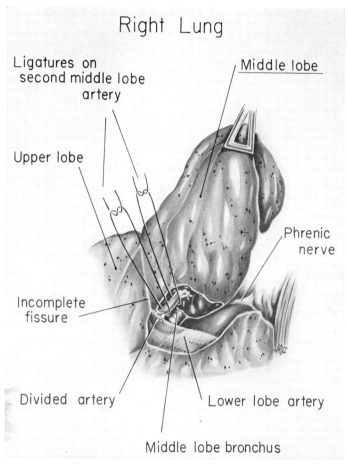

Fig. 83. Right middle lobectomy. Exposure of the structures at the depths of the fissure between the middle and lower lobes. Bronchus and arteries shown. The fissure between the middle and upper lobes is anatomically incomplete.

usually readily accomplished. This step in the procedure must not be omitted.

As already mentioned, the phrenic nerve should be crushed in order to allow the maximum elevation of the diaphragm to assist in the obliteration of the pleural cavity. Drainage is ordinarily not used.

Comparison of Procedures in Pneumonectomy and Lobectomy. In order to

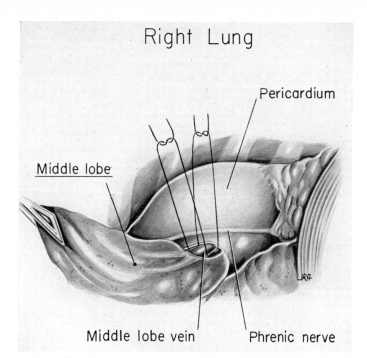

Fig. 84. Right middle lobectomy. Exposure of the middle lobe branch of the superior pulmonary vein on the anterior aspect of the hilus.

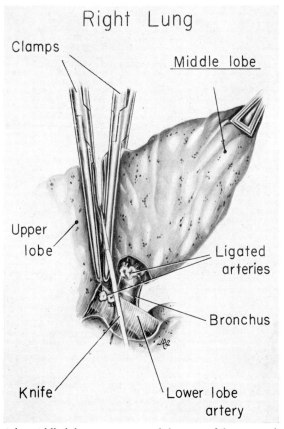

Fig. 85. Right middle lobectomy. Surgical division of the incomplete fissure.

Right Lung

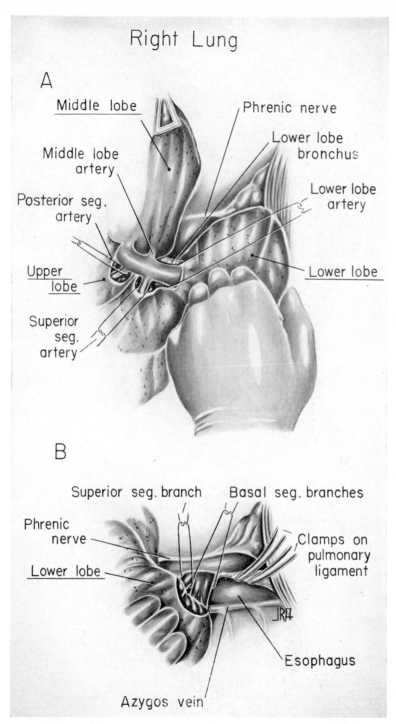

A

Middle lobe

Middle lobe
artery

Posterior seg.
artery

Upper
lobe

Superior
seg.
artery

Phrenic nerve

Lower lobe
bronchus

Lower lobe
artery

Lower lobe

B

Superior seg. branch   Basal seg. branches

Phrenic
nerve

Lower lobe

Clamps on
pulmonary
ligament

JRH

Esophagus

Azygos vein

Fig. 86. Right lower lobectomy. *A*, Exposure of the structures within the fissure showing the relations of the branches of the pulmonary artery. *Note:* In order to avoid occluding the lower middle lobe artery in this case it is necessary to divide the superior segment branch of the lower lobe artery separately. The main artery can then be severed below the middle lobe branch. *B*, Division of the pulmonary ligament and exposure of the inferior pulmonary vein. The large branch which arises in the superior segment is shown. In basal segmental excision this branch must be preserved. In superior segmental excision it is divided, but the remaining branches of the vein must be preserved. In lower lobectomy and pneumonectomy the entire inferior vein is severed.

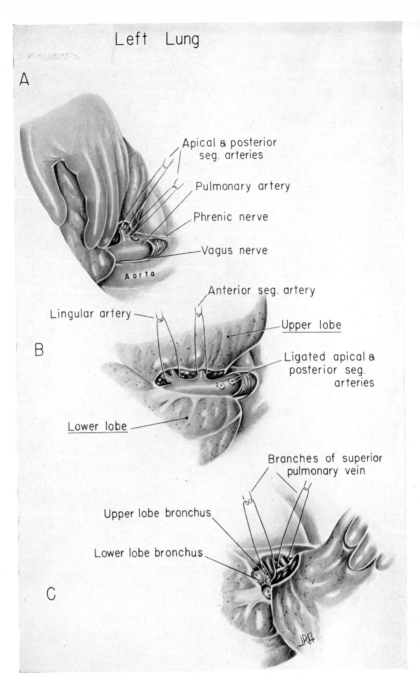

A

Apical & posterior
seg. arteries

Pulmonary artery

Phrenic nerve

Vagus nerve

Aorta

B

Lingular artery

Anterior seg. artery

Upper lobe

Ligated apical &
posterior seg.
arteries

Lower lobe

C

Branches of superior
pulmonary vein

Upper lobe bronchus

Lower lobe bronchus

Fig. 87. Left upper lobectomy. Exposure of the vessels which must be divided in the performance of left upper lobectomy and lingulectomy. *A*, Exposure of the left pulmonary artery and its first branches. In the performance of a pneumonectomy on this side the main trunk can usually be ligated safely proximal to these branches. *B*, Dissection within the fissure to expose the remaining upper lobe arteries for lobectomy or lingulectomy. *C*, Superior pulmonary vein as seen from the anterior aspect of the hilus where it has been made ready for division in the performance of a lobectomy or pneumonectomy. The lingular vein is shown where it is to be divided for a lingulectomy. Separate division of the two principal branches as shown is usually preferable to using a single ligature on the main trunk for lobectomy or pneumonectomy.

Left Lung

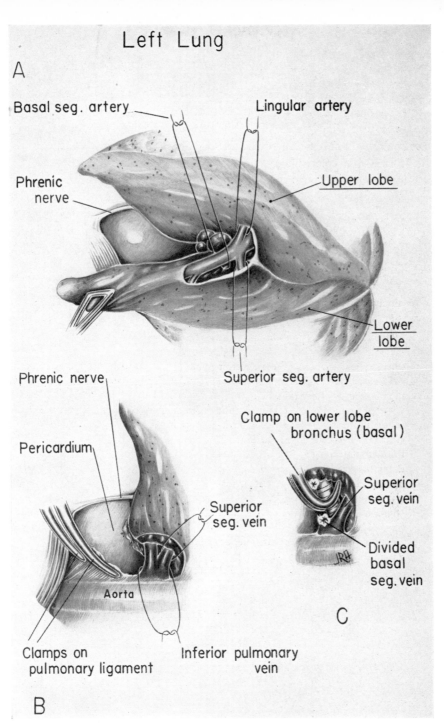

A

Basal seg. artery

Lingular artery

Phrenic nerve

Upper lobe

Lower lobe

Phrenic nerve

Superior seg. artery

Clamp on lower lobe bronchus (basal)

Pericardium

Superior seg. vein

Superior seg. vein

Divided basal seg. vein

Aorta

C

Clamps on pulmonary ligament

Inferior pulmonary vein

B

Fig. 88. *A,* Exposure within the fissure of the lingular and lower lobe branches of the left pulmonary artery. The ligatures indicate points of division of the several vessels for lingulectomy, basal or superior segmental excision, or lower lobectomy. *B,* Division of the pulmonary ligament and exposure of the inferior pulmonary vein and its major segmental branches for a basal or superior segmental excision, lobectomy or pneumonectomy. *C,* Technic of basal segmental excision: Division of the basal segmental venous trunk with preservation of the superior segmental vein. Bronchial trunk distal to the superior segmental bronchus clamped and ready for division. (For artery see *A.*)

simplify the understanding of the essential steps in the technic of lobectomy and pneumonectomy as applied to each of the several lobes and of the two lungs, the following outline is submitted along with suggestions for the most convenient utilization of the illustrations (Figs. 82, 83, 84, 85, 86, 87, 88). It must be clearly understood, however, that because of anatomic variations and situations which result from pathologic processes it may be necessary to vary the sequence of the steps as outlined. The decision in each instance must be made by the surgeon, depending upon the exigencies of the case. In using this outline it will be found helpful to make frequent reference to Figures 16, 17, 18, 19, 20, 21, 22, 23, 24, 25, 26, 27 and 28 in Chapter 1.

OUTLINE OF PROCEDURE

A. Pneumonectomy

Right Lung	*Left Lung*
1. Incision and reflection of perihilar pleura.	1. Same
2. Ligation and division of the superior pulmonary vein to gain better access to the pulmonary artery (Fig. 82).	2. Ligation and division of the main trunk of the pulmonary artery proximal to its first upper lobe branch (Fig. 87).
3. Ligation and division of (a) first branch of pulmonary artery (to apical and anterior segments) and (b) the main trunk below this branch (Fig. 82). *Note:* Sometimes the artery proximal to the first branch is long enough to permit safe division at that level.	3. Ligation and division of the superior pulmonary vein (Fig. 87).
4. Division of the pulmonary ligament (Fig. 86).	4. Same (Fig. 88).
5. Ligation and division of the inferior pulmonary vein (Fig. 86).	5. Same (Fig. 88).
6. Ligation and division of the bronchial arteries close to the level of severance of the bronchus.	6. Same.
7. Section of the bronchus and closure of the bronchial stump (Fig. 78). *Note:* These steps in the procedure are performed simultaneously.	7. Same (Fig. 78).
8. Covering the bronchial stump (Fig. 79, *A, C, D* and *E*).	8. Same (Fig. 79, *A, C, D* and *E*).
9. Crushing the phrenic nerve.	9. Same.
10. Injection of antibiotic solution into pleural cavity.	10. Same.
11. Closure of incision without drainage.	11. Same.

B. Upper Lobectomy

Right Lung	*Left Lung*
1. Ligation and division of the apical, anterior and posterior branches of the superior pulmonary vein. These are usu-	1. Ligation and division of the superior pulmonary vein (Fig. 87).

ally secured separately but may at times be ligated as one or two trunks. *Note:* The middle lobe vein which enters the superior vein must be preserved. Thus the main trunk of the superior vein cannot be ligated singly (Fig. 82).

2. Ligation and division of the apical and anterior segmental branches of the pulmonary artery. *Note:* These arise usually as a single branch but may come off separately. Thus it may be necessary to ligate only one or sometimes two arteries at this point (Fig. 82).

2. Ligation and division of the first one or two branches of the pulmonary artery (Fig. 87). See also Figures 24 and 25, Chapter 1.

Note: Steps 1 and 2 are carried out on the anterior aspect of the hilus of the lung.

3. Ligation and division of the posterior segmental artery (Fig. 86, *A*).

3. Ligation and division of the remaining upper lobe arteries including the lingular artery (Figs. 87 and 88). *Note:* Numerous variations of arrangement and number of the upper lobe arteries on the left side are frequently found (Fig. 28).

4. Ligation and division of the lobar bronchial arteries.

4. Same.

5. Section of the bronchus and closure of the bronchial stump (Fig. 78). These steps are performed simultaneously.

5. Same (Fig. 78).

6. Covering the bronchial stump (Fig. 79, *C, D* and *E,* rarely in lobectomy *B*).

6. Same (Fig. 79, *C, D* and *E,* rarely *B*).

7. Reexpansion of the middle and lower lobes.

7. Reexpansion of the lower lobe.

8. Injection of antibiotic solution into the pleural cavity.

8. Same.

9. Insertion of a drainage catheter (sometimes omitted) (Figs. 32, 33 and 34).

9. Same (Figs. 32, 33 and 34).

10. Closure of incision.

10. Same.

C. Middle Lobectomy and Lingulectomy

Note: Because of the anatomic similarity between the right middle lobe and the lingular segment of the left upper lobe, these procedures are arranged together although lingulectomy is almost always technically a segmental excision. Rarely the lingula comprises a separate lobe (see Chap. 1).

Right Lung: Middle Lobectomy

1. Ligation and division of the middle lobe arteries (or artery) (Fig. 83). This step is accomplished within the fissure.

Left Lung: Lingulectomy

1. Ligation and division of the lingular artery (Fig. 88, *A,* also Fig. 81, *A*). This step is accomplished within the fissure.

2. Ligation and division of the middle lobe vein. This step is sometimes performed before the artery is dealt with (Fig. 84). *Note:* This vein may be a tributary of

2. Ligation and division of the lingular vein (Fig. 87, also Fig. 81, *A*). *Note:* This vein may empty into the inferior pulmonary vein instead of the superior

the inferior pulmonary vein (Fig. 21) or it may enter the heart independently. This step is accomplished on the anterior aspect of the hilus.

vein. This step is accomplished on the anterior aspect of the hilus.

3. Ligation and division of the bronchial arteries.

3. Same.

4. Section of the bronchus and closure of the bronchial stump (Fig. 78). These steps are performed simultaneously.

4. Same (Fig. 78).

5. Covering the bronchial stump (Fig. 79, B, C, D or E).

5. Same (Fig. 79, B). Note: Method B, whereby the stump is buried within the contiguous portion of the remainder of the upper lobe, is usually sufficient in lingulectomy.

6. Separation of partially or entirely incomplete fissure between the middle and upper lobes (Fig. 85). Note: This step is frequently accomplished before Step 4. Either sequence is satisfactory.

6. Severance of the parenchyma of the lung along the intersegmental plane (Fig. 81, B). Occasionally there is a partial fissure between the lingular and adjacent segments. Rarely this fissure may be complete.

7. Reexpansion of the upper and lower lobes.

7. Reexpansion of the remainder of the upper lobe and the lower lobe.

8. Injection of antibiotic solution into the pleural cavity.

8. Same.

9. Insertion of a drainage catheter (sometimes omitted) (Figs. 32, 33 and 34).

9. Same (*Rarely* omitted) (Figs. 32, 33 and 34).

10. Closure of the incision.

10. Same.

D. Lower Lobectomy

Right Lung

1. Ligation and division of the pulmonary artery below the middle lobe branches (Fig. 86, A). Note: In order to preserve the lower middle lobe artery it is sometimes necessary to divide the superior segmental branch of the lower lobe artery separately; the main trunk can then be severed below the middle lobe vessel.

Left Lung

1. Ligation and division of the lower lobe artery (Fig. 88). Note: If the origin of the lingular artery is unusually low on the main trunk or if it actually arises from the lower lobe artery, it is necessary, in order to preserve it, to divide the superior segmental branch and the main trunk of the lower lobe artery separately.

2. Division of the pulmonary ligament (Fig. 86, B).

2. Same (Fig. 88, B).

3. Ligation and division of the inferior pulmonary vein Fig. 86, B).

3. Same (Fig. 88, B).

4. Ligation and division of the lower lobe branches of the bronchial arteries.

4. Same.

5. Section of the bronchus and closure of the bronchial stump (Fig. 78). These steps are performed simultaneously. Note: Because of an unusually high origin of the superior segment bronchus opposite or actually proximal to

5. Same (Fig. 78). Note: In the rare situation where the lingular bronchus arises independently from the main bronchial trunk, a relation to the lower lobe bronchus similar to that which frequently prevails with the middle lobe

the origin of the middle lobe bronchus, it may be necessary to sever this bronchus independently of the main lower lobe bronchial trunk which must be divided separately. In this instance two bronchial stumps must be dealt with if the middle lobe bronchus is to be preserved. Otherwise the middle lobe must be removed with the lower lobe. This is sometimes unavoidable.

bronchus in the right lung may be encountered. The same treatment is then required as on the right side.

6. Covering the bronchial stump (Fig. 79, C, D or E).

6. Same (Fig. 79, C, D or E).

7. Reexpansion of the upper and middle lobes.

7. Reexpansion of the upper lobe.

8. Injection of the antibiotic solution into the pleural cavity.

8. Same.

9. Insertion of a drainage catheter. (Figs. 32, 33 and 34) (sometimes omitted).

9. Same (Figs. 32, 33 and 34) (sometimes omitted).

10. Closure of the incision.

10. Same.

Tourniquet Method of Lobectomy. Before the technic of hilar dissection was well developed, it was sometimes thought best in the presence of intense inflammatory reaction within the hilus to abandon the attempt to isolate the pulmonary vessels for separate ligation and division and to resort to the use of the tourniquet method of lobectomy. Although rarely needed nowadays, a lung tourniquet should always be available. The necessity for its use, however, bears an inverse relation to the experience and skill of the surgeon.

In case it should be necessary to use the tourniquet method of lobectomy, a brief description of the technic follows.

After its peripheral attachments have been freed and the fissure is completely developed, the lobe is held up by means of a lung forceps (large Duval forceps) and the tourniquet is passed over it and down as far as possible around the hilar pedicle of the lobe. This pedicle consists of the bronchus, the bronchial arteries, the pulmonary arteries and veins and the lymph nodes, all of them matted together by inflammatory adhesions and infiltration. The tourniquet is then tightened so that there is no doubt that the pulmonary artery to the lobe is occluded. This necessitates a very considerable degree of compression. A second tourniquet is applied to the lung several centimeters distal to the proximally applied tourniquet. If there is danger of its slipping, a large clamp can be used distally instead of the second tourniquet. Using a knife, the lobar pedicle is then cut in a V-shaped manner with the depths of the V directed centrally toward the proximal tourniquet. The diseased lobe is then removed from the chest.

From this moment on the members of the operating team must be careful not to trip the ratchet which holds the tourniquet tight. This accident would result promptly in the escape of the pulmonary artery with grave consequences because of the difficulty of securing the severed vessel in a mass of inflammatory lymph nodes and other hilar structures.

The en masse closure of the hilar stump is begun by passing numerous mattress sutures of catgut across the divided tissues, starting at the depths of the V-shaped surface and ending with a series across the edges. It is well to leave several of the outer sutures uncut with hemostats attached so that the stump can be controlled. After the last of these sutures has been tied, the tourniquet is released gradually. As the compression of the stump is diminished, bleeding will occur from any vessel which may not have been secured by the mass suture ligatures. In this event the tourniquet is tightened once again and another suture is applied at the point whence the blood was seen to emerge. The adequacy of the hemostasis is then tested again and further bleeding is stopped by sutures until it has been controlled completely. The tourniquet is then removed and the lobar stump is released.

Healing of such a mass of partially devitalized tissue compressed by ligatures is naturally slow and often incomplete because of the necrosis and sepsis which usually result. A bronchial fistula develops in many such cases and empyema is a frequent complication. The tourniquet method is to be condemned except for emergency use or in exceptional instances of inflammatory fixation of the hilus.

Technical Problems Presented by Certain Diseases

Bronchiectasis. The ease with which a lobe or a lung can be removed for bronchiectasis bears a direct relation to the severity of the complicating infection and the duration of the resultant inflammatory changes. The manifestations of infection in this disease consist of adhesions between the lung and the parietal pleura and the diaphragm, or between the lobes, and enlargement and inflammatory fixation of the hilar lymph nodes.

In some cases the element of infection is negligible and there is therefore almost no inflammatory reaction. Such lungs are not adherent and the hilar lymph nodes are only moderately enlarged. In fact, it would often be difficult to determine just where the diseased segments of the lung might be if it were not for the benefit of preoperative roentgen studies of the bronchial tree after the injection of iodized oil.

Certain guides to the identification of the abnormal areas are helpful in these relatively uninfected lungs. In the first place, the bronchiectatic portion of the lung is often much more free of anthracotic pigmentation than the other segments or lobes. This difference is sometimes very striking and, if not understood by the surgeon, might lead him to the erroneous conclusion that the diseased portion is actually uninvolved. Secondly, in the majority of cases it is possible to palpate the abnormal terminal bronchi which are more obvious to the sense of touch than in the normal lung and impart to the examiner's fingers the sensation that they are thickened and drawn closely together. A third important aid to the identification of the abnormal portion is the observation of areas of atelectasis or of trapped air in emphysematous regions. Atelectasis of the alveolar portion of the diseased segments is, of course, a frequent and helpful finding. A less well-recognized phenomenon which, when found, is also characteristic of the lung in a bronchiectatic segment before atelectasis has supplanted it, is a tendency of the alveolar portion of the diseased segment to retain its air after the pressure within the bronchial tree has been reduced. This is sometimes so pronounced that for many minutes after the air has left the remainder of the lung, the bronchiectatic segment remains air-filled or even emphysematous. This is spoken of as "obstructive emphysema."

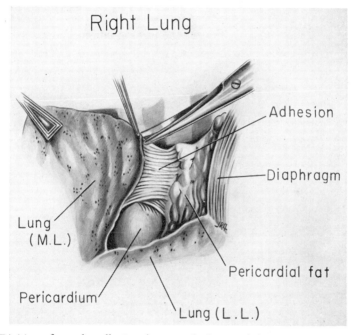

Fig. 89. Division of vascular adhesions between the lung and the pericardial sac in a case of bronchiectasis of the right middle lobe.

In patients who have experienced infection in the bronchiectatic portion of the lung one finds at operation evidences of inflammation which vary in degree depending upon the extent and duration of the infection. The technical difficulty of the operation in such cases naturally varies with the manifestations of inflammation. In some the adhesions of the lung to the chest wall and diaphragm are very dense and exceedingly vascular. Adhesions to the diaphragm and pericardial fat tabs in particular are notably vascular and often difficult to divide (Fig. 89). It is in such cases that transillumination with a small operating light is valuable to avoid cutting into the diaphragm or the lung itself during the dissection.

The hilar lymph nodes in bronchiectasis are frequently much inflamed and adherent. In some cases this tendency is so pronounced that it is difficult to free the pulmonary vessels for individual ligation and division. However, by painstaking work and with a thorough knowledge of the anatomy of the hilus of the lung it is usually possible to accomplish the desired result. In order to find the vessels to a given lobe or segment it is frequently necessary to dissect between the enlarged lymph nodes which are so swollen and adherent as to make a confluent mass of inflammatory tissue completely surrounding the vessels which are to be divided. Once the dissection has been accomplished and the vessels have been severed, the management of the bronchus does not usually present any special problem. However, after its closure the bronchial stump is almost completely surrounded by swollen lymph nodes and the covering flap of pleura must sometimes under such circumstances be sutured to the nodes rather than to the bronchus itself.

Lung Abscess. In lobectomy or pneumonectomy for lung abscess the technical problems are essentially the same as in the cases of bronchiectasis with associated inflammatory changes. The peripheral adhesions, though dense and often exceedingly vascular, are usually confined to a smaller area than in bronchiectasis. The inflammatory reaction at the hilus of the lung in abscess cases is likely to be very pronounced and the presence of enormously swollen inflamed lymph nodes is characteristic.

The technical difficulty of performing a lobectomy in a case of lung abscess is sometimes greatly magnified by the fact that the process has crossed the septum and involved the contiguous portion in an adjacent lobe. This occurrence takes place only when the abscess lies in certain segments and near the fissure. Abscesses located in the middle lobe, in the lateral aspects of the upper lobe, and in the superior segment of the lower lobe are the most frequent offenders in this manner. The fact that an abscess may have crossed the septum to involve an adjacent lobe may make it necessary to excise a portion of the lobe which has been involved secondarily. This is a potentially dangerous procedure because of the possibility that the surgical trauma might cause the propagation of a necrotizing infection in the remainder of the lobe. This occurrence may be prevented by the prophylactic utilization of the antibiotics, penicillin and streptomycin; if these drugs are not available it is unwise to perform a local excision of the process. Under such circumstances it is far safer to resort to a pneumonectomy than to temporize with the attendant serious risk of gangrene of the remainder of the residual lobe, of empyema and of bronchopleural fistula, all of which are likely to develop once the spread of infection has begun.

Another serious difficulty which may interfere with the successful performance of a lobectomy for abscess is the sudden flooding of the bronchi and trachea with pus from an abscess which has not emptied previously through the bronchus or has not been drained as a preliminary phase of the surgical treatment. The dangers of such an accident are spread of infection in the opposite lung because of inhalation of pus into the bronchi or the sudden asphyxiation of the patient before the anesthetist is able to aspirate the material from the trachea. Under these circumstances the surgeon may prevent a fatal outcome in one of two ways. He may, if the dissection of the hilus has been carried far enough, occlude the bronchus by applying a large clamp to it. If the bronchus is not sufficiently exposed to allow the application of a clamp, the alternate procedure is to open the cavity in the lung and aspirate or wipe out its contents as quickly as possible so as to avoid spilling into the bronchial tree. After the cavity has been emptied in this manner, it can be closed with several sutures or merely stuffed with gauze to prevent continued contamination of the pleural space with pus and the escape of pressure from the anesthesia system during the remainder of the operation. The protection afforded by the use of the antibiotics makes it possible to carry out this maneuver without serious danger of postoperative empyema.

Tuberculosis. In the extirpative surgery of pulmonary tuberculosis the most frequent technical difficulty arises from the presence of unusually dense peripheral adhesions. As would be expected, the regions where these adhesions are usually most impervious are over the upper and posterior aspects of the upper lobe and along the posterior surface of the superior segment of the lower lobe. In the average case the lower and anterior surfaces of the lung are not particularly adherent unless there has been a complicating chronic empyema. In many cases where it is impossible to find a plane of cleavage between the visceral and the parietal pleural membranes, it is easier and safer to enter the extrapleural fascial plane and remove the fused parietal layer over the most adherent area along with the lung itself. In this way it is possible to avoid the contamination which results from opening into the diseased area within the lung.

Once the periphery of the lobe or lung has been freed, however, the remainder of the operation in tuberculous cases is not likely to cause unusual difficulty. Envelopment of the structures of the hilus by inflammatory tissue and matted lymph nodes is rarely excessive except in a few cases where caseation of some of the perihilar lymph nodes may have occurred. In rare instances the structures of the hilus may be buried in a mass of caseous material or surrounded by a tuberculous abscess. In such a situation it is probably wiser to abandon the operation than to run the risk of disseminating the infection or of postoperative opening of the bronchial stump. Occasionally, also, when there is predominant bronchial involvement, there may be considerable thickening of the bronchus itself and some degree of peribronchial infiltration. This may be sufficiently pronounced to make the isolation of the pulmonary vessels difficult, but the condition is very unusual and the difficulty in such cases rarely insurmountable.

Benign Tumors. Benign tumors of the lung arise either in the periphery or, as in the case of the tumor known as adenoma of the bronchus, in relation to the primary bronchi. Those in the first category can usually be removed by local or segmental excision. A lobectomy may occasionally be necessary if they are large or have begun to encroach upon a major lobar bronchus.

In the case of adenoma of the bronchus, however, it is practically always necessary to perform a lobectomy or even a pneumonectomy because of the location of the growth. (For exception see section on Bronchotomy.) There is also often the additional factor of bronchiectasis in the lung distal to the tumor. Technical difficulties in such cases have to do more with the results of secondary infection in the bronchiectatic lobe than with the presence of the tumor per se. As would be expected, they follow the same pattern as in any other case of bronchiectasis.

On the other hand, the adenoma itself may offer some difficulty, especially in the decision as to the level at which the bronchus is to be divided. The decision depends upon the conditions found in each individual case.

Malignant Metastatic Tumors. Under certain conditions the removal of a metastatic malignant tumor from the lung may be indicated. There are enough reports of long survival of the patient to make extirpation a rational method of treatment when the evidence points to the possibility that the lesion in question may be a single metastasis. That a given lesion is actually the only one present, of course, can never be proven. Furthermore, it is not always possible to be certain before operation that the pulmonary tumor is not actually primary in the lung itself. Certain malignant tumors, on the other hand, have been known to produce single metastases more frequently than others. These are renal cell carcinoma of the kidney, carcinoma of the thyroid gland, sarcoma of the breast, fibrosarcoma of the soft parts, and occasionally carcinoma of the colon.

In many cases of presumed single metastatic tumor of the lung the location of the growth is in the lung parenchyma at a point where a local wedge-shaped excision of a portion of a lobe is sufficient to remove the lesion. In other cases, however, it may be necessary to perform a lobectomy because of the proximity of the growth to a major bronchus. For the same reason a pneumonectomy is required in rare instances. In a very few cases the metastasis is located in the wall of a major bronchus. When this occurs the surgical problem is essentially that presented by a primary bronchogenic carcinoma, and a lobectomy or a pneumonectomy must be performed. The only significant difference from primary carcinoma is that there need be no concern about lymph node metastases from the pulmonary lesion.

Bronchogenic Carcinoma. In bronchogenic carcinoma of the lung the technical problem may be threefold, depending upon the location and extent of the tumor. In the first place, the tumor may be adherent to the parietal wall, if located in the periphery of a lobe of the lung. In some such cases it is possible to free it by entering the extrapleural fascial plane for the dissection. In that event a portion of the parietal pleura must be excised with the adherent growth. In other cases, however, the growth has actually invaded the structures of the chest wall, even the overlying ribs. In some of these it is still possible to remove the lesion by excising en bloc a section of the parietes including portions of the ribs, the intercostal muscles, the nerves and the vessels. In the apex of the chest this can rarely be done because of the early involvement of the sympathetic nerves and the cords of the brachial plexus by direct invasion (Pancoast tumor).

Inability to complete the operation may result also from invasion of the pericardium or envelopment of the pulmonary artery or veins in such a manner that these vessels cannot be divided and ligated with safety. In a few such cases, however, it may be possible to proceed by opening the pericardium so that the vessels may be ligated closer to the heart and so that the invaded section of the pericardium may be excised with the diseased lung. Such heroic attempts to eradicate a carcinoma of the lung, however, are rarely crowned with ultimate success.

Peripheral adhesions in carcinoma of the lung are sometimes merely inflammatory because of the pneumonitis which frequently occurs as a complication of the partial obstruction of a major bronchus by the growth. It is almost always possible to differentiate between these inflammatory adhesions and the fixation which results from direct extension of the tumor. They are divided in the usual manner, often with the aid of transillumination as described previously.

The second factor of importance in the removal of a carcinoma of the lung is the degree of involvement of the regional lymph nodes. The nodes within the hilus itself are usually involved first, but metastases may occur to the nodes of the mediastinum, neck or abdomen in the absence of hilar node involvement. Ideally the operation should make provision for the removal of as large a number of the nodes as possible. In order to do so, it follows that all hilar nodes, those in the pulmonary ligament, and as many as possible from the adjacent region of the mediastinum, especially in the subcarinal area, be excised. If this is done, it is obvious that a pneumonectomy would be required in every case. In the management of carcinoma of the lung, however, other factors must be considered, such as the pulmonary and cardiac reserve of the patient. If there is no evidence of lymph node metastases in the hilar region either by gross examination or by frozen section biopsy, it is preferable in some poor risk patients to be content with the performance of a lobectomy instead of the theoretically ideal pneumonectomy.

The final consideration which has a bearing upon the technical problem in carcinoma of the lung is the location of the tumor in the bronchus. It is necessary if possible to cut the bronchus as far away from the tumor as

8

practicable in order to diminish the possibility of a recurrence of the disease in the bronchial stump. This makes it necessary in many instances in which the lesion is primary in a lobar bronchus to perform a pneumonectomy even when the lymph nodes appear to be uninvolved. Furthermore, when the tumor lies within the primary bronchus it is not always possible to perform a pneumonectomy because of proliferation of the growth too close to the carina. This occurrence may occasionally defeat the efforts of the surgeon to complete the operation even in the absence of extensive lymph node involvement.

Emphysematous Blebs. Serious impairment of the respiratory function in patients who have emphysematous blebs may occur either because of the development of tension pneumothorax as a result of the rupture of a bleb or because of the pressure produced by overinflation when the bleb is large. Although the usual course of spontaneous pneumothorax resulting from the bursting of an emphysematous bleb is benign and healing is permanent, there are cases in which surgery is useful or necessary to effect a cure. The most frequent indications for operation in this condition are the failure of the lung to remain expanded or the frequent recurrence of pneumothorax. Many times the lesion is a small one and a simple procedure is sufficient. This consists in the excision of the outer portion of the bleb down to the substance of the lung followed by an over and over suture of the area from which the bleb arose, including the small bronchial opening. In some cases more than one opening is found, while in others there are multiple con- fluent blebs. However, the compression of a continuous suture of fine catgut usually suffices to control the air leakage. Before the chest is closed the lung should be expanded completely in order to test the efficacy of the repair. It is wise also in all such cases to insert a catheter through an intercostal space as a precautionary measure to prevent the development of tension pneumo- thorax.

Cases exist where a giant emphysematous bleb may become so enormously distended with air that it encroaches to a serious extent upon the space re- quired for the proper functioning of the remainder of the lung. In some the lesion may occupy the entire hemithorax and may even push across the mediastinum to compress the opposite lung. In certain of these extreme cases removal of the overdistended bleb is required. When this becomes necessary, it is rarely possible to excise the bleb alone either because of the distortion and compression of the remainder of the lobe in which it lies or because the adjacent lung tissue is diffusely involved by the same process and is actually valueless from the functional point of view. In the majority of examples of giant emphysematous bleb, therefore, nothing short of a lobectomy or in some cases a pneumonectomy is sufficient to correct the condition. Unless an intercurrent infection has developed, there are no peripheral adhesions and the hilus is usually free. It is often quite striking, however, that the pulmonary artery and veins in such cases are relatively small. The vessels of the bronchial circulation, on the other hand, may be unusually well developed.

No particular technical difficulties are encountered, but the surgeon should keep in mind the fact that in all these cases the bleb becomes inflated immediately as the lung is expanded by the anesthetist, and the expansion of the remainder of the lung lags behind. If an opening has been made in such a bleb, therefore, there is danger that the rapid escape of the anesthetic gases will cause a relative deflation of the remainder of the lung on the operated side and also of the opposite lung. Such an occurrence would, of course, interfere with the maintenance of the proper level of anesthesia and also give rise to a serious degree of relative anoxia if long continued. The difficulty can be overcome by the temporary application of hemostatic forceps to the leaking area or, if possible, by putting a clamp across the lobar bronchus.

Postoperative Care Following Pulmonary Surgery

The care of patients who have been the subject of an operation upon the lung demands the exercise of judgment and skill based upon a knowledge of the possible complications which might ensue. It should be intimately supervised by the surgeon himself. Although a detailed consideration is not the subject of a volume which deals chiefly with operative technic, mention should be made of certain important aspects of the after-care.

Infusions and Transfusions. The avoidance of shock resulting from blood loss depends upon the routine utilization of blood transfusions during the course of the operation and in the first few hours of the postoperative period. Enough blood should be administered to replace the amount lost. The additional intravenous infusion of solutions of glucose and sodium chloride must be used with caution because of the possibility of overloading the circulation with the resultant danger of precipitating pulmonary edema. This precaution is more necessary in older patients than in young adults or children, and particularly in those who have had the amount of available lung volume greatly reduced, as by a pneumonectomy. There is little reason why patients who have had operations upon the lung should be given parenteral fluids after their recovery from the effects of the anesthetic. They can usually take an adequate amount by mouth and the dangers of embarrassing the circulation are thereby minimized.

Intrathoracic Pressure Changes. The pressure relations within the thorax should also be the subject of concern to the surgeon during the early convalescent period. There is always the possibility that an undetected leak of air from the lung parenchyma in cases of local or segmental excision, or from the stump of the bronchus in cases of lobectomy and pneumonectomy, may lead to the development of tension pneumothorax. Such an occurrence is manifested by the development of dyspnea and by signs of the shifting of the mediastinum to the opposite side. The most obvious objective signs are a shift in the apex impulse of the heart and deviation of the trachea to the nonoperated side. Immediate correction by the aspiration of air is indicated. If the leakage of air persists, a small catheter should be introduced through an intercostal space for the application of suction or to provide a valvular escape of air by the use of a water-seal apparatus. In the majority of instances the leak, which is usually from the lung parenchyma, will seal over in a few days and the catheter may then be removed. Leakage from a carefully closed and properly covered bronchial stump is an exceedingly rare occurrence.

When a catheter has been inserted at operation, as in the average case of lobectomy or segmental excision, the danger of developing tension postoperatively exists only if the catheter should become obstructed. This possibility must, however, be kept in mind.

Sometimes after a pneumonectomy has been performed without drainage, an increase in the intrathoracic pressure may develop on the side of the operation as a result of the rapid effusion of fluid during the first few days after the operation. A moderate shifting of the mediastinum may result from this because the absorption of air from the pleural space on the operated side takes place more slowly. When this difficulty arises, an adjustment of pressure should be made by aspirating some of the air. If the serosanguineous effusion becomes excessive, some of the fluid should be removed also. One should remember that in such a case a large amount of protein and red cells may be lost from the volume of circulating blood, and appropriate measures, including transfusions of blood, should be taken to overcome this loss. This observation applies likewise chiefly to cases of pneumonectomy.

Administration of Oxygen. Oxygen should be administered routinely to all patients who have had extirpative pulmonary surgery. The duration of its use, however, should depend upon the volume of lung which remains and upon other factors such as the amount of available hemoglobin in the circulating blood and the presence or absence of certain complications, such as tension pneumothorax and atelectasis of portions of the remaining lung. Every effort must be made to make the utilization of the inspired oxygen effective by clearing the respiratory passages and by improving the oxygen-carrying capacity of the circulating blood with transfusions if the hemoglobin level is below normal.

The technic used to administer the oxygen depends upon the preference of the surgeon and the apparatus available. In general three methods are useful. For short periods of time, as, for example, during the transfer of the patient from the operating theatre to his room, a face mask such as the

Boothby type may be used. When conscious, the majority of patients object to the mask and a shift should be made to one of the other two methods as soon as practicable.

For the great majority of patients the use of the intranasal catheter is the best. The catheter is introduced so that its tip lies at the choana so that the oxygen is delivered into the nasopharynx. It is held in place by a narrow strip of adhesive tape. This method is tolerated well by the majority of patients, except young children, and it has the advantage of simplicity. No apparatus is required except a tankful of oxygen and a connecting unit which consists of a humidifier and a valve with a meter attached to indicate the volume flow of the gas. One of the greatest advantages of this method over the oxygen tent is the fact that it greatly simplifies the problem of nursing care. Furthermore, there is reason to believe that it is more efficient than the average oxygen tent. Two possible drawbacks, however, must be mentioned. Both of these can be avoided by the use of the proper precautions. First, the nasal catheter frequently becomes occluded by the presence of inspissated secretions on the tip. This may occur in spite of the fact that a continuous flow of oxygen has been maintained at all times. It is wise, therefore, to change the catheter at eight hourly intervals in all cases. Advantage should be taken of this opportunity to relieve the patient's discomfort by shifting to the opposite nostril.

The second difficulty which may on occasion assume serious proportions is the danger of introducing oxygen into the gastrointestinal tract under certain conditions. This may result from the fact that the catheter has been unskillfully introduced and pushed too far into the pharynx. Furthermore, when a Levin tube has been introduced into the stomach for some reason through the other nostril, an inexperienced attendant may unknowingly connect the oxygen to the stomach tube instead of to the nasal catheter. In either event the rapid inflation with oxygen may produce a sudden rupture of the overdistended stomach. This rare accident is easily recognized by the sudden pain experienced by the patient and the development of the signs of pneumoperitoneum with characteristic tympanitic enlargement of the abdomen. The occurrence of this complication obviously calls for a prompt laparotomy. The site of rupture of the stomach is usually on the lesser curvature, just distal to the cardia. Deflation of the peritoneal cavity and suture of the injured stomach serve to prevent serious consequences.

The third method of administering oxygen, namely by means of a tent over the entire bed or a hood over the head and shoulders of the patient, is the least efficacious of all three. By actual measurement it has been shown that it is very difficult, even by using all possible precautions against the escape of the gas, to obtain an increase of more than a few volumes per cent of oxygen in the inspired air over the room air concentration. This method must be used, however, in place of the easier and more efficient intranasal catheter technic in uncooperative adults and in children.

In the average case the administration of oxygen to patients who have had a segmental excision or simple lobectomy can be discontinued after twenty-four to forty-eight hours. After a pneumonectomy its use will be required usually for a longer period, but rarely more than four or five days. It is wise to give a patient a preliminary trial of a few hours without it before stopping the oxygen permanently.

Prevention of Atelectasis. It is of special importance to avoid the accumulation of secretions in the tracheobronchial tree. This is done by encouraging the patient to cough, by frequent changes of position, by early rising after operation, and by other measures as the indications occur. If the patient is unable to expectorate by coughing, either because of pain or because the secretions are too viscid, intratracheal aspiration through a catheter connected to a suction apparatus may be effective. If this should fail, however, it is wise to resort to bronchoscopic aspiration rather than run the risk of the development of atelectasis from plugging of one or more bronchi. This procedure can be carried out in the patient's bed without moving him from his room and may be a life-saving measure in certain instances. It will at least avoid the retardation of recovery which sometimes follows the delayed expansion of an atelectatic portion of lung.

Management of Fluid Accumulations in the Pleural Space. After lobectomy and segmental excision it is usually wise to employ closed drainage of the pleural cavity during the first forty-eight hours postoperatively. This removes the majority of the fluid which may accumulate after the operation. If drainage has not been used, and sometimes when the effusion is prolonged with reaccumulation after the catheter has been removed, it may be advisable to remove the fluid by thoracentesis subsequent to the withdrawal of the catheter. This depends upon the amount of fluid present and its probable effect upon the remainder of the lung. If no embarrassment of respiration is caused by the effusion, however, it will usually be absorbed spontaneously. In general, large effusions should be removed. After pneumonectomy, unless there is evidence of infection or shifting of the mediastinum, it is best not to remove the fluid because of the part it plays in the obliteration of the pleural cavity on the operated side.

Early Ambulation. The advantages of early ambulation are as obvious in the field of thoracic surgery as in abdominal surgery. It is important to remember, however, that in the care of patients who have had a pneumonectomy there may be a profound physiologic disturbance having to do chiefly with the circulatory system; such patients must not be forced out of bed too soon. Much depends upon variable factors such as the presence or absence of emphysema of the remaining lung, the maintenance of a good expansion of this lung, the prevention of mediastinal deviation, and also the underlying integrity of the heart function. Many patients have a partially damaged myocardium as the result of previous infarctions or are in a potentially precarious state because of arteriosclerosis of the coronary arteries even though no occlusion has yet occurred. The decision as to when such patients may be allowed out of bed and how rapidly they are to be encouraged to resume physical activity must be based upon the exigencies of the individual case, and no general rule can be supplied. On the average, few patients who have had a pneumonectomy are able to be much out of bed before the fourth or fifth postoperative day unless they are young and have an unusually sound heart. A left pneumonectomy is better tolerated than a right because of the relatively smaller volume of lung tissue removed.

SPECIAL PROCEDURES

Biopsy of the Lung

When carcinoma is suspected, a biopsy may be required in order to plan the roentgen ray treatment in cases which appear to be inoperable, or to make certain of the diagnosis at the operating table in order to decide upon the amount of lung to be removed.

In patients presumably inoperable because of the obvious extent of the disease or who because of age or poor general condition are not suitable candidates for surgery, a diagnosis may be made by the aspiration method sometimes used in other fields of surgery. An accurate localization of the tumor is determined by means of fluoroscopy or a study of the roentgen ray films. A large caliber (No. 16) sharp needle attached to a glass syringe is thrust through the chest wall into the tumor. Traction is then exerted upon the plunger of the syringe and at the same time the syringe is rotated in an attempt to cut loose a small bit of tissue in the tip of the needle. These forces are continued as the needle is withdrawn, when a few bits of tumor tissue will be seen to pass into the barrel of the syringe as the needle leaves the chest wall. These should be placed immediately in a fixative and sent to the laboratory.

This method should never be used when the growth is resectable because of the definite danger of implanting carcinoma cells in the needle track within the thoracic wall.

In certain patients, especially where the chest wall seems to be invaded, a direct approach through a short incision may be preferable. Local anesthesia can be used. The advantage of this method lies in the fact that larger pieces of tissue are obtained directly from the growth with a greater certainty of establishing an accurate diagnosis.

In other patients, when a positive diagnosis cannot be made beforehand it may be advisable to obtain tissue by biopsy from a suspicious lesion in the lung during the course of an exploratory thoracotomy. If the mass is peripheral, it is no problem to excise a small portion with a knife. From this a frozen section diagnosis may be made by the pathologist. If the mass is located more centrally, it is necessary to incise the lung parenchyma to reach it. In this instance, if bleeding or leakage of air from the incised area becomes troublesome, a temporary closure of the area should be made with interrupted sutures. It is wise whenever a pulmonary biopsy must be obtained at the operating table to provide extra protection of the operative field with gauze pads to prevent soiling if an area of infection is encountered. When an abscess or tuberculous area is thus inadvertently opened, the pulmonary incision should be closed as thoroughly as possible with sutures or by applying hemostatic forceps. The instruments and gloves of the operator which were used during the biopsy procedure should be discarded in favor of clean ones for the completion of the operation.

Bronchotomy

The direct opening of a major bronchus may be necessary to remove a pedunculated tumor or a foreign body which cannot be extracted through a bronchoscope. The operation is performed using a standard thoracotomy incision with intratracheal inhalation anesthesia. The bronchus is exposed by reflecting the pleura from the posterior surface of the hilus of the lung. The exploratory incision through the noncartilaginous posterior bronchial wall can be made either longitudinally or transversely. In general the transverse incision is preferable. Through such an incision, by bending the bronchus slightly, the proximal and distal portions of its lumen may be inspected and the object within it extracted with an appropriate instrument. Closure of the bronchial wall is made by edge-to-edge approximation with interrupted sutures of fine silk. The needles should be small. The best method is to use a swedged-on suture of silk such as those intended for arterial anastomoses. Air leakage is prevented by fastening the hilar pleural flap over it with fine sutures. The lung is then expanded and the chest wall is closed. The danger of developing tension pneumothorax from an unsuspected leakage of air is minimized by inserting a catheter intercostally before closing the chest wall. After the patient is returned to his bed, a connection is made with a water-seal bottle or a three bottle suction apparatus.

Closure of Bronchial Fistulas

Fistulous communications between a bronchus and the exterior of the chest may be grouped under three headings depending upon the etiology. The details of treatment may vary slightly from one type to the other.

Bronchopleural Fistula as a Complication of Empyema

A fistulous communication with a bronchus is a frequent cause of chronicity in cases of empyema, no matter what the etiologic agent may have been. The condition may be treated either by a direct attack upon the opening with an attempt to close it by suture or in an indirect manner by suturing a flap of muscle against it or by obliterating the empyema cavity with a thoracoplasty of the Schede type.

A direct closure of the fistulous opening by suture made through the empyema cavity is rarely successful unless it is done in combination with a decortication and expansion of the partially collapsed lung. A wide incision is made into the empyema cavity and the restricted thickened pleural membrane is removed according to the method previously described (Chap. 5). Once the lung has been released, it resumes its normal pliability. The thickened edges of the fistula are excised so that a closure can then be made with fine suture material. The closed opening is then infolded into the lung substance with a row of sutures of the Lembert type. With the leakage of air controlled, the lung remains expanded and the usual tight closure of the thoracic incision is made.

When the empyema cavity is small and a decortication and expansion of the lung may not seem necessary, the fistula may be closed by filling the cavity with a flap of muscle. The interior of the cavity is exposed by resecting a portion of the rib on either side of the drainage opening. A rectangular or rounded flap is developed from whichever muscle happens to lie in the most convenient location to allow the flap to be placed in the cavity. This is often the latissimus dorsi. It may be, however, the trapezius, the serratus anterior or the pectoralis major muscle. Sometimes portions of two or more muscles may be used to fill the same cavity. The pedicles of the flaps must be broad enough to preserve an adequate blood supply. A portion of muscle large enough to fill the cavity completely must be freed. This flap of muscle is swung over the edge of the cavity and stuffed tightly into it. There it is held firmly in place by means of interrupted sutures around the periphery. If the fistula opening is large, it is wise to incise the tissue around its edge and close it with fine sutures before inserting the muscle flap. Catgut sutures and ligatures should be used throughout the operation because of the possibility of developing infection in the wound which might be prolonged as a result of the foreign body reaction around nonabsorbable suture materials such as silk or cotton. A tight closure should be made, however, unless it is impossible to leave a sufficiently dry operative field. If oozing of blood persists, a small rubber drain may be inserted. This should be removed after twenty-four to forty-eight hours. The occurrence of infection is unusual, especially if advantage is taken of the prophylactic use of antibiotics.

Bronchopleural Fistula as a Complication of Lobectomy or Pneumonectomy

As a result of the abandonment of the tourniquet technic in favor of individual ligation of the vessels and closure of the bronchial stump, the occurrence of a bronchopleural fistula after extirpative pulmonary surgery is now a rarity. It is almost never encountered except as a result of infection due to postoperative empyema which in itself is now an unusual occurrence. The closure of such a fistula is, however, unusually difficult. Because of its large size the use of muscle flaps for obliteration of the empyema cavity is rarely practicable. The most universally applicable method for the management of such cases is a direct closure of the secondarily opened bronchial stump by suture followed by the performance of a thoracoplasty of the Schede (intrapleural) type (See Chap. 5).

Bronchocutaneous Fistula as a Complication of the Drainage of a Lung Abscess

A certain percentage of lung abscesses do not heal after drainage. Although the acute infection is overcome, the cavity persists and becomes epithelized. If the drainage tube is left in place for a long period of time in such a case, the process of epithelization may extend into the chest wall sinus and ultimately communicate with the ingrowing dermal epithelium from the exterior. This results in a persistent bronchocutaneous fistula which will not close spontaneously when the drainage tube is removed.

A fistula of this type can be closed surgically by a local procedure or it can be eliminated along with the extirpation of the chronic abscess cavity, which is the most satisfactory treatment in such a case. If because of age or otherwise the patient's condition does not allow the removal of the diseased portion of the lung, the patient can be saved the annoyance of the fistula by the simple expedient of closing it by sutures. The chest wall is incised through the external fistula opening and sufficient lengths of regenerated rib are removed to expose the surface of the lung in the region of the fistula tract. The tract is excised down to the lung. The opening in the lung is closed with sutures and infolded with another layer. It may be necessary to free extensively the adhesions of the lung in order to obtain sufficient mobility to make an infolding possible. The thoracic incision is closed in layers consisting of muscle, fascia, fat and skin in order to eliminate any dead space which might collect fluid and lead to infection. Catgut should be used for all buried sutures.

Elimination of the fistula by lobectomy or segmental excision is the most effective method of treatment when the condition of the patient permits.

Removal of Foreign Bodies from the Lung

The technic for the removal of foreign bodies lodged in the substance of the lung depends upon the amount of injury to the lung and to some extent upon the kind and size of the object. A standard thoracotomy incision is used in all cases. In the least complicated situation it is necessary merely to extract the foreign body and to close the laceration in the lung after débridement of devitalized tissue, ligation of vessels and suture of any bronchial openings which may be found. In other cases it may be necessary to excise large segments and, if the damage to the lung substance is great or if large vessels have to be ligated, a lobectomy or in extreme cases a pneumonectomy may be necessary. The technics of these procedures have been described elsewhere.

CHAPTER 7

OPERATIONS WITHIN THE MEDIASTINUM

GENERAL PRINCIPLES

Before undertaking an operation which entails an exposure of the structures within the mediastinum, the surgeon should become familiar with the topographic anatomy of the region. He must keep in mind also the mechanics of the thorax and the physiologic principles which must be understood in order to manage successfully any intrathoracic operation. Certain considerations deserve special emphasis.

Effect of Diminished Pulmonary Volume. When it is necessary to work with the lung partially collapsed in order to carry out any procedure within the mediastinum, it is essential for the anesthetist to reinflate the lung at intervals of twenty to thirty minutes in order to insure continuous adequate oxygenation of the blood and also to make full expansion at the end of the operation easier. Elderly patients are particularly sensitive to prolonged diminution of the pulmonary volume during the course of an operation, especially when the opposite pleural cavity has been opened across the mediastinal space. The evidences of disturbance are a fall in blood pressure, sometimes cardiac arrhythmia, and often the development of slight cyanosis. These changes are usually corrected by total reexpansion of the lungs. In certain patients the untoward effects of partial atelectasis are so alarming that the surgeon must work with the lung almost completely expanded at all times or else abandon the operation.

Effect of Stimulation of Heart and Aorta. Another important consideration in mediastinal surgery is the effect of stimulating the heart and aorta. Pressure upon the heart by retractors or the hands of the surgeon and assistant must be avoided at all times. In some patients the heart seems to be unusually irritable and responds immediately to local stimulation by developing extrasystoles or other manifestations of disturbed rhythm such as auricular flutter. In the majority of instances a normal rhythm is resumed as soon as the local pressure is removed. Sometimes, however, especially with auricular flutter, the disturbance may be long continued. In a few such cases it is necessary to abandon the operation if the arrhythmia cannot be controlled by the intra-muscular injection of quinidine or by the use of procaine hydrochloride injected intravenously or within the pericardial sac. Excessive irritability of the heart may be prevented in the great majority of patients by the routine prophylactic use of quinidine one hour before the operation is begun and sometimes also, if it seems necessary, during the course of the operation.

Effect of Stimulation of Cardiac Regulatory Nerves. Disorders of the cardiac function manifested by a drop in the peripheral blood pressure are seen frequently when it is necessary to perform an extensive dissection in the region of the aortic arch, as, for example, during an esophagectomy. Marked arrhythmia may be observed, due probably to a reflex disturbance resulting from stimulation of cardiac regulatory nerves in that region. When this occurs, it may be necessary to interrupt the operation temporarily in order to favor a return to a more normal function. The anesthetist should take advantage of these brief intervals of delay in the progress of the procedure in order to reexpand the lung. The increased oxygenation of the blood which results from this tends to favor a restoration of the heart to a normal rhythm. Several interruptions of this sort may be required before the dissection in the region of the aortic arch can be completed.

Effect of Stimulation of Vagus Nerves. Contrary to the opinion of certain surgeons, there is rarely any demonstrable disturbance as a result of stimu-lating the vagus nerves during the course of any operation within the medi-astinum. The only important effect which might be attributed to such stimulation is an activation of the cough reflex observed in certain suscep-tible patients when the plane of anesthesia is fairly light. Whether this reflex is mediated primarily by way of the vagus nerves is open to debate. How-ever, this tendency is usually overcome promptly by infiltrating the peri-bronchial tissues with a solution of procaine hydrochloride (1 per cent) or by deepening the plane of anesthesia. The so-called "vago-vagal" reflex which is said to occur as a result of handling the vagus nerves within the mediastinum and which is held responsible for a sudden cessation of the heart beat in some patients does not occur even when the nerve is crushed, pulled upon, cut or otherwise traumatized, at least when a patient is under general anesthesia. A careful investigation of cases of cardiac arrest observed during the course of a thoracic operation, whether mediastinal or otherwise, will almost invariably bring to light the fact that the patient had been labor-ing under a state of relative anoxia of the circulating blood for a prolonged period of time. Sudden cardiac arrest occurring during manipulations within the tracheobronchial tree in a conscious patient is another matter and does not apply to the subject under consideration.

Effect of Injury to Structures Within the Mediastinum. RECURRENT LARYNGEAL NERVES. It should be kept in mind that it is possible to cause a paralysis of one or both vocal cords by accidentally injuring the recurrent laryngeal nerves. Because of its greater accessibility the recurrent branch of the left vagus nerve is more vulnerable than the corresponding nerve on the right. This nerve may be injured in dissections beneath or behind the arch of the aorta as well as during mobilization of the upper portion of the esophagus or in the removal of a tumor from the posterior region of the superior mediastinum. It is possible also, under the latter condition, to injure the right recurrent laryngeal nerve. This is especially true in dealing with intrathoracic goiters which have descended into the posterior mediastinal space.

BLOOD VESSELS. It is relatively easy to avoid injury to the pulmonary vessels in the performance of an operation in the mediastinum, but certain other vessels such as the veins of the azygos system and the intercostal, esophageal and bronchial branches of the aorta may be torn. A knowledge of the course of these vessels will aid the surgeon in the control of bleeding resulting from such an accident.

THORACIC DUCT. A structure of great importance in any dissection within the mediastinum is the thoracic duct (Fig. 1). This vessel may be injured at any point along its course, but because of its less sheltered position there, it is frequently encountered in the superior mediastinum at the point where it crosses the left side of the esophagus to assume a position near the trachea along which it ascends into the neck. The serious consequences of leakage of chyle from the injured thoracic duct make it imperative to expose and identify this structure to be certain that it remains intact in every case when the dissection must be performed in the region where it lies. If the duct has been torn, if a portion of it has been excised with a malignant tumor or if there may be doubt as to whether it has been injured or not, it is necessary to ligate it at a point above and below the level of actual or possible injury. In this way the leakage of chyle is avoided. There are usually enough collateral lymphatic vessels to take over the function of the interrupted channel. Ligation of the duct, therefore, is of no consequence, but leakage of chyle leads to the death of the patient in a large percentage of cases.

ESOPHAGUS, TRACHEA, BRONCHI AND LUNGS. Injuries to the esophagus, trachea and bronchi are readily avoided except in the case of adherent or invasive tumors. Injury to the lung during the performance of a mediastinal operation may be the result of excising a portion of this organ with an invasive tumor, but more often it arises from the necessity of freeing pulmonary adhesions to the chest wall or diaphragm in order to gain access to the mediastinum. While it is usually possible to identify and suture any areas where the lung may be traumatized in this manner, the surgeon may not always succeed in preventing a slight leakage of air which will almost certainly give rise to tension pneumothorax after the chest has been closed. Therefore, in any patient where such a probability exists, it is judicious to insert a catheter through an intercostal space so that air may be allowed to escape under a water seal.

DRAINAGE OF MEDIASTINAL ABSCESS; POSTERIOR MEDIASTINOTOMY

An accumulation of pus within the mediastinum usually occupies the posterior portion of the space and is most easily reached by an approach from behind. The operation can as a rule be performed under local anesthesia, but a skilled anesthetist should be at hand in case the pleural cavity is opened. A vertical incision is made not far from the spine at the level where the abscess is most prominent, as depicted in the roentgen films. Short segments of two or three ribs are resected. The rib segments to be removed should extend from the articulation with the transverse process of each corresponding vertebra to the angle of the rib. An aspirating needle is inserted close to the side of the vertebral column and if pus is obtained, the parietal pleura is pushed gently away from the spine until the bulging mediastinal tissues are reached. By spreading cautiously with a pair of blunt scissors, the abscess is entered and the pus is removed with an aspirating apparatus. Soft rubber drains are then inserted. It is usually sufficient to establish drainage on one side of the vertebral column only.

EXCISION OF PRIMARY TUMORS

Inhalation anesthesia with positive pressure through an intratracheal tube is required.

The type of incision used depends upon the location of the tumor and the degree of exposure desired. In the majority of cases a standard thoracotomy incision, placed either high or low depending upon the necessities of the case, provides the best access to mediastinal tumors. The only exception to this generalization is in the case of certain tumors in the anterior portion of the mediastinum, especially if they are small and therefore not easily found, which may be reached best through a sternum-splitting incision. This applies particularly to parathyroid tumors and small thymomas. It is to be noted that substernal goiters can usually be removed through a thyroidectomy incision in the neck.

The majority of mediastinal tumors tend to bulge more into one side of the chest than the other. Advantage should be taken of this fact in choosing the side for the incision. In the case of tumors which seem to arise in the anterior mediastinum it may be necessary to carry the incision as far forward as possible. This can be done best when the incision is made through an intercostal space instead of through the bed of a resected rib, although if the cartilage is removed along with the bony portion, the same result may be obtained with the rib resection technic.

The problem presented by the removal of a mediastinal tumor depends, of course, upon its location, its size and its pathologic characteristics. It is convenient for the purpose of discussion to differentiate between the cystic and the solid types.

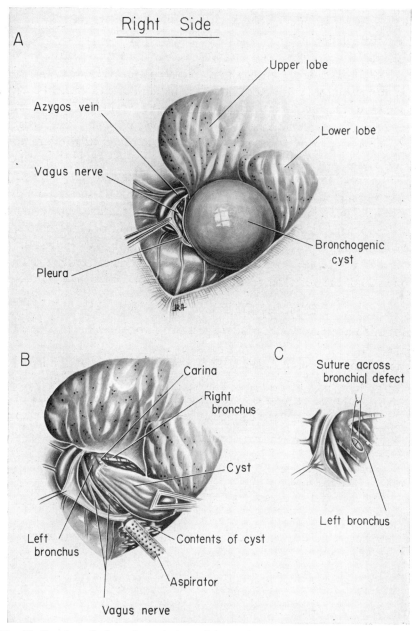

Fig. 90. Excision of a bronchogenic cyst of the mediastinum. *A,* Exposure of the cyst as it lay behind the right main bronchus. *B,* View obtained after emptying the cyst of its mucilaginous contents, showing its attachment to the left main bronchus where it arose, bulging as it developed into the subcarinal area and finally behind the right main bronchus. *C,* Detail of the closure of the defect in the outer layer of the posterior bronchial wall after removal of the cyst.

Cysts of the Mediastinum. The four types of cyst most frequently found in the mediastinum are the simple, the dermoid, the bronchogenic or tracheal, and the enterogenous or esophageal reduplication varieties. As a rule, *simple* or *"clear water"* *cysts* present no problems. They are almost never adherent and can be freed easily once the proper plane of cleavage has been entered. *Dermoid cysts,* on the other hand, are sometimes firmly adherent to the surrounding structures. The fact that they arise in the anterior portion of the mediastinum may make it necessary to free these cysts from the pericardium, the ascending aorta, sometimes from the innominate veins, and often from the structures of the anterior aspect of the hilus of the lung. The phrenic nerve is frequently adherent to such a cyst. Dermoid cysts sometimes become firmly attached to a bronchus and may actually develop a fistulous communication, with ultimate evacuation of some of their contents into the bronchial system. When such a condition is found, measures must be taken to close the bronchus; otherwise it may be necessary to combine a lobectomy with excision of the cyst. The avoidance of accidental injury to pulmonary vessels or important mediastinal organs during the removal of an adherent dermoid cyst depends upon finding a safe plane of cleavage for the dissection. This is done by working continuously against the cyst wall as the procedure progresses and sometimes penetrating deeper and deeper layers of the pericystic tissues until the proper plane is reached.

The technical problem presented by the *bronchogenic* and *enterogenous cysts* varies greatly from case to case, depending upon the location of the tumor and the presence or absence of infection. When such a cyst lies free in the mediastinum, no special difficulty is encountered. When the cyst is adjacent to or actually a part of the wall of the trachea, a bronchus or the esophagus, its removal may present a problem which taxes the ingenuity and skill of the surgeon (Fig. 90). This is true particularly when a complicating infection has developed within the cyst. This occurrence results from the intimate adherence of certain of these cysts to the wall of the organ against which they lie. The inflammatory process makes it almost impossible in some instances to find a safe plane of cleavage for the dissection. If this difficulty promises to lead to accidental perforation of important vessels or the bronchus, trachea or esophagus, it is usually advisable to open the cyst, aspirate its contents, and then, with the finger inside as a guide, to complete the dissection, often removing the cyst wall in pieces. Sometimes as a result of complicating infection there is a fistulous communication between one of these cysts and the bronchus or esophagus. The opening is usually small, however, and may be closed with a few interrupted fine sutures. The closure should always be reinforced with a flap of the adjacent mediastinal pleura sutured over it to make a seal. If it is large, the opening may be closed with a pleural flap alone. The sutures must be placed close together to prevent leakage.

Congenital cysts of the type under discussion sometimes develop within the wall of the tubular organ in which they arise. When this occurs, although the cyst expands peripherally into the surrounding mediastinal tissues in an eccentric manner and ultimately appears merely to lie beside the organ to which it is attached, it is actually an integral part of its wall. In this small area of attachment, the wall of the trachea, bronchus or esophagus is incomplete and consists merely of the mucous membrane to the outside of which a corresponding small surface of the cyst wall is attached (Fig. 90, C). In the removal of such a cyst this fact must be kept in mind and if possible the integrity of the mucosa should be preserved by peeling the cyst wall from it. If the cyst is one which has been infected, this may be impossible. In any event, if the mucous membrane is opened, a careful closure must be made. In the esophagus it is relatively easy to accomplish this with a layer of sutures in the mucosa and an outer layer in the muscular coat for reinforcement. In the trachea or bronchus, however, it may be difficult or impossible to secure a tight closure because of the rigidity of these organs. Recourse must then be had to other measures. In the case of the trachea, after drawing the edges of the defect together as completely as possible with a single layer of sutures, the adjacent wall of the esophagus can be sutured over the tracheal defect with two longitudinal layers of delicate sutures. The two organs will then become adherent and air leakage from the trachea is prevented. Sometimes it is possible to accomplish the same result with a flap of the mediastinal pleura which can be turned in over the defect. The latter method is almost always the only one available to reinforce a bronchial opening, although in some locations an adjacent portion of one of the lobes of the lung can be utilized.

Solid Tumors of the Mediastinum. With solid tumors of the mediastinum the technical problem of removal depends upon whether they are benign or malignant. Usually a benign solid tumor has little or no tendency to become adherent, and once it has been exposed by the incision of the overlying pleura, it can be removed with relative ease (Fig. 91). The blood supply to these tumors is sometimes extensive, but it comes from mediastinal vessels which can be controlled readily by ligatures. These tumors may reach an enormous size before they are discovered. Large tumors of this sort acquire a considerable weight which may lead to an unexpected complication when the chest is opened. As soon as the pleural space is exposed to the atmospheric pressure, the heavy tumor falls suddenly into the mediastinum. This may lead to alarming disturbances of the heart action with a drop in blood pressure almost to the point of circulatory collapse. However, if the surgeon is alert to this possibility, he will waste no time in enlarging the incision completely to obtain a wide exposure. It is then necessary merely to grasp the tumor with the hand or with a large tenaculum and exert traction upon it in order to relieve the mediastinal structures of its weight. The tumor must be supported in this way throughout the course of the dissection and until it can be removed from the chest in order to prevent a recurrence of the circulatory disturbance.

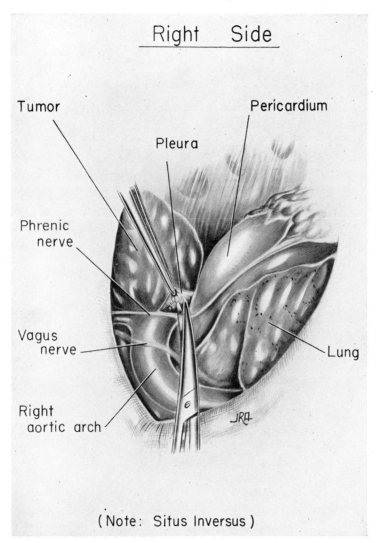

Right   Side

Tumor   Pericardium

Pleura

Phrenic
   nerve

Vagus
   nerve   Lung

Right
   aortic arch

(Note: Situs Inversus)

Fig. 91. Removal of a solid tumor of the mediastinum. The view is of the right thoracic cavity with exposure of the right side of the mediastinal structures in a patient with complete situs inversus. The apex of the heart, the aortic arch and the descending aorta are shown. The right recurrent laryngeal nerve (not shown) passes beneath the aortic arch. The start of the dissection for the removal of the tumor is shown.

A special difficulty is sometimes encountered in the removal of the neurogenic fibromas which are found in the costovertebral gutter where they arise from the fibers of the intercostal or sympathetic nerves. Such tumors are not, strictly speaking, mediastinal, although for the purpose of simplicity they are usually grouped under the general heading of mediastinal tumors. The exposure of these chest wall lesions may be made easily through a standard thoracotomy incision. Their removal usually presents little difficulty, but in some instances they tend to send projections along the course of the nerve from which they arise into the intercostal space or even through the corresponding intervertebral foramen. When this occurs it is sometimes necessary to leave some of the tumor behind to be removed by a spinal approach posteriorly at a later time if symptoms arise. In the apex of the chest they may present difficulties from local extension behind the great vessels at the base of the neck.

Malignant solid tumors of the mediastinum may be removed only if local invasion has not yet occurred or become extensive. The operability of such a tumor depends upon the extent of adherence or actual invasion of vital structures which cannot be sacrificed by en masse excision of the growth. The surgical problem, of course, varies from case to case.

A special difficulty is presented by certain vascular tumors which, though benign, envelop and surround the structures of the mediastinum to such an extent that they cannot be removed completely. They sometimes extend from the mediastinum into the neck so that a separate cervical approach is necessary if the entire growth is to be removed. These tumors often arise from the lymphatic vessels and are related to the so-called "cystic hygromas" of the neck. Sometimes, however, they contain blood and are therefore hemangiomas. A communication with a large vein, such as the azygos or the innominate, may be found.

The after-care following the removal of a mediastinal tumor does not differ from that of any post-thoracotomy patient.

THYMECTOMY

The attempt to alleviate the severity of symptoms in a patient with myasthenia gravis is the most frequent indication for the removal of the thymus gland. Certain details of the management of the case which are of particular importance in this disease should be mentioned. Every effort should be made to shorten the length of time during which the patient must be under the influence of the anesthetic agent. This is accomplished in part by using cyclopropane, from which the recovery of consciousness is rapid, and in part by an expeditious conduct of the operation. There is evidence also that cyclopropane does not have as lasting an effect on the myoneural mechanism as ether seems to exert. Furthermore, it is of great importance to have the dosage of prostigmine properly adjusted to the needs of the individual patient and to continue the administration of this drug intravenously during the course of the operation. In patients with myasthenia gravis, therefore, it is expedient to have two intravenous infusions running simultaneously in different veins. One is to be used for the prostigmine in dilute solution and the other is for the transfusion of blood as indicated by the needs of the patient.

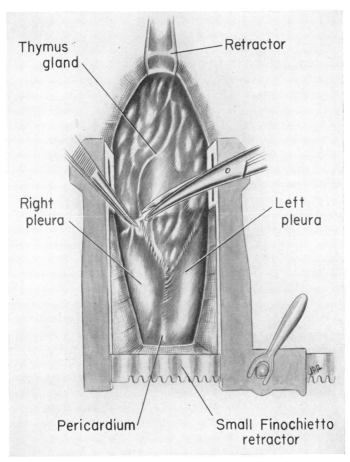

Fig. 92. Exposure of the thymus gland for thymectomy. View of the anterior mediastinum obtained through a median sternotomy incision with transection of the gladiolar portion at the level of the fourth intercostal space. *Note:* The retractor should be of small size.

Technic. The technic of the sternum-splitting incision, which gives the best exposure for the excision of the thymus gland, has already been described in Chapter 3. The thymus lies immediately beneath a thin layer of areolar tissue and is recognized by its characteristic pink color. It consists of two lobes or halves which are joined in the middle and extend in a bilateral fashion downward over the pericardium and upward into the base of the neck (Fig. 92). Its principal blood supply enters from each side as branches of the internal mammary vessels. However, there are other small vessels which must be ligated as well, some in relation to the upper poles and some from the pericardial region. The lateral lobes often extend deeply into the mediastinum around the ascending aorta. Here they must be separated from the mediastinal reflection of each pleural sac. The dissection must often be carried as far posteriorly as the phrenic nerves. As the gland is freed, search should be made for the two veins which lead away from its posterior surface to enter the left innominate vein. There is sometimes only a single thymic

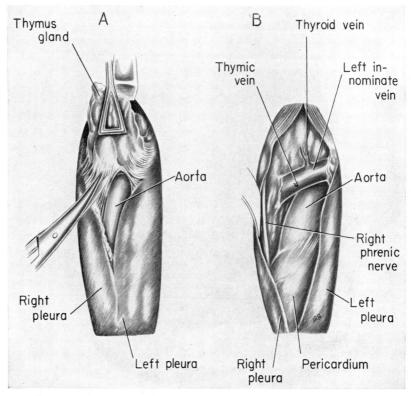

Fig. 93. Thymectomy: Stages in the removal of the thymus gland. *A*, Dissection of the inferior portion of the gland. *B*, Structures observed after the gland has been removed.

vein (Fig. 93, *B*). The gland is usually not adherent and if the locations of the vessels are anticipated so that they can be ligated quickly, very little time is consumed in its removal.

If either pleural sac has been opened inadvertently during the dissection, one need only have the anesthetist maintain full expansion of the lung during the closure of the incision to avoid any subsequent respiratory embarrassment.

The after-care is the same as that of any post-thoracotomy patient, with particular emphasis upon maintaining a correct level of prostigmine at all times. Intimate cooperation with the internist is of particular importance.

OPERATIONS ON THE PERICARDIUM AND PERICARDIAL CAVITY

Pericardial Paracentesis

Aspiration of the pericardial sac may be indicated either to obtain fluid for diagnostic purposes or as a method of treatment to overcome the effects of cardiac tamponade resulting from the extravasation of blood or from excessive effusion of fluid of an inflammatory character. The same type of apparatus used in the performance of thoracentesis is recommended. There are two satisfactory approaches. One is to insert the needle directly into the chest through the fourth or fifth intercostal space close to the left side of the sternum. At this point there is usually no pleural reflexion over the pericardium, so that injury of the lung is avoided. The operator must keep in mind the course of the internal mammary vessels. Another approach is through the upper abdominal wall at the junction of the left costochondrium with the left side of the xiphoid process. The needle is inserted at the proper angle and pushed upward and to the left in an oblique direction, penetrating the subpericardial portion of the diaphragm and the inferior reflexion of the pericardial sac. The choice between the two methods rests with the individual operator. The direct intercostal approach is simple but perhaps more likely to be attended by accidents than the paraxiphoid method.

Pericardiostomy for Drainage of the Pericardial Cavity

The operation comprises almost wholly the making of an incision through the chest wall to expose the pericardium for drainage. The previously described incision involving the excision of the left fifth costal cartilage usually provides adequate drainage (Chap. 3, Fig. 53). In opening the pericardium caution must be exerted to avoid injury to the anterior coronary vessels. Drainage may be provided by inserting soft rubber tubes (such as the Penrose drain) which are held in place by sutures to the skin edges. If a prolonged period of drainage is indicated, the edges of the pericardial opening can be sutured either to the fascia or to the edges of the skin incision.

No particular problem of after-care need be anticipated unless an opening has been made accidentally in either pleural sac. In that event empyema or pyopneumothorax may have to be dealt with as the occasion demands. Usually the only important decision required is to know how long drains are to be left in place. This depends upon the circumstances of each case.

Pericardiectomy for Constrictive Pericarditis

Intratracheal inhalation anesthesia is used because of the possibility that one or both pleural cavities may be opened either accidentally or intentionally during the course of the operation. The accidental opening of the pleural sacs is of no importance if it is recognized so that the anesthetist may keep the lungs properly expanded. The deliberate opening of one or both pleural cavities may be required in some patients either to aspirate an effusion of fluid in order to increase the pulmonary volume or, on the left side occasionally, to assist in the enlargement of the incision.

Improvements in diagnostic methods have made it possible in recent years to predict with some accuracy whether there is a preponderance of constriction of the heart over the right or the left side. This may be of some importance in planning the thoracotomy incision for the exposure of the pericardium and especially in deciding how far to carry the denudation over the chambers of the heart. Experience has demonstrated that in the majority of instances, no matter which side seems to be most constricted, the *classical anterior approach* described in Chapter 3 is adequate. If the right ventricle and right auriculoventricular groove need extensive liberation, a larger than usual segment of the sternum can be excised. If, on the other hand, the left ventricle and the left side of the auriculoventricular groove need special attention, the same incision can be used if the ribs are divided somewhat further to the left than usual and if the inferior end of the incision is enlarged laterally. As an alternative the *sternum-splitting incision* may be used with the advantages that less deformity is produced and postoperative paradoxical motion of the precordial area of the chest wall is avoided. The exposure provided by this means is somewhat greater over the right side of the heart than the left, but adequate denudation of both sides is accomplished readily. A larger experience with its use may demonstrate that this approach is superior to the older method, at least in the management of the average case.

Under unusual circumstances, especially when the classical anterior incision has already been used unsuccessfully, it may be necessary to use a *left transpleural approach*. A long anterolateral intercostal incision is made through the fourth intercostal space. This gives good access to the left posterior aspect of the pericardium provided it is carried as far forward as the sternum. When employed for a secondary operation following the original use of the usual anterior approach, the fact that the cartilages have already been removed makes a wide anterior separation of the ribs possible. If used as the primary incision, it may be necessary to enlarge it by cutting the fourth and fifth costal cartilages close to the sternum. It is wise, when this is done, to ligate and divide the internal mammary vessels at the upper and lower limits of the operative field.

Technic of Pericardiectomy. The principal secret of success in the denudation of the heart for constrictive pericarditis is to find the correct plane of cleavage in which to carry the dissection between the heart and the membrane which is to be removed (Fig. 94). Using a sharp knife, the incision into the pericardium is started at some convenient place on the anterior surface, usually

over the left ventricle. Often one or two possible planes for dissection may
be found, but none is correct until as the incision is deepened cautiously,
the heart muscle begins to bulge between its edges at each systole. As soon
as this is observed, the edges of the pericardium are grasped with small
hemostatic forceps and the incision is enlarged. This is sometimes done easily
with the scissors. At other times the heart muscle may be so densely adherent
that a slow and tedious dissection is required. In some cases the pericardium
is glued to the heart everywhere. In others, however, there may be rela-

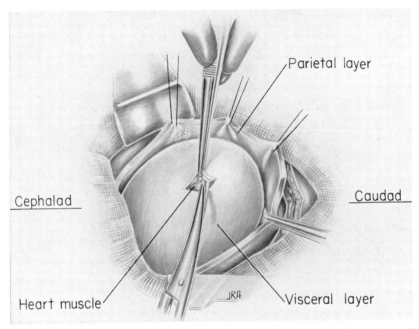

Fig. 94. Pericardiectomy. The operation in this patient was performed through a median
sternotomy incision extending from the xiphoid attachment to the level of transection opposite the second intercostal spaces. In the drawing the patient's head lies to the left and his
feet to the right. In this case the visceral and parietal layers, though much thickened, were
not adherent to each other. The visceral layer was thickened and densely adherent to the
myocardium. The beginning of the separation of the visceral layer from the heart in the
correct planes of cleavage is shown.

tively free areas which make the operation much easier. At times there is a
large amount of calcium deposit which may present technical difficulties.
Sometimes the calcium is wholly or partly amorphous, consisting of a soft
chalky or putty-like substance lying between the heart muscle and the pericardium. At other times it is so firm that it must be cut with a bone shears.
It usually makes up a part of the layer which is being removed. Occasionally
in certain areas the calcium is so intimately adherent to the epicardium that
a thin shell of it must be left behind because of the danger of injuring the
muscle if a deeper dissection is attempted. The calcium deposit is often par-

ticularly dense over the auriculoventricular groove where in some cases it forms a firm constricting ring. Merely dividing this annular band will frequently permit a very noticeable improvement in the filling of the ventricles. As much of the thickened or calcified pericardium as possible should be excised from this area.

A difficulty which may be troublesome in some patients is an unusually irritable condition of the heart muscle which responds to touching or to the gentle pressure which is necessary during the dissection by developing extrasystoles. This tendency may be overcome to some extent by the topical application of procaine hydrochloride solution (2 per cent) applied with a large flat pledget of cotton or gauze which has been soaked in the solution.

If the heart muscle should be injured during the process of freeing an unusually adherent area, the laceration may be closed with sutures of fine silk. The myocardium is often unusually fragile in chronic pericarditis so that it cannot be relied upon to hold sutures well. When such is the case, it may be necessary to suture a small flap of the pericardium back against the injured area to provide additional reinforcement. Special pains should be taken to avoid injury to the coronary vessels.

The extent of denudation which should be carried out varies to some extent, depending upon how much of the heart is affected, but in general it is advisable to perform as wide an excision of the adherent pericardium as possible. In the average case this should include the surface of the right ventricle, the auriculoventricular groove from right to left, the left ventricle including the apex, and the entire left side to a point behind the left phrenic nerve, often as far back as the entrance of the left inferior pulmonary vein. As the left side is freed, the corresponding phrenic nerve is retracted along with the overlying pleural reflection. If necessary the pleura may be incised to gain greater access to the posterolateral aspect of the pericardium on that side. Inflation of the lung is maintained by the anesthetist. It is usually necessary also to reflect the right pleural membrane over the lateral aspect of the right ventricle.

Sometimes there is oozing of blood from the surface of the heart which cannot be controlled completely. This leads to a large effusion of serosanguineous fluid, the effects of which may be prevented by leaving a small catheter in the lower part of the mediastinum to be brought out through the lateral end of the incision. An alternative method of preventing the accumulation of such an effusion about the heart is to make an intercommunicating opening between the mediastinal space around the heart and the left pleural cavity by incising the mediastinal pleural reflection. The fluid will then accumulate in the left hemithorax away from the heart and drainage of the mediastinum to the exterior can be avoided. If the amount of effusion is excessive, it is removed by thoracentesis.

After-care. The after-care of patients who have had a pericardiectomy for constrictive pericarditis demands extraordinary vigilance to protect the heart from any unusual strain which might result from the complications sometimes encountered after thoracotomy. It is important to avoid the accumulation of a large effusion of fluid around the heart itself which tends, when excessive, to reproduce the effects of cardiac tamponade. This occurrence is suggested by the development of the usual symptoms of compression and also by a bulging of the precordial region. Prompt aspiration with a needle and syringe is indicated. As already mentioned, making an opening in the left pleural sac before closure of the incision, so that the fluid which forms around the heart will pass into the pleural cavity, may prevent serious difficulty.

Embarrassment of the respirations by pleural effusions should be prevented by thoracentesis. The patient should be encouraged to cough and raise secretions to prevent pulmonary atelectasis. If he is unable to do so, aspiration should be provided either through a catheter inserted directly into the pharynx and trachea or by means of a bronchoscope. These manipulations may be carried out with the patient in bed in the semisitting position.

The possible embarrassment of the respirations caused by paradoxical motion of the chest where the rib cartilages and a section of the sternum are lacking should be avoided by means of a firm dressing, consisting preferably of a thin layer of gauze covered by a limited anterior plaster shell or plaque to give support. This is necessary only during the first few days after operation. The use of a median sternotomy incision makes it possible to avoid this complication.

Supportive medication for the heart should be provided as indicated.

Excision of Cysts and Diverticula of the Pericardium

The diagnosis of pericardial cyst or diverticulum can rarely be established definitely before the operation. These cysts usually bulge laterally on the side from which they arise and cannot often be distinguished by roentgen examination from primary mediastinal tumors or sometimes from hernias of the sinus of Morgagni, although the latter may be discovered in many cases by roentgen ray studies of the gastrointestinal tract. As for any mass arising in the anterior mediastinum, a long intercostal incision extending anteriorly as far as the internal mammary vessels usually provides sufficient exposure. The actual removal of a cyst or diverticulum of the pericardium is a simple matter which does not involve any particular technical problems and demands no detailed description.

CARDIAC RESUSCITATION

Before the subject of cardiac surgery is begun, it is convenient to present at this point a discussion of the treatment of cardiac arrest. Sudden cessation of the heart beat may occur as a complication of any operative procedure, whether thoracic or otherwise. It has been observed occasionally during the induction or the excitement stage of anesthesia even before the operation is begun. No situation throughout the entire field of surgery demands more prompt and effective treatment. The loss of even a few minutes of time may mean the death of the patient. The surgeon, the anesthetist and all other members of the operative team must know beforehand what is to be done in such an emergency and must carry out the necessary procedures in a calm and deliberate manner. Excitement at such a time may diminish or even abolish the effectiveness of the team with disastrous consequences.

Causes of Cardiac Arrest. Although the important indications for the management of such an accident are obvious, it is helpful in a given case to have at least some knowledge of what may have been the inciting cause of its occurrence. Various factors may be involved. Hypoxia is of enormous importance, and may account for some of the cases which develop early in the course of an operation although the majority of these are due to ventricular fibrillation. Usually the cardiac arrest which results from hypoxia occurs during the course of the operation, often near its termination. Under these conditions it is due apparently to the cumulative effects of a relative degree of anoxia prolonged over a period of one or more hours. The use of certain anesthetic agents such as cyclopropane, a potential myocardial irritant, seems to be complicated by sudden cessation of the heart beat more frequently than the employment of others such as ether.

Other important controllable aspects of the case such as the volume of the circulating blood must be considered. Excessive blood loss without adequate replacement during the course of the operation is a frequent inciting cause. This situation can be avoided usually if the technical difficulties of the procedure have been foreseen and if sufficient compatible blood has been prepared. The necessity for efficient control of the rate of administration of the blood to compensate for that being lost during the operation is obvious.

Disturbances of cardiac rhythm due to underlying myocardial disease can frequently be anticipated if proper preoperative study of the patient has been made. Although not always successful in preventing major accidents, the prophylactic preoperative administration of quinidine or digitalis as the indications may suggest may prevent serious disturbances of rhythm in many patients.

It must not be forgotten also that sudden cardiac arrest may be the result of a massive coronary occlusion with irreversible changes.

Treatment of Cardiac Arrest. In the treatment of cardiac arrest the two indispensable indications are to maintain the circulation of the blood by effective manipulation of the heart and to bring about the exchange of oxygen and carbon dioxide through the lungs by continuous artificial respiration. A third aspect of the treatment which may have to be added to the others is to overcome the disturbed rhythm of the heart, usually ventricular fibrillation, which may have been the cause of the cessation of heart beat or which may be the type of cardiac activity developed as the heart resumes independent action. Ten cc. of 1 per cent aqueous solution of procaine hydrochloride injected intravenously may be employed to desensitize the myocardium in certain instances.

TECHNIC OF CARDIAC MASSAGE. Various methods of cardiac massage have been advocated, but in complete cardiac arrest only one is actually successful in the maintenance of a sufficient circulation of the blood. This consists in the steady forceful squeezing of the ventricles of the heart by the surgeon's hand. This cannot be done adequately by introducing one or two fingers through a hastily made intercostal incision or by pressing against the heart beneath the diaphragm through an abdominal incision. The whole hand must be introduced into the left thoracic cavity either through an adequate thoracic incision or, if the abdomen is already open, through an incision made in the left leaf of the diaphragm. The heart is then grasped and compressed, as the rubber bulb of a syringe is squeezed. This manipulation expels the blood from the ventricles. The pressure of the hand is then relaxed and the heart chambers will be observed to fill again, whereupon the ventricles are forcefully squeezed once more. By alternately squeezing and releasing the ventricles, at the rate of approximately 40 times per minute, a satisfactory circulation of blood can be maintained for a prolonged period of time. If a faster rate of squeezing the heart is adopted, the heart does not fill sufficiently between each compression and the circulation of blood is therefore inadequate. Likewise if a slower rate of squeezing is used, the efficiency of the propulsion of the blood is not so great.

From time to time during this procedure the hand should be removed momentarily to observe any tendency of the heart to start spontaneous contractions. If contractions occur, the heart should be given an opportunity to pick up its activity again. Frequently, however, the first few beats are weak and irregular and more often than not the heart will stop beating in a few moments. The manual control of the circulation is then resumed until spontaneous beats are observed again. This procedure is continued until the heart resumes its normal activity or until it becomes obvious that the patient is dead.

MAINTENANCE OF OXYGENATION. The second essential part of the treatment of cardiac arrest is the maintenance of adequate oxygenation by mechanical means. This is done easily by alternate compression and relaxation of the oxygen-filled rubber bag of an anesthesia machine with the usual equipment in the closed system for the absorption of carbon dioxide. This maneuver can be begun instantly and effectively when an intratracheal tube is being used for the administration of the anesthetic agent. Otherwise such a tube may be inserted if one is at hand and the anesthetist is skilled in its introduction. However, no more than a brief moment should be devoted to the attempt to insert a tube because of the urgent haste required to obtain effective oxygenation of the blood which is already being circulated by the hand of the surgeon. If an intratracheal tube is not already in place and if such a tube cannot be inserted with dispatch, resort must be made to the use of a tightly fitting face mask with an ordinary mouth airway in place in order to maintain a closed system with which to inflate the lungs. It is in a time such as this that the employment of a skilled anesthetist equipped with the knowledge and experience required to handle such an emergency may be instrumental in saving the life of the patient.

STIMULATION OF HEART MUSCLE. Once the circulation of blood has been resumed by manipulation of the heart and with the oxygenation of the blood maintained by artificial means, consideration may be given to the employment of methods to stimulate the heart muscle to resume its contractions or to induce a normal rhythm if ventricular fibrillation should begin. The only method likely to be available in the average operating room is the injection of adrenalin or neosynephrin solution into the heart. It is important, however, to avoid the use of a concentrated solution. One or 2 cc. of adrenalin solution (1 to 10,000 in saline) is safer than the same or even smaller volume of a 1 to 1000 solution. This should be introduced into the chamber of the right ventricle through a needle of small caliber. Sometimes it is helpful, especially if irregular contractions of the heart occur, to add to this solution 9 cc. of procaine hydrochloride solution (1 per cent) to desensitize the irritable myocardium. The stimulating effect of the adrenalin may induce contractions of the heart and as these are felt by the surgeon during his manipulation of the heart, he should begin the alternate interruption and resumption of manual compression until the heart takes up its regular rhythm again.

If the proper electrodes should be available to stimulate the heart electrically, the conversion of ventricular fibrillation into a normal rhythm can be accomplished with reasonable certainty. Until such equipment becomes available for use in every operating room where this emergency may be encountered, the method remains inapplicable in the vast majority of cases.

Criteria for Postponement of Operation. Once the heart has been resuscitated and the normal propulsion of the blood has thereby been resumed, the surgeon must use his judgment as to the advisability of continuing or interrupting the operation. Under certain circumstances, as when the esophagus is partially resected or when the circulation of a lung is interrupted by ligation of the pulmonary artery, there is no choice but to proceed. On the other hand, whenever the operative procedure has not been carried too far before the accident occurs, it is probably wise, if a long operation is contemplated, to close the incision and postpone the completion of the surgical intervention until another day.

OPERATIONS ON THE HEART

There is no branch of thoracic surgery which is more unsettled at the present time than that of the heart. New technics are being tried and older methods are being modified in an effort to overcome the crippling effects of certain cardiac disorders. With a few outstanding exceptions these efforts have been relatively unsuccessful or at least disappointing. Some progress has been made, however, and as more effort is applied to these problems, there is reason to believe that in the not too distant future a significant measure of success may be obtained. No useful purpose would be accomplished by an effort to describe and illustrate all of the operations which have been proposed or tried; therefore, only those which appear to have an established value will be described. Those whose value remains uncertain or whose technic is still in the early phase of development will merely be mentioned.

Operations for Congenital Disorders of the Heart

Established Procedures. No operations on the heart itself for the relief of congenital anomalies have yet been devised which can fairly be considered as established procedures. Those which have been attempted will be mentioned below. For pulmonic stenosis (Tetralogy of Fallot type), however, much relief may be obtained by creating an extracardiac shunt by means of anastomosis between the pulmonary artery of one lung and the aorta or one of its major branches. This method is described in the section dealing with operations on the major vessels (see p. 209).

Unestablished Procedures. VALVULOTOMY FOR PULMONIC STENOSIS. This procedure was attempted unsuccessfully before the principle of the extracardiac shunt between the aorta or one of its branches and the pulmonary artery was developed. Efforts are being made to revive it, however, with some promise of success in favorable cases.

CLOSURE OF SEPTAL DEFECTS. Progress has been made towards the development of a technic for the closure of a patent interventricular septum by means of sutures passed through the heart in the septal plane. Several patients have been operated upon and the procedure gives promise of becoming a useful one under favorable circumstances which remain to be defined.

Operations for Acquired Disorders of the Heart

Established Procedures. In this category it cannot be said that any procedure yet devised has acquired an established place in the treatment of diseases of the heart. On the other hand, a large amount of experimental work has been done and some progress has been made, especially in the field of improving the vascularity of the heart muscle and, more recently, in the management of mitral stenosis by valvulotomy.

Unestablished Procedures. Some of the procedures used more or less experimentally to date are mentioned in the following pages. They may be arranged in two groups.

OPERATIONS TO IMPROVE VASCULARITY OF THE MYOCARDIUM. In the first group are those operations intended to improve the vascularity of the myocardium after the development of insufficiency of the coronary artery circulation.

INTRAPERICARDIAL POUDRAGE. The method which consists of abrading the epicardium, followed by the application of powdered asbestos, seems to bring about a limited collateral circulation or to increase that already being developed between the branches of the coronary arteries.

FLAP GRAFTS TO THE EPICARDIUM. Equivocal results have been reported from attempts to improve the vascularity of the heart muscle by suturing pedicled flaps of omentum or skeletal muscle to its surface.

LIGATION OF THE CORONARY VEINS. In experimental animals which have had one of the coronary arteries occluded by ligature, an improvement in the circulation in the heart muscle has been reported as a result of ligation of the coronary veins. A limited trial has been made in human beings.

CARDIAC NEURECTOMY. Interruption of the sympathetic nerve fibers at the base of the aorta and around the origin of the left coronary artery has been tried sometimes in conjunction with ligation of the coronary veins.

DIRECT ANASTOMOSIS OF BLOOD VESSELS. A few attempts made to direct blood from a systemic artery such as the internal mammary by anastomosis with a coronary artery have been reported. Attempts have been made also to use an arterial graft between the aorta and the coronary sinus.

OPERATIONS TO OVERCOME HYPERTENSION IN THE PULMONARY CIRCUIT. In the second group are operations intended to overcome hypertension in the pulmonary circuit produced by stenosis of the mitral valve.

VALVULOTOMY. For many years sporadic attempts have been made to enlarge the constricted orifice in mitral stenosis by intracardiac manipulation. The idea of dilating the valve with a finger was soon abandoned. Efforts to incise or actually to excise a portion of the stenotic valve were at first unsuccessful, largely because of the creation of an insurmountable burden for the heart in the form of mitral regurgitation. Recent revivals of this method show more promise as new instruments and an approach through the auricle instead of the ventricle are being tried. The procedure is not yet on a sound basis either from the standpoint of the perfection of its technic or from the aspect of its effects upon the mechanics of the circulation. The regurgitation which usually results from the excision of a portion of the stenotic valve cannot as yet be adequately controlled and may produce a serious load upon the heart muscle. Valvulotomy has been advocated chiefly in mitral stenosis, but a few patients with aortic stenosis have been treated by this method as well. With few exceptions the operative mortality thus far has been prohibitive.

CREATION OF AN INTERAURICULAR SEPTAL DEFECT IN MITRAL STENOSIS. The knowledge that those patients with mitral stenosis who have a congenital interauricular septal defect do not develop attacks of pulmonary edema because of the relief from hypertension in the pulmonary circuit which the intracardiac shunt provides, has led certain surgeons to attempt to create such a defect by surgical means. The procedure appears to be a relatively hazardous one and the results in the very few patients on whom the operation has been tried are still uncertain.

CREATION OF AN EXTRACARDIAC SHUNT TO RELIEVE THE PULMONARY CONGESTION OF MITRAL STENOSIS. The relief of congestion in the hypertensive pulmonary circulation has been accomplished by performing an anastomosis between the cardiac end of the divided superior segment branch of the right inferior pulmonary vein and the cardiac end of the azygos vein after division. This is a procedure which can be carried out with relative ease and greater safety than the intracardiac manipulations. It has produced striking amelioration of symptoms in a few patients and perhaps should be given further trial.

Although this operation does not involve a direct attack upon the heart itself, it is described at this point because it has nothing to do with the surgery of the great vessels to be considered subsequently. A brief description of the technic follows.

A standard thoracotomy incision is made on the right side. The pleural cavity is opened through the sixth intercostal space (or through the bed of the sixth rib if the rib resection technic is adopted). The lung is held forward by the hand of the first assistant and the pleura is reflected from the inferior pulmonary vein. The superior segment branch of this vein is identified and freed from the surrounding areolar tissue by sharp and blunt dissection. Any small tributaries which may be found must be ligated with fine silk and divided. The vein is followed upward into the lung as far as its origin where two or three fairly large tributaries join beneath and slightly anterior to the lower portion of the superior segment bronchus. The vein is not divided until the freeing of the azygos vein has been accomplished (Fig. 95).

The mediastinal pleura and retropleural fascia over the azygos vein are incised longitudinally. The azygos vein is freed from a point 2 or 3 cm. below the level opposite the superior segmental vein upward as far as its junction with the highest intercostal vein. In freeing the azygos it is usually necessary to ligate and divide a large number of its tributaries. These include the accessory hemiazygos, sometimes the hemiazygos, most of the right intercostal veins above the level of transection of the azygos vein, and many small esophageal and other mediastinal branches. Occasionally, in order to gain sufficient length for the performance of the anastomosis, it may be necessary to divide the right highest intercostal vein, but the right bronchial vein should be preserved.

A bulldog clamp is placed across the azygos vein at the upper limit of the

9

dissection and the vein is ligated and divided at the lower limit approximately 2 cm. below the level of the pulmonary vein.

A Blakemore-Lord vitallium tube having a diameter of proper size to permit cuffing back the azygos vein upon it is then applied to the upper or cardiac end of the azygos vein. The average size is 4 mm., occasionally 3 mm. The end of the azygos vein is passed through the tube and turned back to the ferrule near the flange where it is tied with heavy silk.

A short clamp ("bulldog type") is applied to the superior segment vein as close as possible to its junction with the basal segment branches of the inferior pulmonary vein. A hemostatic forceps is then applied as far into the

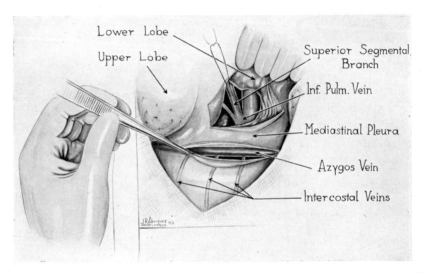

Fig. 95. Operation for the relief of pulmonary hypertension due to mitral stenosis by creating an anastomosis between the superior segmental branch of the right inferior pulmonary vein and the azygos vein. Exposure of the two veins.

lung as necessary to avoid sacrificing any of its length, and the vein is cut close to the hemostat. A suture ligature of heavy silk is used to tie the pulmonary end of the vein (Fig. 96, *A*).

Three strands of arterial silk suture material are passed through the end of the pulmonary vein at equidistant points. Short hemostatic forceps are fastened to these strands about 2 inches from the end of the vein. A curved hemostat attached to the flange of the tube is used to hold the end of the azygos vein and direct it into the open end of the pulmonary vein which is drawn over it by exerting traction on the three strands of silk. The pulmonary vein is drawn up over the proximal ferrule on the tube where it is held with a silk tie. A second ligature is then applied to hold the veins together close to the tip of the tube (Fig. 96, *B*).

The bulldog clamp is removed from the azygos vein first, and then that from the pulmonary vein. In a moment the blood can be observed flowing briskly from the high pressure area in the pulmonary vein to the low pressure

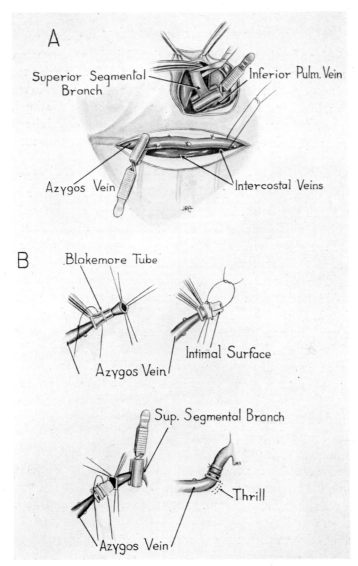

Fig. 96. Anastomosis between the pulmonary vein and the azygos vein; details of technic. A, The superior segmental branch of the right inferior pulmonary vein is about to be severed to make ready for the anastomosis. The level of transection of the azygos vein is indicated by the silk ligature passed around it ready for tying. B, Details of the anastomosis by the Blakemore-Lord vitallium tube method.

region in the azygos vein. Palpation of the latter beyond the anastomosis reveals the presence of a soft thrill.

A small incision is made in a lower intercostal space posteriorly and a large catheter is inserted for drainage. The lung is then expanded fully and the chest wall is closed.

Operations for Cardiac Injury

The majority of patients who sustain serious injuries to the heart and great vessels die so promptly of hemorrhage or the effects of cardiac tamponade that there is no opportunity for the surgeon to apply his skill in an attempt to save them. In a few cases of cardiac injury, however, the opening is so small that leakage is not excessive or there is a foreign body or missile which remains to plug the hole temporarily. Under such circumstances surgery may be applied.

Cardiorrhaphy for Penetrating Wounds of the Heart. The approach to the heart already described (Chap. 3) is used. It consists in making a transverse incision through the fourth intercostal space, supplemented occasionally by transection of the adjacent cartilages. As soon as the pericardium has been opened and the blood within it evacuated, the surgeon should be prepared to deal with a fresh spurt of bleeding from the heart wound. The index finger should be laid over the laceration to check the escape of blood, taking care to avoid inserting the finger through the opening because of the danger of enlarging it. A strand of heavy silk should be passed through the apex of the left ventricle and held by an assistant so as to steady the heart for the placing of the sutures. The details of management of a penetrating wound vary to some extent depending upon whether it is in the auricle or the ventricle. In the case of a wound of the ventricle, the silk sutures threaded on fine needles and held in readiness during the early phase of the operation are now used to close the opening. As each suture is passed it may either be held in such a way as to approximate the wound edges until all the others have been inserted or it may be tied by an assistant, the surgeon keeping his finger over the opening meanwhile. The sutures should not be tied so tightly that there would be danger of cutting the heart muscle. Mattress sutures are preferable when the muscle is unusually friable. This holds true especially in the auricle.

Lacerations of the auricle may be sutured directly, using mattress sutures, or a flexible clamp may be applied beneath the wound to hold the wall of the auricle steady and to stop the flow of blood while the sutures are being applied. If the auricular appendage is injured, it may be excised and the cut edges approximated with sutures of fine silk.

Penetrating wounds which are so close to a coronary artery that the sutures cannot be applied in the usual manner should be closed by means of mattress sutures which are carried through the myocardium beyond the artery on the side nearest the vessel.

After suture of the laceration, the pericardium should be closed loosely to allow a few spaces for the escape of fluid in case a postoperative effusion or further leakage of blood should occur. This will usually prevent the recurrence of cardiac tamponade.

The necessity for adequate blood replacement by transfusion during and after the operation need only be mentioned. The use of autotransfusion may be a life-saving expedient if large enough quantities of donor blood are not available.

Extraction of Foreign Bodies from the Heart. The extraction of metallic foreign bodies from the chambers of the heart may be necessary either as a part of the procedure for closure of a penetrating wound or as an elective procedure once they have been carried into the heart by the circulation after penetrating a major vessel. Such an occasion is unusual. Before planning the incision it is important to determine by roentgenographic studies in which chamber the object lies. The exposure of the heart may be made by a transpleural incision on the right or by a classical anterior incision over the precordial region, depending on which heart chamber is to be explored. In the case of foreign bodies which have penetrated directly through the cardiac muscle, their extraction should if possible be a part of the procedure used to close the opening. After the foreign body has been extracted, the closure of the opening in the heart muscle is carried out in the manner described above, no matter whether it be traumatic or surgical in origin.

No such operation should be undertaken without large quantities of compatible blood available for replacement of the large volume which is likely to be lost during the intracardiac manipulation required to extract the foreign body.

OPERATIONS ON THE GREAT VESSELS

Established Procedures

Extracardiac Shunt for Congenital Pulmonic Stenosis. The effects of congenital stenosis of the pulmonary valve can now be greatly relieved by the production of an extracardiac shunt between the pulmonary artery and the aorta or one of its primary branches. Congenital stenosis of the pulmonary valve may be of either the pure type, without an interventricular septal defect and without cyanosis, or the more frequent type spoken of as the tetralogy of Fallot, with cyanosis resulting from the admixture of blood from the ventricles produced by the interventricular septal defect. An accurate preoperative diagnosis must be established in each case. It is especially important also to bear in mind that there are frequent combinations of anomalies and variations in the course and distribution of the aorta and its primary branches which may make major alterations in the exposure and technic necessary. The details of diagnosis are not the subject of this treatise. Two satisfactory methods of increasing the flow of blood into the pulmonary artery are available.

Direct Anastomosis Between the Pulmonary Artery and the Descending Aorta (*Potts-Smith Operation*). The simplest method of directing a flow of blood from the aorta into the pulmonary artery is to make a direct anastomosis between these vessels. In the average case in which the aorta descends in the normal manner along the left side of the mediastinum, this procedure can be accomplished with relatively little technical difficulty by using the ingeniously contrived special aortic clamp devised by Potts and Smith (Fig. 39). On the left side the direction and length of the pulmonary artery make a lateral anastomosis between it and the aorta relatively easy to perform. The operation is, therefore, suitable for use in the usual case of tetralogy of Fallot or simple pulmonic stenosis. If, however, the aorta happens to be one which arches to the right and descends in the right side of the mediastinum, great difficulty is experienced because of the unfavorable direction of the right pulmonary artery in relation to the aorta and also because of the fact that the right pulmonary artery is so short. It is wise, therefore, to limit the use of direct anastomosis between the aorta and the pulmonary artery to the cases where the aorta descends on the left side.

TECHNIC. A standard thoracotomy incision is made on the left side through the fourth intercostal space. The lung is retracted anteriorly. A longitudinal incision is made in the pleura of the mediastinum midway between the aorta and the pulmonary hilus (Fig. 97, *A*). The vagus nerve is dissected free and retracted with a strand of silk passed distal to the origin of the recurrent laryngeal branch. To gain ready access to the left pulmonary artery several pulmonary branches of the vagus nerve must be divided. The perivascular areolar tissues are dissected away from the vessel. This necessitates the ligation of several small vessels which are frequently engorged by the perihilar collateral circulation of blood which is observed in these cases. The greatest possible length of pulmonary artery is denuded of its surrounding areolar tissue and strands of heavy silk are passed twice around the vessel, both proximally and distally, for temporary occlusion during the performance of the anastomosis. It is frequently necessary to isolate and occlude the first branches of the artery distally in order to gain sufficient length for the anastomosis (Fig. 97, *B*).

The next step is to prepare the portion of the descending aorta opposite the pulmonary artery for the anastomosis. This requires the freeing of 4 to 5 cm. of its length. In order to accomplish this it is usually necessary to ligate and divide several intercostal arteries as they arise from the aorta (Fig. 97, *C*). One should be careful to avoid injury to the thoracic duct and esophagus during this manipulation. The Potts-Smith clamp is then applied in such a manner as to isolate a portion of the aorta temporarily in order to make it possible to perform the anastomosis (Fig. 97, *D*). Three sizes of this clamp are available and should be at hand for use. The choice of the correct size is a matter of experience which is learned best by practice on experimenta

animals before attempting to perform the operation on a human being. The
proximal and distal temporary occlusive ligatures are passed one whole turn

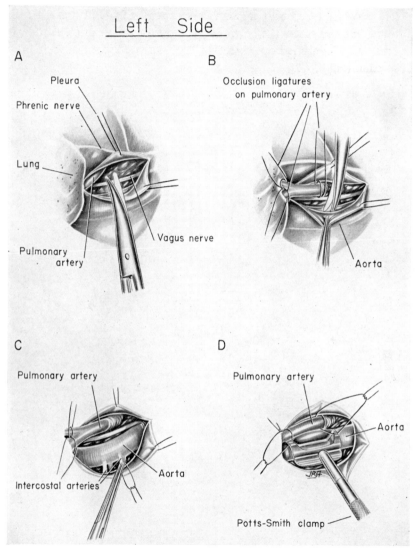

Fig. 97. Anastomosis between the left pulmonary artery and the descending aorta (Potts-
Smith technic). *A*, Beginning of the dissection to expose the pulmonary artery. *B*, Exposure
of the pulmonary artery completed; exposure of the aorta begun. *C*, Both vessels exposed;
division of two pairs of intercostal arteries required to free a length of the aorta sufficient for
the application of the clamp. *D*, Potts-Smith aorta clamp in place showing the method of
drawing the pulmonary artery close to the aorta by passing the ends of the occlusion ligatures through a loop of the clamp.

around the pulmonary artery and the two ends of each are tied together
around the corresponding loop of the aortic clamp so as to draw the artery

close enough to the aorta to make the anastomosis possible. The proximal ligature is tied first after pulling the loop around the artery tight. The distal ligature is then treated in the same manner. In some cases where the artery is short, two distal occlusive ligatures are applied to the primary branches, but only the one nearest the aorta is used to tie to the clamp. If these maneuvers have been carried out correctly, the two vessels will now lie in close apposition (Fig. 98, *E*).

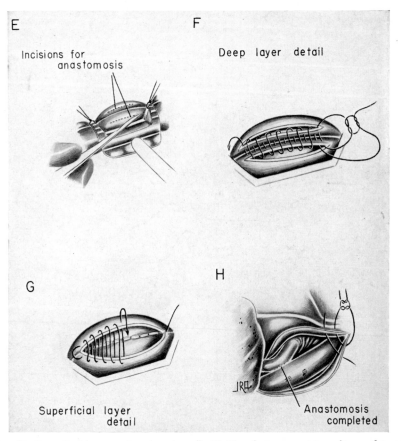

Fig. 98. Potts-Smith operation (continued). *E*, Vessels in apposition; lines of incision shown. *F*, Detail of suture; deep layer of the anastomosis showing continuous suture of fine silk (5–0). *G*, Superficial layer being placed. *H*, Completed anastomosis.

It is important to make certain that every possible bit of perivascular adventitia has been removed before the incisions in the vessels are made. A small sharp knife should be used. If the incision, which should be approximately 4 mm. in length, needs enlargement, a small pair of straight scissors with a lateral angulation of the blades is available for use (Fig. 39). Because of the tendency of the aorta to fracture or tear, these cutting instruments must be sharp so as to avoid unnecessary trauma. A single strand of fine silk fastened to an atraumatic needle is used for the anastomosis (5–0 Deknatel atraumatic). The suture is begun at the proximal (cephalad) end of the incision in the vessels, and after transfixing both aorta and artery it is tied, leaving a short end free. The deep edges of the vessels are then sewed together with an over-and-over continuous stitch until the distal ends of the openings are reached, where the suture may be locked by passing the strand through the last loop before it is pulled tight (Fig. 98, *F*). An alternative method of insuring a tight apposition at this end is to insert a single interrupted suture which is tied before the superficial edges of the vessels are approximated. When the continuous suture has been carried back to the starting point at the proximal end, the two portions are tied together and the excess is cut away (Fig. 98, *G*). The bites of the suture should be placed as close together as possible (not over 1 mm. apart). The temporary occlusive ligatures are then removed from the pulmonary artery, starting with those on the distal end. After the pulmonary artery has been released, the clamp on the aorta is loosened gradually. As the blood begins to flow through the anastomosis into the pulmonary artery, there may be a small amount of leakage through the suture line. If this seems to be excessive at any point, the clamp is tightened again and a single suture may be applied at the weak point. This must be done with the utmost gentleness because of the danger of tearing the vessels, especially the aorta. The clamp is finally removed. A slight amount of leakage is frequently observed, but it usually stops after a few minutes. A thrill will now be felt in the pulmonary artery as the blood from the aorta rushes into it through the completed anastomosis (Fig. 98, *H*).

The lung is expanded fully and the chest wall is closed. It is advisable to insert a small catheter through an intercostal space in the lower part of the chest to provide egress for the postoperative pleural effusion which in some cases may amount to several hundred cubic centimeters.

Anastomosis Between the Pulmonary Artery and a Major Branch of the Aortic Arch (Blalock Operation). By this operation blood from the aorta is directed into one of the pulmonary arteries through a shunt produced by an anastomosis with a branch of the aorta. The vessel which is usually chosen for this purpose is the subclavian branch of the innominate artery. This means, therefore, that the operation is performed typically on the right side because in the majority of instances the aorta descends on the left. However, when the aorta descends on the right the innominate branch lies in the left side and the operation must therefore be done in the left side of the chest. As a matter of fact, experience has shown that the left subclavian artery can be employed equally well no matter on which side the innominate artery may lie. This makes it advantageous to employ a left thoracotomy in all cases because if conditions are unsuitable for the performance of a Potts-Smith procedure, a Blalock operation can still be carried out, and vice versa. The subclavian artery on either side can be freed far enough distally in the majority of instances to obtain sufficient length for the performance of the anastomosis. In a few cases it may be necessary to use the proximal (cardiac) end of the common carotid or the innominate artery if not enough length can be obtained from the subclavian. When vascular anomalies are found, other vessels may have to be employed. For a detailed consideration of these possibilities, one should consult the current surgical literature.

TECHNIC. The operation as originally performed on the right side is described. An anterolateral incision is made through the second intercostal space. The lung is retracted laterally and the mediastinal pleura is incised. The right pulmonary artery is identified and dissected free of surrounding tissue. The azygos vein is divided between ligatures and the dissection is carried upward behind the superior vena cava to the innominate artery. The right vagus nerve and its recurrent branch are identified. The subclavian artery is found. It is wise to make certain also of the location of the carotid artery to be sure that the correct vessel has been found. The subclavian artery is followed distally as far as possible and a rubber-shod bulldog clamp is placed across it close to its origin. It is then divided at the farthest possible point distally and the distal cut end is ligated. The adventitial tissue is excised from the proximal end, which is pulled out from the loop formed by the recurrent laryngeal nerve and turned down for the anastomosis. The pulmonary artery is temporarily occluded as far proximally as possible with a rubber-shod clamp (Blalock type, of which there are three sizes) (Fig. 39). The distal portion of the artery is likewise occluded, but sometimes, in order to gain a sufficient length for the performance of the anastomosis, the first branches are occluded separately instead of the main artery. Bulldog clamps are used. A short transverse incision is made in the pulmonary artery (Fig. 99, *A, B* and *C. Note:* The left side was used in the patient whose operation was the subject of these drawings.)

An end-to-side anastomosis is made, using a continuous suture of fine silk (5–0 Deknatel on an atraumatic needle). The best manner of applying the suture is as an everting continuous mattress stitch to turn the intima outward (Fig. 99, *D*). The posterior row is inserted before drawing it up. After this row has been drawn tight, a single stay suture is inserted at each end of the anastomosis. The anterior row is then applied and the strand is tied to the stay suture at the starting point. The clamp and occlusive ligatures are removed from the pulmonary artery, and finally the clamp is removed from the subclavian artery. A thrill should be felt in the pulmonary artery if the anastomosis is patent.

Division of Vascular Ring Produced by Anomalous Double Aortic Arch. Constriction of the trachea and esophagus by an arterial ring consisting of a persistent double aortic arch can be relieved by ligation and division of one of the two component vessels. The exact arrangement of the anomalous vessels, including the origins of the various branches going to the head and upper extremities, cannot always be anticipated with accuracy although angiographic studies are helpful. There is usually a large channel which passes posteriorly behind the trachea and esophagus and a small anterior vessel which communicates on either side with the ascending and descending

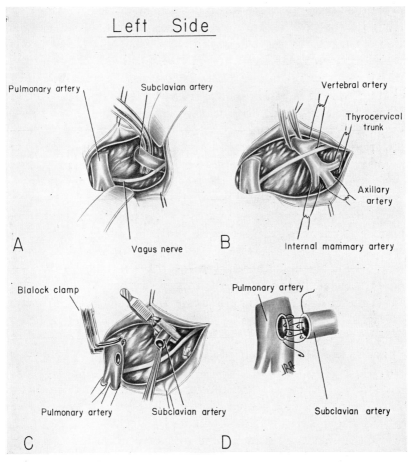

Fig. 99. Anastomosis between the subclavian artery and the pulmonary artery (Blalock technic); left side. *A,* Exposure of the left pulmonary artery and the subclavian artery. *B,* Dissection of the subclavian artery with ligation of its branches (vertebral, thyrocervical, internal mammary and axillary). *C,* Occlusion of the two arteries in preparation for the anastomosis. *D,* Detail of the continuous everting suture used in the performance of the anastomosis. (*Note:* Many surgeons, including Blalock, prefer the right side.)

portions of the posterior arch. The anterior component may be partially or completely obliterated, but in many instances an appreciable volume of blood passes through it. This vessel can usually be divided without interfering to any noticeable extent with the circulation. In an occasional case the larger vessel may be the anterior one, making it necessary to divide the lesser posterior arch. Angiography may be of assistance in deciding which vessel passes behind.

The usual standard thoracotomy incision is used. The chest is opened through the fourth intercostal space. The choice of side depends upon the position of the descending aorta. The anterior vessel always presents toward the side of the mediastinum in which the aorta descends. This is usually the left, but if as a result of roentgenographic investigation the descending portion of the aorta is found to be in the right side of the mediastinum, a right-sided approach may be preferable.

After the chest has been opened, the lung is retracted downward by the hand of an assistant and an incision is made through the mediastinal pleura so as to expose the vessels. The identification of the anomalous vessel and a survey of its branches are completed (Fig. 100, *A*). There is usually a patent ductus arteriosus which may require division. The relation of the recurrent laryngeal branch of the vagus nerve to the anterior arch must be observed. Heavy silk ligatures are then tied around the small anterior vessel at whatever point seems to be advisable to avoid interference with circulation through important branches. As soon as the vascular ring is interrupted by cutting the anterior arch, the trachea and esophagus rise forward in response to the release of the constriction (Fig. 100, *C*). A groove can usually be identified extending obliquely across the lower end of the trachea at the point where the constricting vessel was. It may be necessary also to divide the patent ductus or ligamentum arteriosum in order to produce the maximum relief (Fig. 100, *A*).

The incision in the mediastinal pleura is closed with interrupted fine silk sutures and the chest wall is closed after the lung has been expanded completely.

Interruption of Patent Ductus Arteriosus. Either the anterolateral or the standard thoracotomy incision may be used. The latter is preferred because it avoids interference with the mammary gland, provides an exceptionally wide exposure, and makes it possible to approach the ductus in a more direct manner. The incision is made through the fourth intercostal space on the left side. The upper lobe of the left lung is retracted downward and forward to expose the surface of the mediastinum above and behind the hilus of the lung. A vertical incision is made through the pleura about midway between the vagus and phrenic nerves. This is extended downward behind the lung hilus. The subpleural layer of areolar tissue is divided to expose the aortic arch and pulmonary artery. Several small vessels, sometimes including the highest intercostal vein, must be severed. Several lymph nodes must be dissected away from the pulmonary artery. In children these are frequently large and may show evidence of inflammatory changes. The vagus nerve below the origin of its recurrent laryngeal branch is retracted posteriorly by means of a strand of silk passed around it. It is necessary to sever some

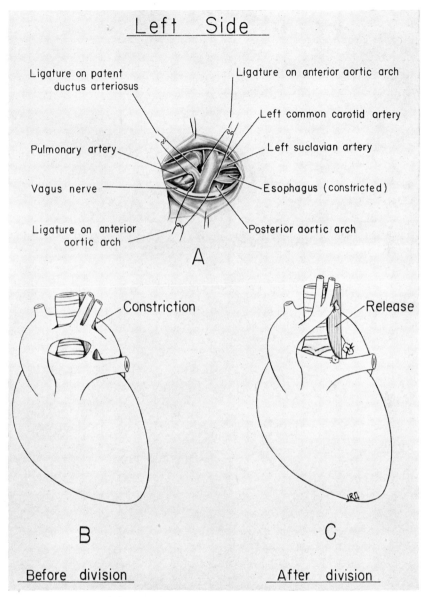

Left Side

Ligature on patent ductus arteriosus

Ligature on anterior aortic arch

Left common carotid artery

Pulmonary artery

Left suclavian artery

Vagus nerve

Esophagus (constricted)

Ligature on anterior aortic arch

Posterior aortic arch

A

Constriction

Release

B

C

Before division

After division

Fig. 100. Division of the vascular ring produced by an anomalous double aortic arch. A, Drawing made at operation in a typical case, showing the anatomic relations of the vessels as they were exposed ready for division. B, Diagram to show the constriction of the trachea and esophagus by the double aortic arch in the case illustrated in A. C, Diagram to show the release of the constricted trachea and esophagus after division of the anterior component of the double aortic arch.

of its pulmonary branches in order to retract it sufficiently. The ductus is readily found by identifying the recurrent laryngeal nerve, which always passes around beneath it to ascend behind the aortic arch. The palpation of a thrill in this region gives further evidence of its location.

In order to render the freeing of the ductus easy, it is essential to start the dissection in the deepest possible plane over the vessels. It is wise to begin on the anterior surface of the aorta, sweeping the areolar tissues of the adventitial layer forward against the pericardial reflection over the ductus.

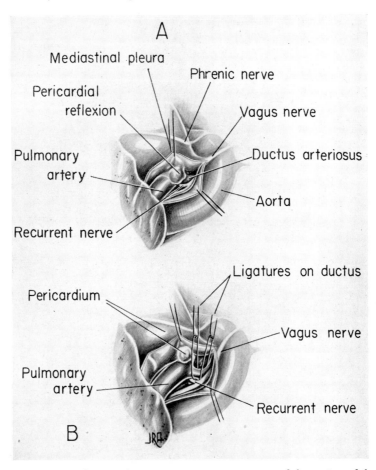

Fig. 101. Ligation of patent ductus arteriosus. *A,* Exposure of the region of the ductus after reflecting the mediastinal pleura. *B,* ductus completely exposed and ready for double ligation.

This reflection sometimes extends onto the aorta itself. Sharp dissection with scissors and occasional wiping with gauze are used. As the pericardial reflection becomes obvious, it should be lifted from the ductus (Fig. 101, A). This makes it possible to approach the junction of the ductus with the pulmonary artery safely. With the anterolateral surface of the ductus exposed, the dissection is carried beneath and behind, using the same technic. For this part of the procedure additional assistance is obtained by gently spreading the surrounding tissues with a curved hemostatic or cystic duct forceps. In doing this, however, there is danger of tearing the pulmonary artery at the point where the ductus is attached. This is the most vulnerable region. In fact, in the majority of instances where hemorrhage is encountered, the leaking point is at the angle between the artery and the ductus along the inferior surface. When freeing the deep surface of the ductus, also, the tip of the dissecting instrument should be directed as much as possible toward the aortic side to avoid the fragile pulmonary artery. A part of the deep dissection can be done also from above. By working in turn first from below and then from above, the entire circumference of the ductus is freed. If it is difficult to free the pericardial reflection because of inflammatory fixation, it may be necessary to open the pericardial sac in order to find the way around behind the vessel. However, the anatomic relations of the region are such that it will be necessary to find an exit from the pericardial sac behind the ductus in order to pass an instrument completely around its pulmonary artery end. This maneuver is rarely necessary.

Certain anatomic variations should be mentioned. The pericardial reflection over the ductus may be large and long, extending sometimes onto the aorta itself, or it may be very small or even nonexistent. The ductus varies greatly from patient to patient in length, diameter and direction. It tends to be relatively longer in children than in adults. Sometimes it leaves the pulmonary artery and joins the aorta almost at right angles. At other times it joins these vessels at acute angles. Finally there is in some instances marked, almost aneurysmal bulging of the aorta at the site where the ductus is attached. This does not occur at the pulmonary artery end.

The interruption of the flow of blood through the ductus may be accomplished either by double ligation in continuity or by division and closure of the divided ends. Ligation has the advantage of safety and simplicity. If carried out properly it gives completely satisfactory results. The possibility of recanalization must be mentioned, but the reports which have described this complication may have been based upon developments in cases where the ligation of the ductus was not thoroughly done. A good method is to tie the ductus as closely as possible to the major vessel at each end, using very heavy braided silk (Deknatel No. 2 to No. 4). If heavy material is used, there is practically no danger of cutting through the vessel wall by the ligature to cause immediate hemorrhage or of damage which might lead to aneurysmal dilatation at a later time. Care must be exerted to avoid pinching the recurrent laryngeal nerve while setting the knot of the ligature nearest the aorta (Fig. 101, B).

An alternative method is to divide the ductus between two pairs of straight hemostatic forceps, the serrations of whose jaws have been modified so as to prevent sidewise slipping. The distal clamp is removed from each side and the edges of the end of the vessel are sutured over and over with a continuous strand of fine silk. The proximal clamp is then removed and the suture is carried back again through the end of the vessel to the starting point where it is tied. So far as can be determined at the present time, this method does not provide enough superiority of ultimate result to make justifiable the additional risk it entails in the hands of the average surgeon.

As soon as continuity has been interrupted, the thrill in the ductus and the pulmonary artery can no longer be felt. It should be remembered, however, that many of the patients who are operated upon because of a patent ductus arteriosus also have other congenital anomalies such as septal defects. These may cause a thrill and a murmur which do not depend upon the existence of a patent ductus and which persist after the ductus has been ligated. This fact must be kept in mind when evaluating the results of the operation. Differentiation, however, is not usually difficult.

To complete the operation the incision in the mediastinal pleura is closed loosely with interrupted sutures, the lung is expanded and the chest wall incision is closed in the usual manner. Drainage of the chest cavity is optional, depending upon the amount of oozing from small mediastinal vessels and the thoracic incision.

Operations for Coarctation of the Aorta. A standard thoracotomy incision is used on the left side. In an adult the fourth or fifth rib should be resected. In a child the incision may be made through the fourth intercostal space. In either case it may be necessary to divide adjacent ribs posteriorly in order to gain a sufficiently wide exposure. The enormous enlargement of the vessels in the chest wall usually prolongs this portion of the operation because of the difficulty of securing satisfactory hemostasis. The intercostal vessels are not only very much enlarged but also unusually fragile.

The principle involved in the surgical correction of coarctation of the aorta is to remove the obstructing barrier by excision and to establish vascular continuity so as to make a direct flow of blood into the descending aorta. The exact method of accomplishing this result depends upon the location and extent of the abnormal segment. In general, three different situations may be encountered, each requiring a different solution of the technical problem. These will be considered separately as follows.

SHORT CONSTRICTION LOCATED IN THE DESCENDING SEGMENT SEVERAL CENTIMETERS AWAY FROM THE SUBCLAVIAN ARTERY. This is the simplest type of case to handle. It is usually possible to resect the short segment in which the constriction lies and to make an end-to-end anastomosis between the proximal and distal severed ends. A long incision is made in the mediastinal pleura over the aorta. The aorta is uncovered from the region of the arch down to a point well below the coarctation. A long segment of the vessel, including several centimeters of normal artery both above and below the constricted area, is mobilized and freed of its adventitial layer so that clamps may be placed a suitable distance away in both directions from the portion which is to be removed. It is usually necessary to divide several intercostal arteries to accomplish this. The clamps are applied and the diseased segment is excised, leaving as much vessel on each side as possible for

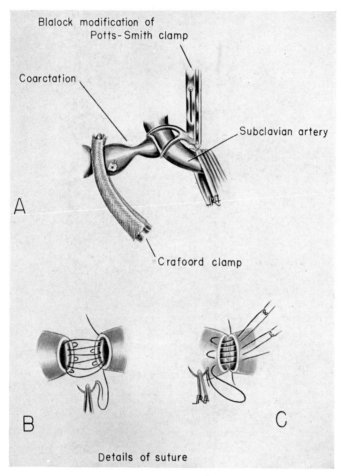

Fig. 102. Coarctation of the aorta. Details of excision and anastomosis of the divided ends. *A*, Coarctation segment ready for excision. Note the use of the Blalock modification of the Potts-Smith clamp used in cases of coarctation near the left subclavian artery; a Crafoord clamp is used on the aorta distal to the constriction. *B* and *C*, Details of the everting suture.

the anastomosis. In some cases it may be necessary to mobilize the divided ends more extensively either by cutting one or two more intercostal vessels below or by freeing the aortic arch above. It is sometimes helpful to divide the ductus arteriosus or ligamentum arteriosum.

When it is apparent that the two ends can be approximated without excessive tension, the anastomosis is begun. The handles of the clamps are swung forward and the posterior sutures are inserted first. The position of the clamps is then altered and the anterior aspect of the anastomosis is completed. The exact method of suturing depends on the preference of the surgeon and to some extent the nature of the case. A simple over-and-over continuous suture which merely approximates the edges of the aorta is

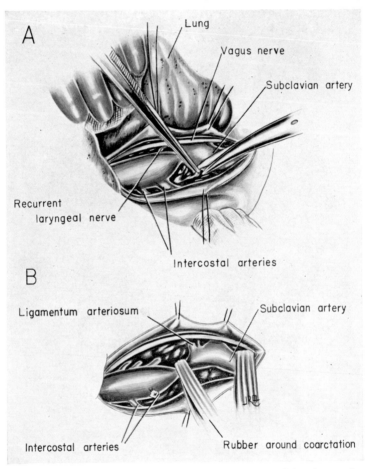

Fig. 103. Coarctation. Preparation of the vessel for excision of the abnormal segment. *A,* Beginning of the dissection. *B,* Start of the division of two sets of intercostal arteries below the coarctation. *Note:* The ligamentum arteriosum had to be divided also in this case.

satisfactory. A better method, which should be used if possible, is to evert the edges of the vessels by either a continuous or an interrupted suture of the mattress type. If the continuous strand is used, reinforcement should be secured by means of two or three interrupted sutures placed at equidistant intervals around the circumference (Fig. 102, *B* and *C*). Another technic is to insert a layer of interrupted everting mattress sutures of silk followed by a second continuous suture passed over and over the everted edges. Such an anastomosis will not leak and is unusually strong.

The distal clamp is removed first. The proximal clamp is then released slowly to detect any evidence of leakage and to prevent too sudden loss of arterial resistance. If necessary the clamp may be tightened again and one or more extra sutures applied. It is advisable to avoid this if possible because of the danger of tearing the fragile aortic tissues. The edges of the pleura are approximated loosely unless they have been torn during the operation so that they will not come together easily. The lung is reexpanded and the chest incision is closed. Drainage of the thoracic cavity is optional.

CONSTRICTION AT OR NEAR THE ORIGIN OF THE SUBCLAVIAN ARTERY (Fig. 103). In many patients the coarctation is so close to the left subclavian artery that it is impossible to place a clamp across the aorta proximal to it in the manner just described. This difficulty may be overcome by clamping the aortic arch proximal to the subclavian branch and by occluding the subclavian separately. A satisfactory proximal end of aorta is sometimes thereby made available after excision of the narrow segment, and an end-to-end aortic anastomosis can be made as in the first type. The technical problem, however, is often almost insurmountable, especially in the placing of the posterior layer of sutures. A modification of the Potts-Smith clamp devised by Blalock is useful in this situation. If this instrument is available, an end-to-end anastomosis can be made in the majority of these cases (Fig. 102, A). Occasionally, however, it is impossible to approximate the ends of the aorta. When this situation arises, the proximal end must be occluded by ligature or by sutures. The proximal end of the subclavian artery may then be swung down after its division to perform an anastomosis with the distal end of the aorta. This is made possible because the diameter of the subclavian artery is unusually large and that of the aorta below the coarctation correspondingly small. The subclavian artery must be handled gently because of the danger of fracture of these unusually fragile vessels. The anastomosis is performed by the method described above.

LONG DEFECTIVE SEGMENT OR UNFAVORABLE RELATION TO THE SUBCLAVIAN ARTERY. In some cases the excessive length of aorta which must be excised or the relation of the abnormal area to the subclavian artery makes it impracticable to attempt to perform an excision and direct anastomosis. It then becomes necessary either to abandon the operation or to adopt some other expedient. Recent experiments have shown that a long defect in the aorta can be bridged successfully by inserting a heterogeneous graft taken from the aorta of another member of the same species. This procedure has been used in a few human beings, but it is still not practicable for widespread use. The difficulty of universal application centers around the problem of obtaining and preserving the necessary material for use in the patient with coarctation.

Procedures Not Well Established

Operations for Aneurysm of the Thoracic Aorta. Thus far no preeminently satisfactory procedure has been developed for the treatment of aneurysms of the intrathoracic portion of the aorta.

The largest experience has been with attempts to bring about clotting in the aneurysm by stuffing its cavity with great lengths of fine wire introduced through an especially constructed needle. The procedure may be carried out by introducing the wiring needle blindly through the chest wall or under direct vision through a standard thoracotomy incision. Relief of pain has resulted from the use of this method in some patients, but there is little evidence that life has been prolonged by it.

Attempts to stay the expansion of a thoracic aneurysm by wrapping it with cellophane have been reported. The method is still in an experimental phase.

Operations for Transposition of the Great Vessels. This rare anomaly which consists in a reversal of the circulation so that the aorta arises from the right ventricle and the pulmonary artery comes off of the left ventricle is not compatible with life unless there is some sort of shunt between the two vessels. In the relatively few infants who have been known to survive, this shunt has been provided by congenital patency of the interventricular or inter-auricular septum. However, this is not usually sufficient for a prolonged existence and attempts have been made, thus far with indifferent success, to better the situation by means of an additional intercommunication between the two circulatory systems. Two methods have been tried. One is to perform an extracardiac shunt by anastomosis between the left pulmonary artery and the descending aorta or some other combination of vessels to increase the mingling of the two streams of blood. This puts a considerable additional strain upon the heart. The other is to create an interauricular septal defect. Recently a combination of an additional intracardiac with an artificial extracardiac shunt has been shown to offer the greatest promise of ameliorating the difficulty. Relatively few survivals have occurred after these operations and the future of such patients is obviously precarious.

OPERATIONS FOR LEAKAGE FROM INJURED THORACIC DUCT

The serious consequences of a continuing leak from the thoracic duct into the pleural cavity make it necessary to attempt to close the opening. The fragile nature of this vessel precludes the possibility of restoring continuity by anastomosis with sutures. Two alternative methods are available, each of necessity requiring a direct approach by open thoracotomy.

Ligation of the Thoracic Duct. A standard thoracotomy incision is made on the side of the chest in which the chyle accumulates. After the fluid has been removed and the lung has been retracted forward, the mediastinal pleura is incised in the region where the leakage occurs. The thoracic duct is identified and freed by sharp dissection. The site of injury or rupture is found and the duct is ligated proximal and distal to that point.

Packing with Gelfoam. If it is impossible to identify the duct itself because of the induration and inflammatory infiltration of the adjacent tissues, leakage may be controlled successfully by stuffing the area with gelfoam and suturing adjacent surfaces of the pleura together over this pack. If the tissues are not flexible, an incision is made on each side of the packed area in order to create two edges of pleura which can be turned toward each other and approximated over the pack with a row of sutures.

TRANSTHORACIC VAGECTOMY

The transthoracic approach provides ready access to the vagus nerves. Its chief advantage lies in the fact that a very long extent of the nerves may be observed so that branches which arise at a high level and do not join the nerves again below may be more readily discovered. In some cases, therefore, it may provide greater certainty of obtaining a complete interruption of all the vagus fibers than the abdominal approach. On the other hand, it must be pointed out that in contrast to the abdominal approach it is more difficult to gain access to the ulcer if it seems necessary to visualize it, although the stomach and duodenum can be explored by opening the diaphragm. There is the additional disadvantage also that postoperative thoracic complications such as tension pneumothorax, resulting from trauma to the lung while severing pulmonary adhesions, and effusions of fluid into the pleural cavity may develop. The performance of a gastroenterostomy at the same operation, although it can be carried out by opening the diaphragm, is more easily done through the abdominal approach.

Technic of the Operation. Although the vagus nerves can be reached through an incision in the right side of the chest, the left side is used for vagectomy because of the possibility that it may be necessary to gain access to the stomach especially if a gastroenterostomy is to be done. A long standard thoracotomy incision is made through the eighth intercostal space or through the bed of the eighth or ninth rib. Adhesions between the lung and the thoracic wall must be freed sufficiently to gain access to the lower mediastinum. The mediastinal pleura is incised from the level of the inferior pulmonary vein to the diaphragm. The lower end of the esophagus is freed by blunt dissection and a long strip of Penrose rubber drain is passed under it for retraction. The two ends of this are held together with a hemostat. The right and left vagus nerves are identified both above and below the periesophageal plexus (Fig. 104).

As they are isolated, the well-known variations in the course and arrangement of the nerves should be kept in mind. It is a frequent occurrence to find several independent trunks in the place of a single nerve. All these nerve trunks are identified and followed down below the esophageal plexus through the esophageal hiatus of the diaphragm into the region of the cardia, where each is divided and tied. The proximal division is made high enough to facilitate the excision of several centimeters of each trunk. These ends are likewise tied, largely to secure the small vessels which may run with them. Proximal ligation or crushing with a dura clip has been advocated for the purpose of preventing regeneration, but no evidence has been brought forth to show that effective regeneration of the vagus nerves ever occurs. Excision of long segments, to prevent restoration of function, is also very likely unnecessary. During the dissection of the nerves and especially as a result of the excision of segments from them, some of the small periesophageal veins must be divided. An effort should be made, however, to avoid injuring any more blood vessels than necessary and to keep from injuring

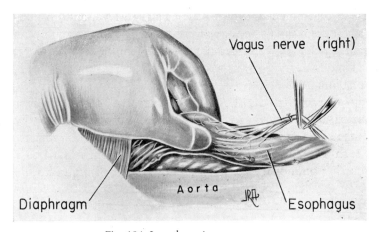

Fig. 104. Intrathoracic vagectomy.

the esophagus by rough handling. Transitory partial dysphagia resulting from swelling of devitalized or traumatized tissues of the esophageal wall will thus be prevented. The mediastinal pleural edges are approximated with fine silk.

If it is desired to perform a gastroenterostomy as an adjuvant procedure, an incision is made through the diaphragm. Through this the ulcer may be visualized and palpated, and a gastrojejunostomy may be performed in the usual manner. This may be made either antecolic or retrocolic and antiperistaltic or isoperistaltic, as the relations of the viscera may suggest, to suit the preference of the individual surgeon. It must be kept in mind that the transthoracic approach provides access to the viscera in a direction different from that with which the surgeon is more likely to be familiar if he is more accustomed to the abdominal approach. This precaution will make it easier to place the anastomosis in a correct position. After the abdominal phase of the operation is completed, the diaphragm is closed with interrupted silk sutures. The lung is expanded and inspected for air leaks if it was necessary to sever adhesions. Leaking points are dealt with either by ligation of a small portion of lung caught in a hemostat or the placing of several fine silk sutures. The chest wall is closed in the usual manner. Closed catheter drainage should be used if a leakage of air is anticipated or if there is reason to believe that an unusually large serosanguineous effusion might occur. When in doubt, it is best to drain.

After-care. Following a transthoracic vagectomy one should be prepared to deal with any of the usual complications which may follow the performance of a thoracic operation. These include pleural effusion, tension pneumothorax and inability to raise secretions with resultant massive atelectasis of some portion of the lung. In addition there is the problem of dealing with the effects of the interruption of the vagus nerves. Excessive gastric dilatation can be avoided in the majority of patients by means of constant suction applied with a Wangensteen apparatus to the end of the inlying Levin tube. The tube should be left in place for at least five to six days. After its removal daily or bidaily aspiration may be required for a brief period.

CHAPTER 8

OPERATIONS ON THE ESOPHAGUS

GENERAL PRINCIPLES

Operations upon the esophagus involve the application of principles which encompass a wide field of biologic and surgical knowledge. The esophagus differs from other portions of the alimentary canal in certain important respects.

Anatomy. From the anatomic standpoint the esophagus is characterized by the fact that it lacks a serosal coat, upon the presence of which some of the methods of anastomosis of the intraperitoneal portions of the digestive tract largely depend. Its fragile muscular coat consists mostly of longitudinal fibers with only a weak circular layer; therefore it is relatively inadequate to hold sutures. The mucosa, on the other hand, is of the squamous cell variety and relatively strong. The blood supply is segmental in origin (Fig. 105). The lymphatic drainage from the esophagus is extensive, with numerous connections in the regional nodes of the neck, mediastinum and upper abdomen (Fig. 105). The topographic anatomic relations of the esophagus are likewise of great importance to the surgeon and must be thoroughly understood before operations upon it are undertaken (Fig. 1).

Physical Characteristics. The physical characteristics of the esophagus are such that it distends circumferentially and shortens by retraction, but does not stretch readily. Therefore, every anastomosis with this organ must be absolutely free from any possibility of tension on the suture line. Mobilization of the esophagus can be accomplished with safety to a limited extent but, with the exception of the lower end, only for the purpose of pulling it upward. Attempts to displace it downward are limited by the pull of the already downward sloping segmental arteries and, in the lower portion, by the suspensory effect of the vagus nerves and their periesophageal plexus in the lower thoracic area. A small degree of downward displacement of the abdominal segment of the esophagus can be accomplished by cutting all these vagus nerve fibers. It is axiomatic that all manipulations involving the handling of this organ must be carried out with the greatest possible gentleness.

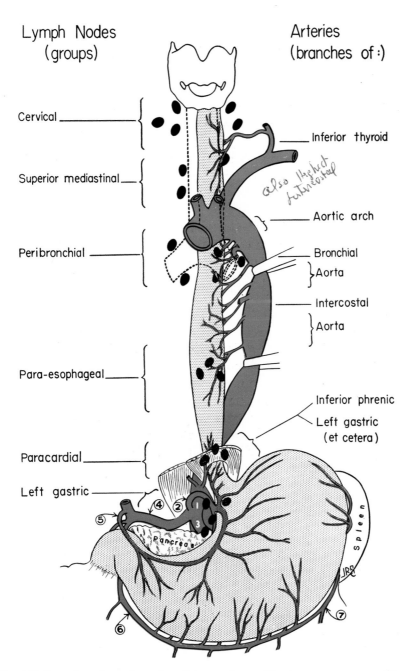

Fig. 105. Lymph nodes and arteries of the esophagus. The important groups of lymph nodes which drain the esophagus at various levels are shown on the right side. On the left are illustrated the principal arteries which supply the esophagus. Several small arteries which contribute to the blood supply of the abdominal segment, including the branch from the superior suprarenal artery, lie posteriorly and are not shown. The arteries which have to do with the blood supply of the stomach are designated by number as follows: (1) celiac axis; (2) left gastric artery; (3) splenic artery; (4) hepatic artery; (5) right gastric artery; (6) right gastro-epiploic artery; and (7) left gastro-epiploic artery. The vasa brevia pass between the hilus of the spleen and the fundus of the stomach.

Bacteriology. From the bacteriologic standpoint it is important to emphasize that the contents of the esophagus are grossly contaminated with the bacterial flora of the mouth, including virulent organisms of the gram-positive coccus group, predominantly streptococci and staphylococci. Because of their effectiveness in inhibiting the growth of these organisms, penicillin and streptomycin are valuable in the surgery of the esophagus. As a method of prophylaxis in elective cases, a satisfactory procedure is to give penicillin intramuscularly during the twenty-four hours preceding operation and a solution of streptomycin orally during the last forty-eight hours before operation. Just before the incision is closed, a solution containing the two antibiotics is inserted in the mediastinum and in the pleural and upper abdominal cavities (in case the diaphragm has been incised). Both antibiotics are administered parenterally during the first few days of the postoperative period, until the possibility of the development of sepsis has been eliminated.

Anesthesia. Anesthesia for esophageal surgery must provide for control of the inflation of the lungs even when only the cervical area is being dealt with. This is accomplished with ether and oxygen, or other suitable volatile agent, administered through an intratracheal tube. This tube should be provided with an inflatable rubber cuff or balloon to prevent the backward escape of anesthetic gases into the pharynx when pressure is applied. If this precaution is not observed, some of the gas may pass down the esophagus and produce troublesome or even dangerous degrees of inflation of the stomach. The potential danger of this occurrence during the inflation of the lung after the completion of an esophagogastric anastomosis is obvious. Even aspiration through a Levin tube lying within the esophagus during the course of the operation may not be sufficient to prevent the disruption of the suture line from overdistention.

Approach to the Esophagus. The approach to the esophagus depends upon the segment which is to be exposed, the nature of the lesion and the type of procedure to be carried out. For operations upon the short cervical segment the patient is placed on his back with the head turned slightly to the opposite side. An incision made parallel to the anterior margin of the sternocleidomastoid muscle provides good access to the cervical segment and upper end of the mediastinal portion (Fig. 112, *A*). To expose the long thoracic portion a thoracotomy incision must be used. In general, the midthoracic segment is dealt with more easily through the right side of the chest than through the left. In all benign lesions such as congenital or inflammatory tracheo-esophageal fistulas, benign tumors to be removed by local excision, and in any case which does not require the use of the stomach for an anastomosis, the right side provides ready access to the esophagus at all levels in the mediastinum. On the other hand, when there is a strong probability that a large portion of the esophagus must be resected, as in the case of a carcinoma, the left side is used in order to make the mobilization of the stomach (or rarely the jejunum) more easily accomplished. In either case the standard thoracotomy incision, usually with a rib resection, is used, the patient lying in the lateral recumbent position. When the growth is high in the thorax, this incision must be enlarged upward by posterior division of adjacent ribs (Chap. 3). For tumors in the superior mediastinal segment a combined thoracic and cervical exposure using two separate incisions is required. Combined right thoracic and left abdominal incisions have been advocated by some surgeons, but this method is unnecessarily complicated. A recent modification of technic involves the use of a long thoraco-abdominal incision which is used to open the right chest and, by crossing the midepigastric region, can be made to provide a reasonably satisfactory exposure of the stomach. In this way a single incision is used for both the resection of the esophagus and the mobilization of the stomach, and a one-stage operation by the right thoracotomy approach can be performed with greater ease than when two separate incisions are used.

Lesions in the short abdominal segment are dealt with through a left transthoracic approach, using a standard thoracotomy incision through the bed of the ninth rib or in the eighth intercostal space.

General Operative Considerations. The *performance of an anastomosis or the closure of an incision* in the esophagus must be carried out with the greatest gentleness and with special precautions to insure prompt and satisfactory healing. Certain details of technic which are acceptable in operations on the stomach or intestine are inapplicable for operations on the esophagus. The most important single aim is to prevent necrosis of the edges which are to be sutured. Thus prompt and accurate healing, especially of the mucous membrane layer, is fostered and the cicatrization which results from delayed or secondary healing is avoided. It is such cicatrization which is responsible for stricture formation at the site of anastomosis. This means that crushing clamps must never be applied, that the esophagus must be cut with a sharp instrument and not with the cautery, and that continuous sutures which cause necrosis because they compress the entire sutured edge must be avoided. In every instance, therefore, an open anastomosis made without the use of clamps is preferred. The esophagus is cut with the knife or scissors, and interrupted sutures of fine material are used. The nature of the suture material is of relatively little importance provided that the smallest size which can be tied without breaking be used. Because of the ease with which it can be handled, waxed silk is highly satisfactory for this purpose (size 5–0).

Under certain circumstances in the closure of an opening in the esophagus or in the performance of an esophageal anastomosis it is possible to obtain a satisfactory result with two layers of sutures, one to approximate the mucosal edges and the second to unite the muscular layers. It is preferable in the majority of cases, however, especially in the making of an anastomosis, to add a third layer to provide additional reinforcement. The sutures of the mucosal layer are inserted in such a way that when tied the knots present within the lumen (Fig. 106, *1*). This is done to avoid the presence of the knots between the layers where the healing is to take place. It also facilitates the separation and sloughing away of the sutures of the inner layer, which is anticipated. Simple sutures applied in the ordinary manner are used to approximate the edges of the muscular layer (Fig. 106, 2). The outer layer should be of mattress sutures, which have less tendency to cut through the fragile muscularis. Each layer of sutures should be placed not more than 2 or 3 mm. from the other so as to avoid infolding too much tissue, which might tend to narrow the lumen too greatly. The individual sutures of each

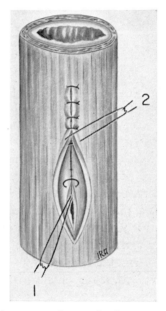

Fig. 106. Technic of esophagotomy (longitudinal incision and lengthwise closure). *1,* Mucosal suture showing the method of insertion of stitches employed in all esophageal surgery. The knot lies within the lumen when tied. *2,* Simple interrupted suture employed for the approximation of the edges of the muscle layer.

succeeding layer should be inserted so as to pierce a different group of longitudinal muscle fibers from those which hold the preceding layer (Fig. 115, *A, B, C* and *D*).

In contradistinction to the small intestine, in which stenosis may result, lengthwise incisions in the esophagus may be closed longitudinally instead of circumferentially. In fact, unless the incision is very short, circumferential closure may be impossible or at least result in excessive tension on the sutures. Lengthwise closure, however, does not produce stenosis because of the ease with which the esophagus expands circumferentially.

With few exceptions, in operations on the esophagus it is expedient to *insert a Levin tube* before the operation is begun, leaving the tip close to the lesion. This is to prevent spilling of the contents while the esophagus is open during the course of the operation. It also provides to some extent for the escape of anesthetic gases which might have been forced into the esophagus during the administration of the anesthetic. The tube is valuable also for the continuous aspiration of fluid during the early convalescent period.

Classification	Procedure	Closure or Anastomosis	Diagram	Application					
				Carcinoma	Stricture	Obliteration	Web	Achalasia	Benign tum.
Esophagotomy	1. Longitudinal incision	Lengthwise closure	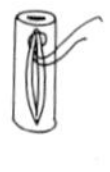	o	o	o	o	o	X
Plastic operations without resection	2. Excision of web	Lengthwise closure	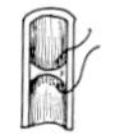	o	o	o	X	o	o
	3. Longitudinal incision & circumferential closure	Circumferential closure	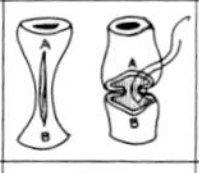	o	X	o	o	X	(X)
Resection with restoration of continuity	4. Segmental resection	End-to-end anastomosis	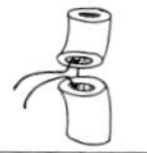	(X)	X	o	o	o	o
	5. Segmental resection	Interposition of skin tube	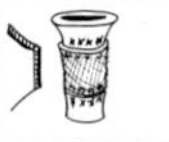	X (cervical)	X	o	o	o	o
	Partial esophagectomy 6. Lower fourth	Esophago-gastric anastomosis supra-diaphragmatic	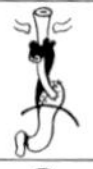	X	X	X	o	o	(X)
	(Same) 7. Lower fourth & part of middle half	(Same) subaortic arch	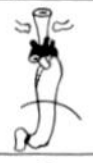	X	X	X	o	o	(X)
	(Same) 8. Lower fourth & all of middle half	(Same) supra-aortic arch	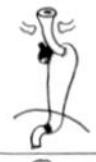	X	(X)	X	o	o	o
	Subtotal esophagectomy 9. Lower fourth, middle half, & superior mediastinal segment (part)	Apical intrathoracic anastomosis	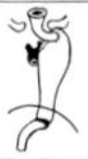	X	o	X	o	o	o
	(Same) 10. Lower fourth, middle half, & all of superior mediastinal segment	(Same) Intracervical (supra-clavicular)	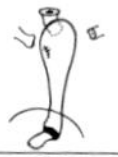	X	o	X	o	o	o
	Total esophagectomy 11. Entire esophagus	Pharyngogastric anastomosis	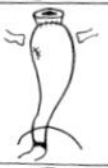	(X)	o	X	o	o	o
	(Same) 12. Entire esophagus	Pharyngojejunal anastomosis	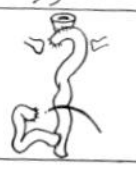	(o)	o	X	o	o	o

Legend:
X Usual indication
(X) Unusual indication
(O) Improbable indication
O Not indicated

Fig. 107. Chart summary of procedures employed in the surgery of the esophagus.

For the latter purpose it is usually sufficient to leave the tube in position with its tip just above the level of the anastomosis. In this way the possibility of injury to the suture line because of pressure by the tube is avoided. When a high intrathoracic or cervical esophagogastric anastomosis has been made, it is wise to pass the tube through the anastomosis to prevent the disturbing consequences of overdistention of the large intrathoracic stomach with air or fluid. In such cases the tube should be left in place for approximately four to five days.

Operations on Esophagus. As an introduction to the various operative procedures which may be employed in dealing with the lesions of the esophagus requiring surgical treatment, the outline presented in Figure 107 is submitted. It represents pictorially and in summary the procedures ordinarily used and suggests their most frequent applications. These may be arranged in groups as follows:

Group 1. *Esophagotomy*
   1. Longitudinal incision for removal of impacted foreign bodies or excision of benign tumors. It is completed by lengthwise closure of the incision.
Group 2. *Plastic Operations Without Resection*
   1. Excision of a web through a longitudinal incision with lengthwise closure.
   2. Esophagoplasty by longitudinal incision followed by circumferential closure; used in achalasia and certain cases of benign stricture.
Group 3. *Resection with Restoration of Continuity (Esophagectomy)*
   1. Segmental resection with
      (*a*) *End-to-end anastomosis* used occasionally for short stricture (benign).
      (*b*) *Interposition of a skin tube* used in cervical segment for resection of carcinoma.
   2. Partial esophagectomy with esophagogastric anastomosis at the following levels:
      (*a*) *Supradiaphragmatic* for carcinoma of cardia and lower esophagus, inflammatory strictures, chemical obliteration (when confined to lower end) and massive benign tumor at lower end (leiomyoma).
      (*b*) *Subaortic* for same lesions as above at a somewhat higher level.
      (*c*) *Supra-aortic* for same lesions as above extending behind the aortic arch.
   3. Subtotal esophagectomy with esophagogastric anastomosis at the following levels:
      (*a*) *Apical intrathoracic* for same lesions as above extending into the lower portion of the superior mediastinal segment of the esophagus.
      (*b*) *Intracervical* (supraclavicular) for same lesions extending into the upper portion of the superior mediastinal or lower portion of the cervical segments of esophagus.
   4. Total esophagectomy with anastomosis as follows:
      (*a*) *Pharyngogastric* for total obliteration of esophagus by chemical burning.
      (*b*) *Pharyngojejunal* for same indication.

Note: In any instance following esophagectomy, whether partial, subtotal or total, the jejunum may be employed for the restoration of continuity instead of the stomach. The stomach is better functionally and mechanically.

OPERATIONS FOR CONDITIONS RESULTING FROM TRAUMA

Suture of Perforations

Perforations of the esophagus may result from instrumental manipulations either during the course of an esophagoscopic examination or in the attempt to dilate a stricture. Many such cases respond favorably to conservative management consisting of the prohibition of oral intake and the administration of penicillin and streptomycin. In a few, however, the prompt resort to surgical exploration with the intent to suture the laceration may be relied upon to save the patient the dangers and annoyances of prolonged mediastinal and pleural sepsis with fistula formation. The decision must be made soon after the injury is sustained.

The same reasoning holds true in cases of penetrating wounds from sharp instruments, projectiles or flying objects such as broken glass. If not too much time has elapsed after the injury, the laceration may be closed in layers, using interrupted sutures of fine material such as 5–0 silk (or catgut). Either the cervical or the thoracic approach is chosen, depending upon the location of the injury. If the thoracic portion of the esophagus is involved as a result of instrumental perforation or the laceration produced by a foreign body such as an open safety pin, a right thoracotomy incision is used. If the source of the injury is a penetrating wound of the chest, the side through which the traumatizing object entered is preferred. In either instance the lung should be inspected for injuries. If any are discovered, suitable débridement and suture of lacerations should be carried out as indicated. After the esophageal laceration has been dealt with, the lung should be expanded completely. Before the chest is closed, a catheter is inserted for continuous suction drainage in order to maintain expansion of the lung and to remove the extravasated blood and plasma which accumulates during the early recovery period. Liberal use should be made of the antibiotics.

Esophagotomy for the Extraction of Impacted Foreign Bodies

The majority of impacted foreign bodies can be removed through the esophagoscope. If they cannot be extracted by this means, they may be pushed into the stomach whence they may be removed through a laparotomy incision if they fail to pass through the gastrointestinal tract in the natural manner. If these measures fail, a direct approach may be necessary through a cervical or a standard thoracotomy incision as the case may require. A longitudinal incision is made with a knife through all layers of the esophageal wall in the area where the foreign body lies. After the object has been removed, the opening in the esophagus is closed by means of interrupted sutures, using a layer in the mucosa, a second layer to approximate the muscle edges, and sometimes an outer layer of mattress sutures to invert the suture line (Fig. 106). It is wise to employ closed catheter drainage of the thorax. In the cervical region a drain is not required.

LOCAL OPERATIONS FOR CERTAIN BENIGN LESIONS

Operations for Webs and Localized Strictures

Strictures of limited longitudinal extent and weblike constrictions are unusual except at either end of the esophagus. The majority of such lesions respond favorably to instrumental dilatation. In a few cases a direct surgical approach must be made and one of three methods of dealing with the condition may be chosen depending on the exigencies of the case.

Excision of an Esophageal Web. In rare instances a weblike stenosis may exist which for some reason cannot be dealt with by instrumental dilatation. These occlusions consist of a diaphragm-like constriction involving the mucosa almost exclusively. They occur most frequently in the cervical segment. The esophagus is exposed in the usual manner and a longitudinal incision is made through all layers near the region where the web lies. The incision is extended sufficiently to open the lumen both above and below the lesion. The web is excised with a curved scissors and the mucosal edges at its base are approximated with sutures of fine silk. The esophagotomy opening is then closed longitudinally as already described (Fig. 106).

Plastic Enlargement of a Stricture (Esophagoplasty). This method applies to sharply localized strictures. The esophagus is exposed and a longitudinal incision is made through its wall in the constricted area. If more than the mucous membrane is involved, the difficulty may be overcome by circumferential closure with three layers of sutures. This procedure is applicable, however, only if the longitudinal extent of the stricture is very limited. The details of the technic are described in the section dealing with esophagoplasty for achalasia (Figs. 114, 115 and 116).

Local Resection and End-to-End Approximation. Sometimes the longitudinal extent of the stricture, although too great for correction by esophagoplasty, is still short enough to permit the excision of a small segment followed by an end-to-end approximation. In order to make the procedure possible, a limited degree of mobilization of the proximal and distal ends of the divided esophagus may be necessary. The availability of an adequate blood supply to each end must be kept in mind and the freeing must be confined to safe limits (not over 3 to 4 cm. each way, depending upon the location of the available arteries). If placed carefully and without any tension on the suture line, two layers of fine silk sutures suffice for this type of anastomosis. The avoidance of tension and the preservation of an adequate blood supply to each sutured end are of such infinite importance that the failure to observe either of these details might mean the death of the patient from separation of the edges. It is unwise to pass a Levin tube through such an anastomosis.

Closure of Acquired Fistulas

Esophagopleural Fistula. A fistulous communication between the esophagus and the pleural cavity may be the result of trauma or it may in rare instances be a complication of empyema of the pleural space. Fistulas resulting from the perforation of an esophageal carcinoma are obviously not amenable to closure and are not included in this discussion. The surgical problem in the noncarcinoma cases varies in degree depending on the size of the opening, a rough estimate of which can be made by observing the kind and amount of esophageal contents which escape.

The first consideration is to establish adequate external drainage of the empyema cavity. If the amount of leakage from the esophagus is excessive, a temporary gastrostomy should be performed. The necessity for the oral intake of foods and fluids is thereby eliminated and the volume of material which might escape through the fistula is greatly diminished. After a suitable period of observation and preparation the patient is operated upon. If the fistulous opening is small, an attempt to close it without the benefit of a preliminary gastrostomy is justifiable.

TECHNIC. Intratracheal inhalation anesthesia is administered, using a cuffed tube. The chest is opened through a standard incision. Except in children, the rib resection method provides the best exposure. The empyema cavity is explored and the fistula opening is found. An incision is made through the mediastinal pleura around the fistulous opening and the esophagus above and below it is identified. The edges of the fistula are freshened and the thickened inflammatory tissue is excised. The esophagus must be mobilized sufficiently to permit closure and infolding of the opening. The closure is made longitudinally with two layers of sutures, one in the mucosa and a second in the muscularis (Fig. 106). Sometimes the tissues are pliable enough to make it possible to reinforce the closure by means of a third layer consisting of mattress sutures. Fine silk is used. Whether or not infolding is impossible, it is advantageous to suture a flap of the mediastinal pleura to the esophagus over the suture line to give additional security.

If the case is one which occurred after pneumonectomy, nothing further is done except to close the incision. If the lung is present and if it is not in itself the seat of a pathologic process which might make it injudicious to do so, a pulmonary decortication should be performed in the hope of bringing about the rapid obliteration of the empyema cavity. In either event drainage should be provided by inserting a catheter through one of the lower intercostal spaces. Protection with antibiotics is highly desirable.

During the postoperative period the patient must be maintained by means of parenteral feeding with intravenous infusions or by means of the gastrostomy which may have been made to improve the preoperative condition of those whose fistula is large. Oral intake should be withheld for several days, after which small amounts of clear liquids taken slowly may be allowed. More nutritious liquids are added as the convalescence progresses, and by the tenth postoperative day very soft solids can usually be tolerated with safety.

The removal of the drainage tube from the chest should follow the principles laid down in the discussion of the management of empyema (Chap. 5).

Esophagobronchial or Esophagotracheal Fistulas. An acquired fistulous communication between the esophagus and the trachea or a major bronchus, other than those resulting from ulceration of a carcinoma, is usually caused by erosion of a calcareous deposit in a mediastinal lymph node. These are almost invariably tuberculous in origin, but the active phase of the disease has in the majority of instances long since disappeared. In many of these patients there is a history of expectorating stonelike objects (broncholiths). The fistulous tract between the two organs is usually small and the orifices are narrow (Fig. 108, *A*).

TECHNIC. Intratracheal inhalation anesthesia is used. A right standard thoracotomy incision usually provides the best access to the diseased area. The mediastinal pleura is incised and the esophagus is dissected free both above and below the region of the fistula. The posterior surface of the

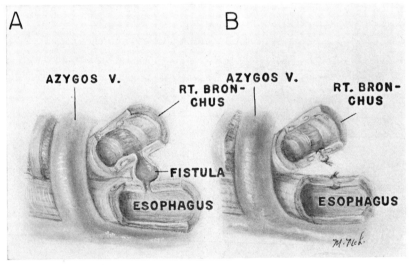

Fig. 108. Acquired broncho-esophageal fistula. *A*, Diagram of the fistula between the right main bronchus and the esophagus. *B*, Diagram illustrating the method of closure. *Note:* There was a history of expectoration of broncholiths in this case. These were calcareous deposits originating in adjacent chronic tuberculous lymphadenitis.

trachea or bronchus is cleared, and the fistula tract is divided. The edges of the orifices in each organ are freshened by trimming any unhealthy tissue which may remain and the closure of each is begun. With the trachea or bronchus only a single layer of fine silk sutures can be used because of the impossibility of inverting the suture line in the semirigid tube. The closure must, therefore, be reinforced with a pleural flap applied with a double row of fine sutures, one on each side of the suture line used to close the opening (see *Excision of Tracheal Cysts*, Chap. 7). When the fistula involves a bronchus, an adjacent surface of the lung may be used. The closure of the esophageal opening is made as described above. This likewise should be covered by a pleural flap if it is available (Fig. 108, *B*). In order to provide drainage into the pleural cavity, the incision in the mediastinal pleura is not closed. The usual closed catheter drainage of the chest should be provided.

The after-care follows the lines set forth above.

Operations for Congenital Atresia of the Esophagus with Tracheo-esophageal Fistula

Although it is necessary to know before the operation is begun which of the several anatomic types of anomaly is present in a given case, their differentiation is not a subject for the present discussion (Fig. 109). In general,

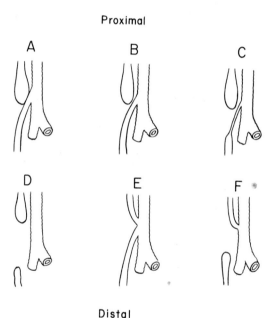

Fig. 109. Diagram depicting some of the anatomic variations observed in cases of congenital tracheo-esophageal fistula with atresia of the esophagus. *A,* Distal end fistula with long proximal pouch attached to the distal segment by means of a membrane of mucosa, suitable for anastomosis. *B,* Distal end fistula; long proximal pouch unattached, suitable for anastomosis. *C,* Distal end fistula, but with elongated area of atresia sometimes reduced to merely a cord without a lumen; long proximal pouch, unsuitable for anastomosis. *D,* No fistula; anastomosis possible if the proximal and distal ends are long enough. *E,* Double fistulous communication, usually suitable for anastomosis, sometimes merely lateral wall closure. *F,* Proximal end fistula; distal pouch, frequently suitable for anastomosis.

the surgeon must be prepared to deal with the condition in one of two ways, either by closure of the fistula and primary end-to-end anastomosis between the proximal and distal segments of the esophagus or by closure of the fistula and the establishment of a cervical esophagostomy and a gastrostomy for feeding, followed later by restoration of continuity by some reconstructive procedure. By adequate mobilization of the lower segment of the esophagus it is possible to perform a primary anastomosis in the majority of the patients.

Only a light anesthesia is required, but some means of inflating the lung must be provided. This can be accomplished by means of a small catheter of suitable caliber passed through the nose into the trachea, with control of the pressure supplied either by a direct connection to the anesthesia apparatus or by means of a tightly fitted face mask especially designed for use on infants.

The incision is made intercostally in the right side through the fifth interspace. The difficulties of maintaining good aeration of the lung are such, however, that it may be preferable to resort to an extrapleural approach unless an anesthetist who has had special training in the anesthetization of such small patients is available. If this method is adopted, several adjacent ribs must be transected posteriorly in order to provide an adequate exposure.

The ensuing description is based upon the use of the transpleural approach.

One-stage Procedure; Closure of Fistula with Primary Anastomosis. The operation should be performed with the lung as completely expanded as possible at all times. Total atelectasis occurs in infants with great rapidity and the surgeon must inform the anesthetist if it should occur so that prompt reexpansion of the lung may be brought about.

The mediastinal pleura is incised and the fistula is identified. It is usually advisable to divide the azygos vein close to the superior vena cava to improve the exposure (Fig. 110, *A* and *B*). The communication may be found between either the proximal or the distal segment and the trachea. The knowledge of the type of condition which is likely to be found can be determined beforehand (Fig. 109). In each instance the attachment of the esophageal segment should be cut absolutely flush with the surface of the trachea in order to preserve every available millimeter of length. The opening in the trachea is closed with interrupted fine sutures (Fig. 110, *C*). Additional protection should be provided by approximating a layer of peritracheal areolar tissue from the mediastinum over the suture line or by the method of attaching a flap of pleura as already mentioned.

The proximal esophageal segment is found and, if long enough to make an end-to-end approximation possible, it is dissected free for use in the anastomosis. If the two ends do not come together easily, additional relaxation may be obtained by extensive mobilization of the distal segment. This maneuver makes it possible to perform a satisfactory anastomosis in almost all cases except those where the proximal pouch does not reach below the neck. The end of the pouch, whether proximal or distal, is opened and a suitable edge is developed for suturing (Fig. 110, *C*). The anastomosis is made without clamps, using two layers of 5–0 arterial silk attached to an atraumatic needle which minimizes the amount of injury to the delicate wall of the esophagus. The mucosal edges are sutured first. A second row of sutures is used to unite the muscle layers edge to edge. No attempt should

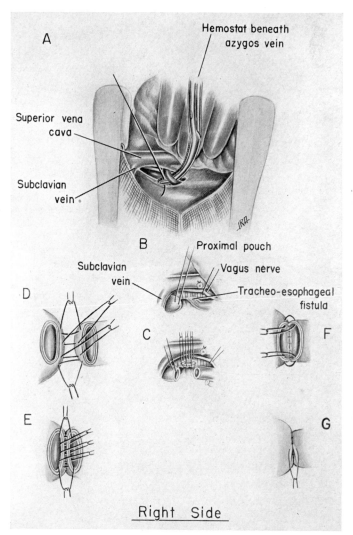

Fig. 110. Congenital tracheo-esophageal fistula with atresia of the esophagus. Operative technic; drawn from a case with long proximal pouch and distal fistula communication. *A*, exposure of the operative field obtained by a right transpleural approach through the fourth intercostal space. The first step in the ligation and division of the azygos vein is shown. *B*, Anatomic relations of the organs before severance of the fistula tract. *C*, Closure of the opening in the trachea. The two ends of the esophagus have been trimmed in preparation for the anastomosis. *D*, Anastomosis; posterior muscular layer of sutures (mattress type). *E*, Anastomosis; posterior mucosal layer of sutures. *F*, Anastomosis; anterior mucosal layer of sutures. *G*, Anastomosis; anterior muscular layer of sutures.

be made to invert the suture line with a third row because of the danger of producing a stenosis or of tearing out the sutures as a result of excessive tension (Fig. 110, *E*, *F* and *G*).

A catheter of small caliber is brought out through a lower intercostal space for continuous aspiration; the lung is expanded completely, and the chest wall is closed in the established manner. If the operation has been excessively time-consuming, it is wise to use continuous chromicized catgut sutures of fine size (3–0 or 4–0) in the muscle layers instead of the customary interrupted silk. This maneuver reduces considerably the time required for closure.

Small amounts of feeding formula can be allowed after forty-eight hours, with gradual increases in volume over the ensuing few days. Continuous vigilance is demanded in these patients to avoid the aspiration into the trachea of fluid or secretions, and repeated recourse to aspiration of the pharynx and trachea is often necessary for this purpose. The usual methods of administering fluids parenterally in infants are employed. A competent pediatrician should be in attendance at all times.

Two-stage Procedure; Closure of the Fistula, Establishment of a Cervical Esophagostomy and Gastrostomy Followed by Secondary Restoration of Continuity. FIRST STAGE. In a few patients, when either segment of the esophagus happens to be too short to permit the performance of an anastomosis, a two-stage procedure must be resorted to. In fact, it is sometimes impossible to determine beforehand whether a primary anastomosis can be made or not. The incision and exposure are the same as in the one-stage operation. The fistulous opening in the trachea is closed and covered in the usual manner (Fig. 110, *A, B* and *C*). If the proximal pouch is too short for the performance of an anastomosis, the end of the distal segment, if it happens to be the open one as is usually the case, is closed by inversion with a purse-string suture. The chest wall is then sutured.

The remainder of the preliminary operative procedure involves the exteriorization of the proximal blind segment of the esophagus and the performance of a gastrostomy for feeding.

The cervical esophagostomy must be made at the time of the closure of the fistula because of the danger of aspiration of saliva by the infant. To accomplish this a short incision is made over the anterior edge of the sternocleidomastoid muscle on the left side. The dissection is deepened in front of the carotid sheath and the prevertebral space is entered. There the proximal segment of the esophagus is found and drawn gently into the wound. It may be necessary to transect the omohyoid muscle. The blind pouch (except in the cases where the proximal segment has a fistulous communication with the trachea) is opened immediately and the edges are sutured to the skin edges of the cervical incision.

The gastrostomy may be established at the same time, but in the majority of cases it is probably better to delay this step of the procedure for a few days, maintaining the infant by parenteral alimentation in the meantime. Because of the fact that the gastrostomy is to be temporary and in order to reduce the amount of distortion of the stomach to a minimum, the rubber catheter method should be used. The tube may be inserted by the Stamm or the Kader technic through a short muscle-splitting incision in the upper portion of the left rectus muscle. There is no objection to suturing the stomach wall adjacent to the catheter to the parietal peritoneum on either side of the incision, but the omentum should not be drawn up.

SECOND STAGE; CLOSURE OF THE GASTROSTOMY AND RESTORATION OF CONTINUITY BY INTRACERVICAL ESOPHAGOGASTRIC ANASTOMOSIS. Formerly, in the unfortunate patients for whom a primary anastomosis could not be performed, attempts to restore continuity of the alimentary canal were made by external esophagoplasty, usually using skin tubes developed from the anterior thoracic wall. A few successes were obtained, but the method is so difficult, time-consuming and ultimately inadequate from the functional point of view that it should be abandoned in favor of esophagogastric anastomosis.

The optimum time for the performance of the second and final stage of the combined procedure cannot be arbitrarily decided. It is probably unwise to do it during the first two years of life because of the fact that the stomach of an infant is relatively so large in relation to the volume of the thorax. Furthermore, the stomach is of necessity distended much of the time by large feedings of liquid and the air which is invariably swallowed in large quantities by infants. During the first eighteen months of life, therefore, the stomach would encroach too much upon the pulmonary volume if it were placed within the chest as the operation requires. Furthermore, if this principle is accepted, it is even more obvious that to perform an intracervical or even intrathoracic esophagogastric anastomosis as a part of the first operation on the newborn infant would be unwise. Therefore, a delay of eighteen to twenty-four months is desirable.

The operation is performed in one stage. It consists of three steps as follows.

FIRST STEP; MOBILIZATION OF THE STOMACH AND EXCISION OF THE DISTAL SEGMENT OF ESOPHAGUS. A standard thoracotomy incision is made through the eighth intercostal space on the left side. A small rib spreader is inserted. The phrenic nerve is crushed. The diaphragm is incised from a point close to its costal insertion through the margin of the esophageal hiatus. The rudimentary distal segment of the esophagus is freed through an incision in the mediastinal pleura, ligated just above the cardia, and removed. The remaining stump is inverted with a purse-string suture of silk reinforced by several Lembert sutures of the same material. The anterior wall of the stomach is then freed from its attachment to the abdominal wall and the gastrostomy opening is closed with two layers of fine silk sutures. The suture line of the closure must be made lengthwise on the stomach so as to avoid longitudinal shortening. The attachments of the fundus of the stomach are divided, including the gastrolienal ligament and the vasa brevia which must be ligated. The left gastro-epiploic vessels are tied and cut and the entire gastrocolic ligament is incised all the way to the level of the pylorus, taking care to avoid injury to the arcade of vessels along the greater curvature which is supplied by the right gastro-epiploic vessels. The left gastric artery and vein are tied and cut. The gastrohepatic ligament is then incised as far as the level of the pylorus. Here likewise the integrity of the vascular arches along the lesser curvature, which are supplied by the right gastric artery and vein, must be preserved. It is important to mention that the left gastric artery should be severed close to its origin from the celiac axis so as to preserve

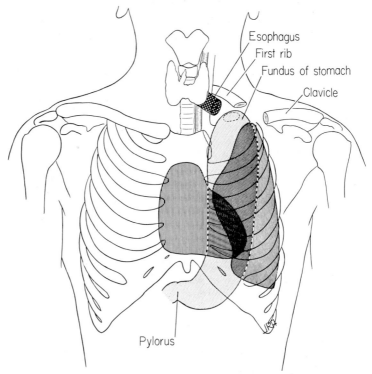

Fig. 111. Congenital tracheo-esophageal fistula treated in two stages. Diagram of the second stage to show the principle involved in the restoration of continuity by esophago-gastric anastomosis. The stomach has been mobilized sufficiently to draw the fundus into the neck through a passageway from the apex of the left thorax to the base of the neck, created by excising the inner end of the clavicle and of the first rib.

the peripheral branches which form the greater portion of the arcade along the lesser curvature. The stomach is now sufficiently well mobilized to allow the fundus to be pulled up through the thorax into the neck (Fig. 111). (*Note:* The technical details employed in this procedure are identical with those described and illustrated in the section dealing with esophagectomy for carcinoma in the superior mediastinal segment [Chap. 9, Fig. 136]).

The stomach is drawn as high as possible into the left thoracic cavity and is prevented from falling back into the abdomen by means of a series of sutures between the antral portion and the adjacent pleural edge overlying the descending aorta. The fundus is allowed to lie free in the upper portion of the chest. The diaphragm is closed around the stomach just above the pylorus. Its edges are sutured to the stomach wall with fine silk. An adequate opening somewhat larger than the size of the normal esophageal hiatus must be provided.

To complete the first step of the operation the lung is expanded completely and the thoracotomy incision is closed in the usual manner. A small catheter is inserted through the ninth or tenth intercostal space for closed suction drainage.

SECOND STEP; PERFORMANCE OF THE INTRACERVICAL ESOPHAGOGASTRIC ANASTOMOSIS. After the closure of the thoracotomy incision has been completed, the patient is turned on his back and a vertical incision is made from the esophagostomy stoma above to the level of the second rib below. The pectoralis major muscle is incised close to its attachment to the sternum and reflected laterally, at the same time separating its insertion on the medial portion of the clavicle. The sternal and medial clavicular insertions of the sternocleidomastoid muscle are severed and retracted laterally. The incision is then carried around the esophageal stoma and enough of the end of the esophagus is freed to make it possible to perform an anastomosis. This mobilization must not be too extensive for fear of jeopardizing the blood supply to the end which must be preserved for the anastomosis.

The medial half of the clavicle and a corresponding segment of the left first rib and costal cartilage are resected extraperiosteally. This produces a large opening from the base of the neck behind the lower end of the sternocleidomastoid muscle into the apex of the left pleural cavity through which the fundus of the stomach can be drawn easily and without danger of compression. The fundus is pulled up behind the apex of the lung into the lower portion of the neck. A short incision is made in the posterior wall of the fundus close to its apex and an anastomosis consisting of three layers of interrupted fine silk sutures is made. Careful approximations of mucosa to mucosa and muscle edge to muscle edge constitute the inner and middle layers. The outer layer is of interrupted mattress sutures. Several interrupted sutures are used to fasten the fundus to the tissues surrounding the region of the anastomosis. The wound is closed by suturing the lower end of the sternocleidomastoid muscle and the cut edge of the pectoral muscle to the sternum and placing a layer of fine silk sutures in the subcutaneous fat and another in the skin. No drainage is used.

THIRD STEP; CLOSURE OF THE ABDOMINAL WALL AT THE GASTROSTOMY SITE. The edges of the former gastrostomy incision in the abdominal wall are excised. The fascia and peritoneum are identified and a layer by layer closure is brought about, using interrupted fine chromic catgut sutures with silk to the skin.

After-care. Following operation the patient is kept in an oxygen tent for the first few days. The pharynx should be aspirated frequently if secretions accumulate. Close watch should be maintained to detect overdistention of the stomach and prompt resort made to deflation by means of a small catheter inserted perorally or intranasally as required. The condition of the patient must be maintained during the first week or ten days by means of the intravenous administration of solutions containing the necessary electrolytes, dextrose, amino acids and vitamins. If the hemoglobin level is low, blood is given. The intravenous alimentation is made continuous so as to avoid frequent piercing of veins with a needle. A polyethylene tube of small caliber inserted through an open incision into a vein such as the saphenous vein just above the ankle is very satisfactory for this purpose.

Fluids may be given orally after five to seven days and the amount increased slowly over the next few days. Soft foods may be allowed in gradually increasing amounts from the tenth day on. It should be kept in mind, however, that the child is not accustomed to eating in a normal manner and he may have to learn how to eat enough to maintain his nutrition. It may take several weeks before he is able to consume enough food to provide for a gain in body weight.

The growth and development of children who have been subjected to this method of restoring continuity proceeds in a normal manner after a period of readjustment to the new situation. There is no apparent limitation of activity or accomplishment, and the function of the left arm and shoulder girdle is not impaired.

Diverticulectomy

True pulsion diverticula of the esophagus occur, with almost no exceptions, either at the junction of the hypopharynx with the esophagus or in the supradiaphragmatic portion. Diverticula observed in other segments are almost invariably of the so-called traction type and are not, strictly speaking, true diverticula. They consist merely of distortions of the wall of the esophagus produced by adhesions to inflammatory areas in the immediate vicinity such as in the case of subcarinal mediastinal lymphadenitis.

Excision of a Diverticulum of the Pharyngo-esophageal Junction. ONE-STAGE PROCEDURE. The success of the one-stage operation depends upon careful attention to the details of technic required in the handling of the esophagus. The most important of these are the utilization of fine suture material, the avoidance of trauma, insistence upon accurate hemostasis and the omission of drains and intraluminal tubes. The prophylactic administration of antibiotics is an important adjunct.

The operation is performed under inhalation anesthesia, using an intratracheal tube. The patient is placed on his back in the position used for thyroidectomy, but hyperextension of the head and neck should be avoided because it tends to decrease the space between the trachea and the vertebral column and interferes to some extent with the ease of access to the diverticulum. The left side of the neck is chosen unless the case is one where the

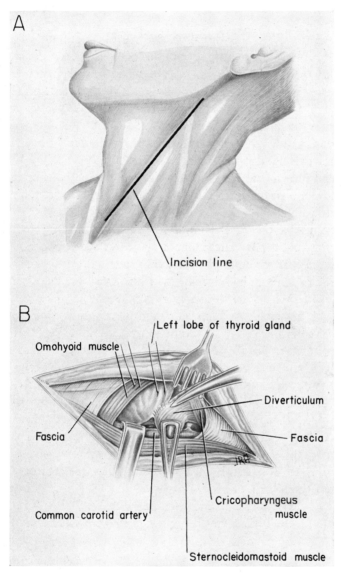

A

Incision line

B

Left lobe of thyroid gland

Omohyoid muscle

Diverticulum

Fascia

Fascia

Common carotid artery

Cricopharyngeus muscle

Sternocleidomastoid muscle

Fig. 112. Diverticulectomy; excision of pulsion diverticulum of pharyngo-esophagea junction. A, Left side of the neck, showing the direction of the incision over the anterior margin of the sternocleidomastoid muscle. B, Details of the exposure of the diverticulum.

diverticulum bulges to the right or unless the surgeon is left-handed, when the right-sided approach is more convenient. An oblique incision is made through the skin, fat and platysma muscle over the anterior border of the sternocleidomastoid muscle. The muscle is retracted posteriorly. The left lobe of the thyroid and the overlying sternohyoid and sternothyroid muscles are retracted medially. The omohyoid muscle is retracted downward and medially, or it may be divided if a larger exposure is desired. The left superior thyroid vessels are usually encountered and may be divided if they interfere with the exposure. The ansa hypoglossi nerve is sometimes in the way and may be cut at the apex of its loop without producing any untoward effects. The carotid sheath and its contents are retracted laterally (Fig. 112, *B*).

By blunt dissection with the scissors the retropharyngeal space is entered and the diverticulum is found by enlarging the field downward in this plane. Gentle dissection frees the fundus of the diverticulum which can be grasped with a mucosa forceps and drawn out through the incision. The neck of the sac is developed by careful dissection (Fig. 112, *B*). In doing this several small pharyngeal arteries and veins are encountered extending from the wall of the pharynx onto the surface of the diverticulum. These should be cut and ligated.

The removal of the diverticulum is now begun. The principle of this maneuver is to cut the diverticulum at its base but without encroaching upon the wall of the pharynx or esophagus, so as to avoid the danger of constricting the lumen. The longitudinal opening which results is then closed neatly with two or three layers of fine silk sutures (Fig. 113, *A, B, C* and *D*). An important detail of technic in this step of the procedure is to cut through the outer layers of the diverticulum at an appreciable distance distal to its base (Fig. 113, *A*). This makes allowance for the tendency of the muscularis of the pharynx to retract and makes it possible to avoid concentric narrowing of this structure after the opening has been closed. After circumcising the outer layer of the diverticulum near its base, stay sutures of fine silk may be placed through the muscularis to outline the upper and lower ends of the longitudinal defect. The incision of the mucosa is then begun and after cutting it part way at the upper end, the first mucosal suture is inserted (Fig. 113, *B*). This is done by passing the needle through one edge from within the lumen and back through the opposite edge in the reverse direction so that after it is tied the knot lies inside. This suture is tied and held until the second has been placed, when it is cut just before the latter is pulled up for tying (Fig. 113, *C*). As this is done, the knot of the first stitch is swept inside the lumen by the tightening of the second stitch. This maneuver is repeated with each succeeding suture, the mucosa being divided further and further across the opening until it has been completely severed. The last mucosal stitch is then put in and tied. No effort is made to invert the edges. If the incision through the outer layer of the diverticulum has been properly placed, the edges of the muscle layer can now be approximated with fine silk sutures without tension (Fig. 113, *D*). In the majority of cases a third layer consisting of mattress sutures may be inserted to invert the suture line. This is desirable as an extra protection against leakage, but it is not absolutely essential. The stay sutures at each end of the incision are removed and the esophagus and pharynx are allowed to drop back in place. As this is done, it will be observed that the line of closure lies on the posterior wall of these structures as they assume their normal position.

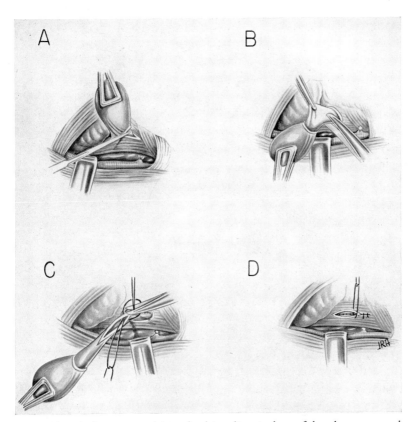

Fig. 113. Diverticulectomy; excision of pulsion diverticulum of the pharyngo-esophageal junction. *A,* Circumcision of the outer layer leaving a muscular edge for subsequent closure. To avoid constriction this incision must not be made too close to the wall of the pharynx. *B,* Outer layer completely divided; mucosa exposed ready for incision and closure. *C,* Placement of the final suture in the mucosal incision before completing the severance of the diverticulum. *D,* Closure of the muscle layer of the hypopharynx by edge-to-edge approximation. (An additional layer of mattress sutures is sometimes inserted to infold the suture line.)

The wound is closed without drainage, using a layer of fine silk sutures in the platysma muscle and another in the skin.

AFTER-CARE. Recovery following operation is usually rapid and the period of hospitalization not over seven to ten days. Every effort should be made, especially during the first forty-eight hours, to avoid retching, vomiting, coughing or swallowing anything which has substance or is large in volume.

A few sips of water are allowed each hour, beginning on the first postoperative day, to prevent excessive dryness of the mouth and to make the swallowing of saliva easier. The necessary amount of fluid containing dextrose, saline and vitamins is administered by venoclysis as indicated. Liquid food is allowed sparingly on the third day, and the amount given at a time is gradually increased each succeeding day until soft solids are begun, usually on the seventh day. From that time on the amount and kind of food are rapidly increased until a normal diet can be tolerated. This is usually by the end of the second week.

The administration of penicillin and streptomycin is continued for a period of four to five days or until any suspicion of sepsis may have subsided.

The patient is allowed out of bed, beginning with the first postoperative day.

Two-stage Procedure. Before the adoption of the present-day improvements in technic and before the advent of the antibiotics, a two-stage operation was preferred. At the first stage the diverticulum was freed and sutured in the upper angle of the cervical incision. The wound was then packed with gauze in order to produce a barrier of inflammatory tissue as a protection against infection of the superior mediastinum. At the second stage several weeks later, the diverticulum was excised. Because the operation no longer has any wide applicability, the details of its technic will not be described here.

Excision of Supradiaphragmatic Diverticulum. Pulsion diverticula in the lower thoracic segment of the esophagus are removed by exactly the same technic as that employed for the one-stage excision of those in the neck. It should be reiterated that the esophagus does not take kindly to the use of crushing clamps, cutting with the cautery and continuous sutures, and all of these should be avoided, The approach to the diverticulum is through a standard thoracotomy incision on either the right or the left side, depending upon which seems to give the better access. In the majority of cases diverticula in this region bulge to the right, making it somewhat easier to get at them from that side, but the left can be used with equal facility in any case. The decision is unimportant.

The after-care presents no specific problems.

Esophagoplasty for Idiopathic Dilatation (Achalasia)

In the little understood condition spoken of as achalasia or idiopathic dilatation of the esophagus and sometimes erroneously called cardiospasm, the segment just above the cardia is anatomically narrowed and relatively atrophic. The lumen is considerably smaller than that of the normal esophagus and the wall is abnormally thin. The principle of the operation is to overcome the effects of this anatomic narrowing. Various procedures have been tried, including longitudinal incision of the muscular coat (Heller operation), lateral anastomosis between the fundus of the stomach and the esophagus above the constriction, and plastic procedures at the cardia similar in principle to the Finney pyloroplasty. The most effective method, as measured by the uniformity and permanence of the relief of dysphagia, is the form of esophagoplasty to be described. This consists of longitudinal incision through all layers of the constricted segment from a wide point on the esophagus above to a correspondingly wide point on the stomach below, followed by circumferential closure of the opening thus produced.

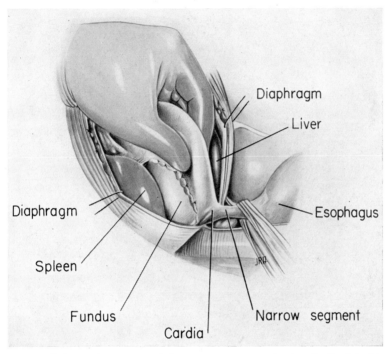

Fig. 114. Achalasia; elimination of the narrow segment by longitudinal incision and circumferential closure. First step: Exposure and freeing of the lower end of the esophagus, cardia and fundus of the stomach. In this, as in the majority of the cases, it was necessary to open the diaphragm in order to mobilize the fundus. The downward pull of the spleen has been eliminated by dividing the upper two thirds of the gastrolienal ligament.

Technic of Longitudinal Incision and Circumferential Closure. Intratracheal inhalation anesthesia is used and a standard thoracotomy incision is made through the eighth intercostal space or through the bed of the ninth rib if the patient is in the older age group.

The mediastinal reflection of the pleura overlying the lower portion of the esophagus is incised longitudinally and the esophagus at that level is mobilized, taking care not to interfere with its blood supply. The pathologically narrow segment is identified and its length is observed (Fig. 114).

A point on the anterior surface of the esophagus at a level where the lumen is sufficiently wide to function well is chosen as the upper limit of the lon-

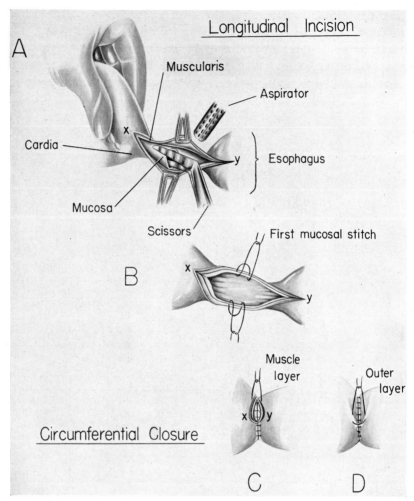

Fig. 115. Achalasia; elimination of the narrow segment by longitudinal incision and circumferential closure. *A,* Incision through the anterior wall of the esophagus from a point at a level of wide circumference on the esophagus (Y) to a point of comparable circumference on the stomach just below the cardia (X). The drawing shows the incision through the muscular layer correctly made and the mucosal layer in the process of being incised. *B,* Commencement of the closure showing the method of inserting the mucosal sutures and the correct starting point on each side of the opening equidistant from the ends (X and Y). *C,* Closure of the muscle layers by edge-to-edge approximation (mucosal layer already closed). Note points X and Y will be drawn together at the completion of this row of sutures. *D,* Insertion of the outer layer consisting of mattress sutures to infold and approximate the esophageal muscularis and the gastric serosa.

gitudinal incision. The lower limit of this incision must lie at or just distal to the cardia where the diameter of the lumen is equivalent to that chosen on the esophagus above the narrowed segment. An incision is then made from the wide upper point to the wide lower point through all layers of the anterior wall (Fig. 115, A). The opening which results is now closed in the opposite or circumferential direction. This maneuver serves to eliminate the long narrow segment of esophagus and substitutes for it a lumen of large size, equivalent to or slightly greater than the actual diameter of the cardia. The technic of the closure is identical with that employed for an esophago-gastric anastomosis or the closure of the defect left after excision of a diverticulum as already described (p. 248). Three layers of fine silk interrupted sutures are used (Fig. 115, B, C and D).

As a result of the circumferential closure of what is often a relatively long longitudinal incision, considerable shortening occurs. This is principally at

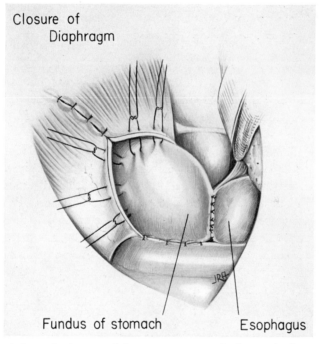

Closure of Diaphragm

Fundus of stomach   Esophagus

Fig. 116. Achalasia; elimination of the narrow segment by longitudinal ncision and circumferential closure. Closure of the diaphragm and fixation of the fundus of the stomach within the chest by means of sutures to the pleura overlying the descending aorta.

the expense of the fundus of the stomach in the region of the cardia and necessitates a moderate amount of mobilization of this portion. If the vasa brevia and upper portion of the gastrolienal ligament are short, a condition which prevails in the majority of patients, it is necessary to incise the diaphragm a short distance from the esophageal hiatus outward so as to gain access to the structures which must be divided. Sufficient mobilization of the fundic and cardiac portions of the stomach can be obtained by dividing the vasa brevia and the peritoneal reflection from the stomach onto the undersurface of the diaphragm (Fig. 115). After the esophageal incision has been closed, the cut edges of the diaphragm are sutured to the stomach in a manner similar to that used in cases of resection of the cardia and lower esophagus as described elsewhere (Fig. 116).

At the completion of the operation a catheter is led out through a short incision in one of the lower intercostal spaces, the lung is expanded fully, and the chest wall is closed in layers, using silk technic.

AFTER-CARE. The after-care is essentially the same as that for any case involving suture or anastomosis of the esophagus. Clear liquids may be allowed at the rate of 30 cc. per hour, beginning on the first postoperative day. The oral feeding program may be advanced at a more rapid rate than in the cases of resection and anastomosis. A normal dietary can usually be resumed by the end of ten to twelve days. (For further details see Chap. 9, p. 290.)

Local Excision of Benign Tumors

Benign tumors of the esophagus are usually intramural and must be removed through a transpleural or transcervical approach, depending upon their location. Occasionally they may be pedunculated and hang down within the lumen. The latter may be removed by means of a snare through the esophagoscope.

Excision of Intramural Benign Tumors. The usual anesthesia is employed. A standard thoracotomy incision is made. The right side may be chosen if one can be certain that there is no possibility that the growth is malignant and would therefore necessitate wide excision and freeing of the stomach for the performance of an esophagogastric anastomosis. If there is reason to believe that a resection of more esophagus than could be treated by end-to-end reapproximation may be required, the left side should be used. The incision is made at whatever level is indicated according to the location of the tumor in relation to the long axis of the chest.

The region of the tumor is exposed by incising the overlying mediastinal pleura, and the tumor-bearing segment of the esophagus is mobilized sufficiently for manipulation. The blood vessels should be disturbed as little as possible. The thinned-out muscular layer over the tumor is incised. If the layer is unusually thin or almost nonexistent, an elliptical incision is made through thicker, more normal tissues, leaving a small amount of thinned-out muscle attached to the growth. The proper plane of cleavage is entered and the mass is dissected free. In the absence of inflammatory or malignant changes, the tumor can usually be shelled out of the surrounding esophageal tissues with about as much ease as a leiomyoma of the uterus in the performance of a myomectomy. In fact, the majority of these tumors are histologically similar to the uterine myomata, arising as they do from smooth muscle cells. The mucosa in the majority of instances remains intact unless it is adherent to the tumor because of attempts made at previous esophagoscopy to obtain tissue for a biopsy. This should be avoided in all cases of benign tumor of the esophagus. If the tumor is an intramural cyst, there is more likelihood of injuring the mucosa because of inflammatory changes resulting from the infection which sometimes develops in such cysts.

The closure of the defect is made in layers, suturing the mucosa (if it has been opened) with fine silk placed so that the knots lie on the side of the lumen, and approximating the muscle layer edge to edge. An additional infolding layer is used if there appears to be no danger of encroachment on the lumen (Fig. 106).

The mediastinal pleural incision is left open. Drainage of the chest is provided with a catheter.

The after-care is the same as that for any patient who has had an incision made in the esophagus. (See Chap. 9, p. 290.)

CHAPTER 9

OPERATIONS ON THE ESOPHAGUS
(Continued)

ESOPHAGECTOMY

Because of recent technical developments in the fields of both anesthesia and surgery, it is now possible to restore the continuity of the alimentary canal after resection of a portion of the esophagus at any level in its course from the hypopharynx to the cardiac end of the stomach. This is accomplished in the cervical region by the interposition of a tube constructed from the skin of the neck. After resection of portions of the thoracic and abdominal segments an esophagogastric anastomosis is performed within the chest or even within the neck after the removal of the superior mediastinal segment. Occasionally the anastomosis may be made between the esophagus and the jejunum.

Although cicatricial stenosis from chemical burns and strictures at the cardia caused by chronic esophagitis with ulceration sometimes require treatment by resection, the most frequent indication for the operation is the necessity for removing a carcinoma. Therefore, the ensuing description is directed toward guidance in the performance of an esophagectomy for carcinoma. Separate consideration will be given, however, to the characteristic findings at operation and the modifications of technic required in the treatment of benign stricture and cicatricial stenosis.

Cervical Segment; Resection with Restoration of Continuity by Means of a Tube of Skin from the Neck

This operation provides for the removal of the cervical segment of the esophagus with a limited number of adjacent lymph nodes. Because of the necessity for preserving the integrity of the blood supply to the large rectangular flap of skin and platysma muscle, it is difficult to perform a sufficiently wide dissection of both sides of the neck to prevent recurrence of the disease from regional node metastases. The scope of the operation is therefore limited and its application should be confined to the earliest and most favorable cases, if possible before any lymph node metastases have occurred. If the growth has arisen on the anterior wall of the esophagus in the retrocricoid region and has invaded the larynx, a laryngectomy can be performed at the same time. Both types of procedure will be described, although the latter has a limited applicability. The operation is performed in two stages.

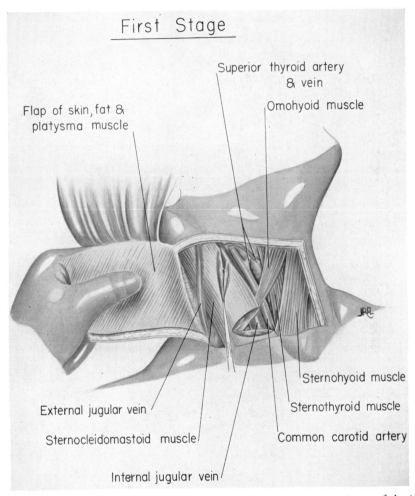

First Stage

Superior thyroid artery & vein

Omohyoid muscle

Flap of skin, fat & platysma muscle

Sternohyoid muscle

Sternothyroid muscle

External jugular vein

Common carotid artery

Sternocleidomastoid muscle

Internal jugular vein

Fig. 117. Cervical esophagectomy without laryngectomy. First stage: Some of the important structures exposed by the reflection of a rectangular flap of skin, fat and platysma are depicted. The excision of a triangular portion of the sternocleidomastoid muscle is shown.

Cervical Esophagectomy Without Laryngectomy. FIRST STAGE. Intratracheal inhalation anesthesia is used. The patient is placed on his back in the position used for thyroidectomy, with moderate hyperextension of the neck. A long rectangular incision is made across the neck, outlining a flap of skin with its base attached on the right and its free end extending to the anterior edge of the left sternocleidomastoid muscle. The upper line of the incision starts just below the angle of the mandible and the lower line just above the clavicle. The two lines are made to converge slightly so that the base of the flap will be approximately 1 inch wider than its free end, which should be about 3 to 3½ inches in the average case. This three-sided incision is deep-

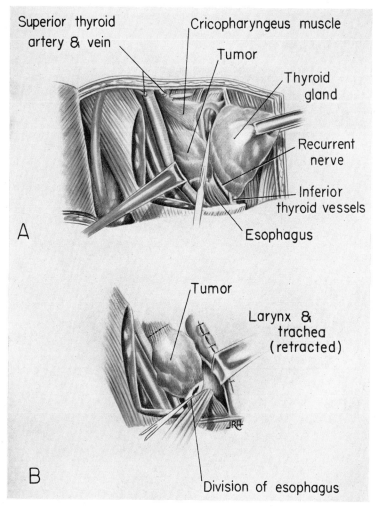

Fig. 118. Cervical esophagectomy. First stage (continued): *A,* Exposure of the tumor in the cervical segment (retrocricoid) and excision of the right lobe of the thyroid gland. *Note:* The remaining edges of the excised sternohyoid and sternothyroid muscles of the right side are shown but not labeled. *B,* Division of the esophagus.

ened through the subcutaneous fat and the platysma muscle. The flap is then dissected back in the layer beneath this muscle to the region of the posterior edge of the right sternocleidomastoid muscle. The flap thus consists of skin, subcutaneous fat and platysma in one thickness (Fig. 117). It is laid between two gauze pads moistened in saline solution. A plane of dissection is developed along the anterior border of the sternocleidomastoid muscle and the prevertebral fascial space is entered, exposing the cervical segment of the esophagus where the growth lies. To obtain an adequate exposure longitudinally it is necessary to transect the omohyoid muscle. If the growth is small and does not invade the larynx and if it is not surrounded by lymph nodes involved in carcinomatous metastases, the way is prepared for its removal. The dissection is carried up as far as the hypopharynx and down to the superior mediastinum. The superior and inferior thyroid arteries and one or two pharyngeal arteries are severed. The corresponding veins are divided. The sternal attachment of the sternocleidomastoid muscle is cut close to its insertion into the bone and a long, triangular-shaped section of the muscle belly is excised (Fig. 117). This is to facilitate the proper fitting of the flap against the prevertebral fascia in that area. The right sternohyoid and sternothyroid muscles are excised and the right lobe of the thyroid gland is removed, cutting across the isthmus just to the left of the trachea (Fig. 118, *A*). During this part of the procedure the right recurrent laryngeal nerve is exposed in the lower part of the field of operation and unless it is invaded by tumor, it should be preserved.

The esophagus is separated from the trachea and a piece of tape or narrow Penrose drain is passed around it to be used for retraction. The dissection between the esophagus and the prevertebral fascia is continued up to the pharyngeal region. The esophagus is cut across as far as possible below the growth but not so low that it will be difficult to suture the lower edge of the flap to the distal end. The lower limit of practicability is approximately at the level of the superior border of the clavicle. The transection above the tumor is usually at the pharyngo-esophageal junction. Rarely it is possible to preserve a very short proximal stump of esophagus, but only in the case of a low-lying small growth. A few small vessels which approach the esophagus from the left must be ligated and cut. A strand of fine silk is passed with a needle through each side of the open end of the lower segment to provide traction (Fig. 118, *B*).

The skin and platysma muscle flap is now turned over into the defect and fastened by means of two rows of fine chromic catgut (5–0) sutures between the platysma and the prevertebral fascia. The right lateral row is inserted first and tied before the left lateral row is put in (Fig. 119, *A*). This maneuver fixes the posterior surface of the flap. The next step is to attach the upper edge of the flap to the pharynx and the lower edge to the esophagus. This is done with two layers of sutures. The outer or peripheral layer approximates the platysma muscle and the muscularis of the pharynx and esophagus. The inner layer joins the skin and the mucous membrane of the two organs. Fine chromic catgut interrupted sutures are used. The posterior muscle layer is inserted first both above and below as far as the left corner on each edge. When this point is reached, the approximation of the skin and mucosa is made. The same suture material is used, but small, fine, cutting point needles are needed to pierce the skin (Fig. 119, *B*).

After the posterior inner layers are completed, the approximation of the anterior edges is begun by continuing the mucosa to skin layer both above

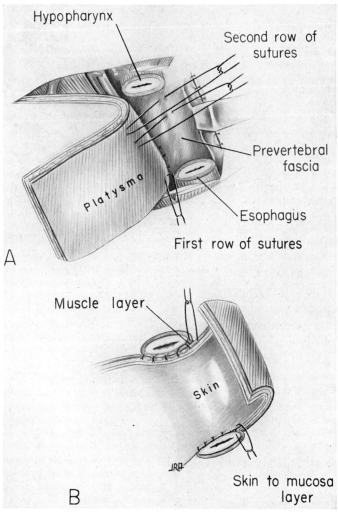

Fig. 119. Cervical esophagectomy. First stage (continued): *A,* Suture of the flap to the prevertebral fascia. *B,* Suture of the edges of the flap to the posterior margins of the hypopharynx above and the esophagus below.

and below. This is continued around to the right as far as the starting point on the circumference of the esophagus and pharynx. The muscle layer is inserted next (Fig. 120, *A*). The remaining free end of the flap is then turned to the left over the larynx and the trachea. Its edges are sutured in layers to the upper and lower edges of the incision as far as the tip of the flap. The defect on the left side of the neck which results from the shortening of the flap produced by folding it into the depths of the neck is covered by a primary Thiersch graft obtained from the skin of the left thigh by an assistant. The superior and inferior edges to the right of the infolding of the flap are sutured, also in two layers. Silk is used in the skin (Fig. 120, *B*).

As a result of the surgical trauma in the region of the pharynx and larynx, a considerable degree of edema and swelling of the tissues develops, reaching a maximum sometime between twelve and forty-eight hours after the completion of the operation. The swelling is sometimes so great that serious obstruction of the airway through the larynx results and an emergency tracheotomy may become necessary. Therefore, it is preferable to perform a tracheotomy as a part of the primary procedure in all cases. This is done through a short incision in the skin just above the suprasternal notch (Fig. 120, *B*). The tube is held in place by means of tapes tied around the neck in the usual manner.

A sterilized Levin tube is inserted into the stomach through the lateral groove produced by the infolded flap.

AFTER-CARE. The after-care following the first stage of the operation presents no special problems. The antibiotics should be continued for five to seven days postoperatively. Feeding through the Levin tube is begun as soon as the patient has recovered sufficiently from the effects of the anesthetic, usually on the subsequent day. The patient's nutrition is provided by a liquid gastrostomy formula during the interval between the stages.

The tracheotomy tube is removed after the danger of obstruction of the airway from laryngeal edema has subsided. This is usually on the third to the fifth day.

SECOND STAGE. The second stage must not be attempted until the wound is completely healed and the subcutaneous tissues are soft and pliable. This also allows enough time to elapse for the implanted skin to acquire a blood supply from the bed in which it lies. The usual interval of time is approximately two months.

The patient is anesthetized in the usual manner. The Levin tube is removed and replaced by a second tube which is inserted through the nose and threaded down the pharynx, through the skin groove, into the esophagus and stomach. An elliptical incision is made around the periphery of the lateral groove, allowing a sufficient margin for closure (Fig. 121, *A*). The inner edges are approximated with a layer of fine catgut sutures inserted so that the knots, when tied, are inside the lumen. A second layer of connective tissue and muscle is brought together over this. The outer edges of the wound are approximated in layers in the same manner (Fig. 121, *B*).

After recovery from anesthesia the patient is fed by means of the Levin tube for a period of approximately seven to ten days. The tube is then

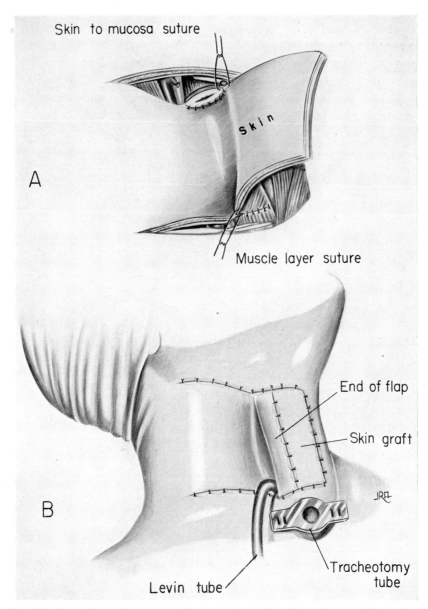

Skin to mucosa suture

A

Skin

Muscle layer suture

B

End of flap

Skin graft

Levin tube

Tracheotomy tube

Fig. 120. Cervical esophagectomy. First stage (completion): *A*, Suture of the edges of the flap to the anterior margins of the hypopharynx and the esophagus. *B*, Completion of the skin closure showing Thiersch graft in place. Levin tube for feeding and tracheotomy tube as a temporary measure to avoid strangulation from laryngeal edema. This is to be removed after the expiration of a few days.

removed and oral feeding is begun. The patient does not as a rule experience any difficulty with deglutition.

Cervical Esophagectomy with Laryngectomy. In the presence of direct invasion of the larynx by the growth, it is justifiable to remove the larynx with the cervical segment of the esophagus if there is relatively little evidence of lymph node metastasis. The number of such cases is small.

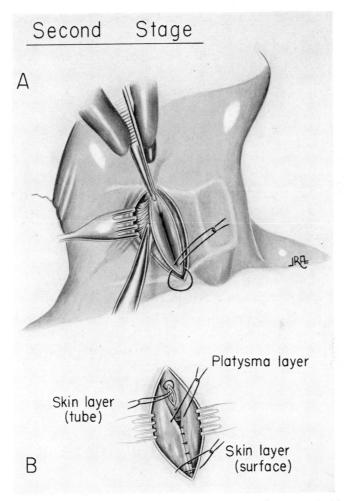

Fig. 121. Cervical esophagectomy without laryngectomy. Second stage: *A*, Incision around the lateral groove as the first step in closure. *B*, Three layers of sutures to close the defect. The innermost layer consists of fine catgut in the edges of the skin tube; the next is of the same material to approximate the platysma over the inner skin layer; the outer is of silk in the skin over the neck.

Intratracheal inhalation anesthesia is used. During the course of the operation it is necessary to remove the original intratracheal tube, and a second one previously sterilized should be available on the nurse's table for use at the appropriate time.

The incision and preliminary dissection are the same as those already described. When it becomes apparent that the larynx must be removed with the esophagus, the steps of the procedure are modified slightly. The pre-tracheal muscles are severed at their sternal attachments. The thyroid isthmus is transected to the left of the trachea and reflected to the right, raising it from the trachea. The right lobe of the gland is left attached to the larynx, but the left lobe is dissected from it and left with its blood supply intact, provided there is no sign of carcinomatous invasion of that lobe. The recurrent laryngeal nerves are cut. The esophagus is transected at the proper level as described previously and the two traction sutures are inserted, one on either side of the open distal end.

At this time the anesthetist is requested to withdraw the intratracheal tube. The trachea is then transected with a knife at as high a level as possible so as to provide a sufficient length to bring the distal end to the surface above the sternum. A second previously sterilized intratracheal tube is inserted by the surgeon into the trachea and its outer end is passed through the drapes over the patient's left shoulder to the anesthetist, who then connects it with his anesthesia apparatus for use during the remainder of the operation.

The way is now cleared for the transection of the pharynx above the larynx and across the pharyngo-esophageal junction. As much length of pharynx as possible is preserved. From this point on the procedure is similar to that described under the technic of cervical esophagectomy alone. A short incision is made through the skin just above the suprasternal notch, as far as possible below the lower transverse incision edge. Through this the end of the trachea is brought out. Its edge is sutured to the skin edges of the short incision with fine silk on curved cutting-point needles. This is done near the termination of the operation because the intratracheal tube must, of course, be removed for the purpose.

The Levin tube is inserted and a light gauze dressing is applied, but the opening of the trachea must be left uncovered. During the early post-operative period the nurse must exert precautions to keep the airway free.

The second stage of the operation is carried out in exactly the same manner as in the simpler procedure. The vertical incisions must be made far enough away from the opening so that the turned-in skin will produce a tube of sufficient diameter.

The after-care is the same as for cases of esophagectomy alone, but the patient will need encouragement regarding the loss of the power of speech. If one is fortunate enough to deal with a favorable tumor so far as freedom from recurrence of the disease is concerned, the patient may subsequently be taught to use an artificial larynx or to employ esophageal speech.

Thoracic and Abdominal Segments; Resection with Restoration by Esophagogastric Anastomosis

The principle of the treatment of carcinoma of the esophagus below the cervical segment involves the widest possible extirpation of the primary tumor and the excision of as many of the regional lymph nodes as can be reached, subject to the anatomic limitations of the region which is involved (Fig. 105). This means that a margin of normal esophagus several centimeters long must be removed above and below the growth, and as many as possible of the regional nodes in the mediastinum and upper abdomen must be excised. The topographic limitations of the region are such that in the superior and middle portions of the mediastinum, only those nodes which lie close to the esophagus can be removed. However, in the lower portion of the mediastinum a larger latitude of dissection makes it possible to remove not only the group of nodes which surround the esophagus in its lower fourth, but also some of the subcarinal nodes and those in the pulmonary ligament as well. In the abdomen it is essential to remove the entire group of nodes which surrounds the cardia and abdominal segment of the esophagus (paracardial) and also, whenever possible (see p. 282 for exception), the important large group which lies along the lesser curvature in relation to the left gastric vessels. Lymph node invasion is observed in over 70 per cent of all patients operated upon.

It is obvious, therefore, that the Torek operation, which was formerly the only method available, is completely inadequate from the standpoint of adequate extirpation of the disease. Furthermore, this operation fails to provide satisfactory palliation. Because of these facts the Torek procedure has been discarded in the management of carcinoma of the esophagus and will not be described.

With minor variations the technical problem involved in the modern treatment of carcinoma of the esophagus is essentially the same for all levels below the cervical segment. It includes extirpation of the growth-bearing segment and the immediate restoration of continuity by esophagogastric anastomosis. The special details required for the management of tumors located in the higher levels represent modifications of the technic employed for those near the cardia. The method as applied to the removal of low-lying tumors will therefore be described first and the modifications required to deal with those in the more proximal segments will be described later. Reference to the chart (Fig. 107) will serve as a review of the technics required at each level.

The usual intratracheal inhalation anesthesia is used. The patient is placed on his right side with the left side arched upward slightly. A standard thoracotomy incision is made, using the rib resection technic. Modifications of the incision which may be required under certain conditions will be mentioned subsequently.

Operation for Carcinoma of the Lower Esophagus and Cardia; Partial Gastrectomy and Esophagectomy with Low Intrathoracic Esophagogastric Anastomosis. For the performance of a resection of the lower esophagus two types of incision may be used, depending almost entirely on the experience and personal preference of the surgeon. The better incision, because it avoids cutting across the costochondral arch, is a standard thoracotomy incision resecting the left eighth or ninth rib. The lung is palpated for metastases, and the lower portions of the esophagus and mediastinum are explored. The diaphragm is then opened by a small incision and the abdomen is explored. The liver, stomach, spleen and regional lymph nodes are observed. If the growth is resectable, the division of the diaphragm is completed through the esophageal hiatus and the resection is begun.

The alternative incision is the abdominothoracic, which is used only when there is a strong suspicion of inoperability of the growth because of its extent within the upper abdomen. A short oblique incision is made through the abdominal muscles lateral to the rectus sheath, inclining upward and outward to the costal margin. Through this incision the region of the growth is explored and the resectability of the tumor is established. If a resection is possible, the incision is enlarged into the thorax by cutting across the costo-chondral margin and extending it posteriorly in the eighth or ninth inter-costal space. The diaphragm is then divided from its costal insertion through the esophageal hiatus. This incision presents the advantage that it avoids the opening of the thorax in case the growth is not resectable. It also provides, of course, an unusually wide exposure of the operative field. However, the division of the costal arch is a distinct disadvantage because of the increased discomfort and interference with deep breathing which results. Furthermore, it requires a longer time for closure than the simple thoracotomy incision. This is an important consideration from the standpoint of the welfare of the patient at the end of a long operation.

The left phrenic nerve is crushed to quiet the left half of the diaphragm and to prevent diaphragmatic pull upon the stomach during the postopera-tive period. When there is doubt about the resectability of the growth it is advisable to inject the nerve with procaine hydrochloride solution to produce a temporary cessation of diaphragmatic motion. The injection of the nerve is made easier if it is steadied by grasping the tissues beyond it in the jaws of a mucosa forceps of the Allis or Babcock type (Fig. 123).

TECHNIC OF DISSECTION. The dissection is begun as follows: Through a longitudinal incision in the mediastinal pleura posterior to the pulmonary ligament, the lower end of the esophagus is freed (Fig. 122). The right and left vagus nerves are severed at a point just above the probable level of section of the esophagus. Small vessels which accompany these nerves must be ligated. The dissection is then carried downward, dividing the attach-ments behind the cardia. In this region several vessels which anastomose with the lower esophageal, left phrenic, left gastric and left superior supra-renal arteries are found. These must be cut and ligated. In the case of a large, locally invasive growth it may be necessary, when the opening in the dia-phragm is enlarged, to remove a rim of the diaphragm along with the tumor. The gastrolienal ligament is incised. This gives access to the lesser omental cavity. If the growth has begun to adhere to the splenic artery or has invaded the tail of the pancreas, the dissection is planned so as to provide for the removal of the spleen or a portion of the pancreas or both. If the growth is not thus invasive, the spleen is not removed. The left gastro-epiploic vessels and the vasa brevia between the spleen and the stomach are

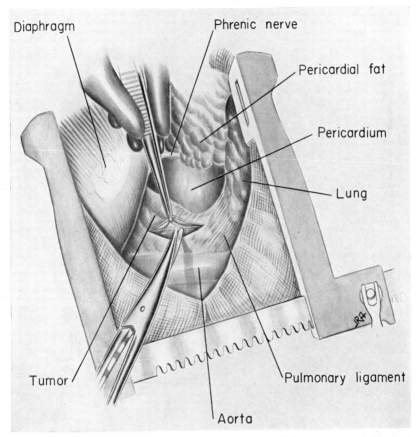

Diaphragm Phrenic nerve Pericardial fat Pericardium Lung Tumor Pulmonary ligament Aorta

Fig. 122. Esophagectomy: Lower segment. Exposure of the operative field obtained through a left standard thoracotomy incision with excision of the ninth rib. Incision of the mediastinal pleura to uncover the tumor-bearing portion of the esophagus. (Note the protection of the wound edges with gauze pads.)

severed and tied. The gastrocolic ligament is divided as far as the region of the antrum of the stomach, taking care to avoid injury to the anastomotic arches of the right gastro-epiploic vessels which lie close to the greater curvature. The gastrohepatic ligament is divided almost to the level of the pylorus, preserving the right gastric vessels which course along the lesser curvature. In the proximal portion of the gastrohepatic ligament an artery is frequently encountered which arises from an ascending branch of the left gastric artery and extends within the ligament to the porta of the liver. It must be divided in order to complete the mobilization of the stomach.

The last attachment which must be freed in order to bring about complete mobilization of the upper portion of the stomach is in the region of the left gastric artery. This vessel should be divided as close as possible to its origin from the celiac axis in order to make it possible to remove the large group of lymph nodes which surround its branches as they approach the lesser

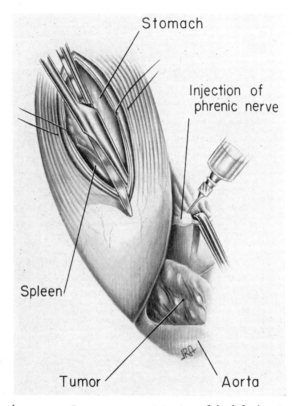

Fig. 123. Esophagectomy: Lower segment. Injection of the left phrenic nerve with procaine hydrochloride to quiet the diaphragm temporarily until the exploration of the abdomen has been completed. Incision and retraction of the diaphragm preparatory to abdominal exploration.

curvature of the stomach. The left gastric vein and the celiac branch of the right vagus nerve must also be severed (Figs. 122, 123, 124, 125, 126, 127 and 128).

A second pair of gauze pads is used to protect the field of operation in anticipation of cutting across the stomach, and two large curved gastric clamps are applied to the stomach as far as possible below the lower extent of the growth (Fig. 129, *A*). The clamps should be placed in such a direction as to leave as long a portion of the greater curvature as is compatible with an adequate excision of the diseased area. The stomach is then cut between the clamps with a knife. A pad of gauze is tied over the proximal cut end and the tumor-bearing segment is turned back over the posterior angle of the incision. Division of the esophagus, however, is postponed until the posterior layers of the anastomosis have been completed. In this way the necessity for the use of a clamp on the proximal portion of the esophagus

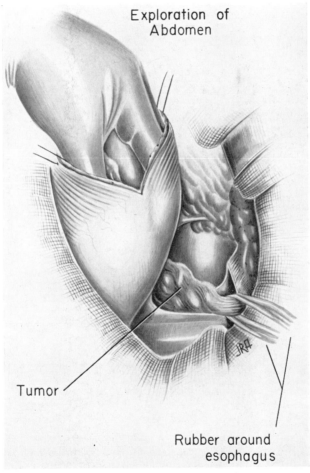

Exploration of
Abdomen

Tumor

Rubber around
esophagus

Fig. 124. Esophagectomy: Lower segment. Growth in the lower esophagus exposed; exploration of the abdomen begun. If resection is to be proceeded with, the left phrenic nerve is crushed at this stage.

is avoided and soiling of the field is postponed until the anterior layers of the anastomosis are begun.

The distal cut edge is closed with two layers of fine catgut reinforced by a row of interrupted Lembert sutures of silk as a third layer. A convenient method of placing the catgut layers is to sew through and through below the distal clamp with a straight atraumatic needle, starting at the greater curvature end. If a clamp with fenestrated blades is available, this suture is passed through the blades (Fig. 129, *B*). When this type of clamp is used, the application of the proximal clamp may be deferred until the through and through suture has been completed. The second clamp is applied and the stomach is cut between. The distal clamp can then be removed without spilling the gastric contents.

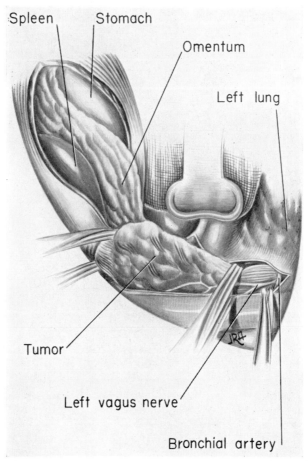

Fig. 125. Esophagectomy: Lower segment. First step in resection: The esophagus is freed to a level several centimeters above the tumor. The diaphragm has been incised through the hiatus and the attachments of the esophagus and stomach in this area are partly severed.

Using the same strand of catgut, the cut edges of the distal portion are sutured over and over from the lesser curvature end back to the starting point at the greater curvature (Fig. 130, *A*). This suture controls the bleeding which arises from the severed intramural gastric vessels. The closure of the end of the stomach is completed with two more layers of sutures, the first consisting of a continuous inverting (Cushing right-angle) stitch and the second of interrupted Lembert sutures of fine silk (Fig. 130, *B* and *C*).

After the end of the distal segment of the stomach has been closed, a circular incision is made through the serous and muscular coats of its anterior wall near the upper extremity, avoiding if possible any injury to the intramural vessels. This incision should be placed where no important branch of the gastro-epiploic vessels may be severed. Furthermore, it should not be made too close to the end of the stomach because of the danger of interference with the blood supply of the bridge of gastric wall which lies between it and the inverted end. The diameter of this incision which is to

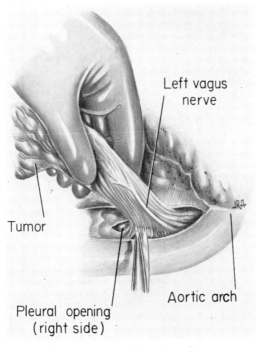

Fig. 126. Esophagectomy: Lower segment. Dissection of the attachments of the esophagus to the right pleura which is shown partially opened. The amount of freeing of the esophagus as shown is sufficient for a carcinoma of the lower portion of the esophagus.

be used for the anastomosis should be approximately equivalent to that of the esophagus when slightly distended. The final excision of this circular portion of stomach wall is postponed until after the first two layers of the posterior aspect of the anastomosis have been placed and tied. This is done to delay the soiling of the field with gastric contents until the last possible moment. After the circular incision has been made, a series of suture ligatures of very fine silk is applied to the small vessels which cross the area in the submucosal layer (Fig. 131, *A*). This facilitates the completion of the anastomosis by diminishing the amount of bleeding which comes from the edges of the gastric wall after the circular piece has been removed.

The anastomosis is now begun with a layer of mattress sutures of fine

(5–0) silk between the muscularis of the esophagus and the seromuscular coats of the stomach wall (Fig. 131, B). After the completion of this layer, a right-angle clamp is applied to the esophagus just proximal to the upper reaches of the tumor. The muscle layer of the esophagus is next incised as far as, but not through, the mucosal layer. This allows the placing of a second row of silk sutures to approximate the cut edges of the muscularis of both organs. The posterior portion of the mucosa of the esophagus is then incised. A small opening is now made through the mucosa of the stomach and

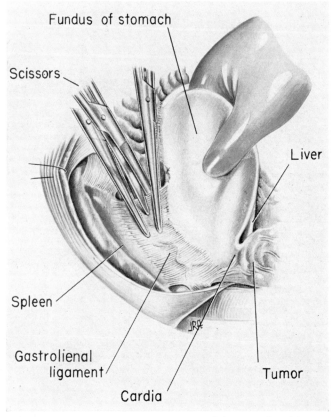

Fig. 127. Esophagectomy: Lower segment. Division of the gastrolienal ligament and vasa brevia.

an aspirator is inserted so as to remove whatever liquid may be within. This maneuver may be accomplished easily as a single manipulation, using a trocar-pointed aspirator if one is available (Fig. 132, B). The circular portion of gastric wall which was outlined by the original incision is now excised and the posterior aspect of the anastomosis is completed with a row of fine silk sutures approximating the mucosal layers. The transection of the esophagus is completed next and the diseased segment, including a portion of the stomach and of the esophagus, is removed. The completion of the anastomosis proceeds from this point by continuing the posterior layers around the circumference anteriorly. The sutures in the mucosal layer are inserted so that the knots are tied on the surface inside the lumen. This is done to allow these sutures to separate and come away with greater ease. The middle and outer layers are placed in exactly the same manner as in the posterior portion of the anastomosis but in reverse order. On its completion

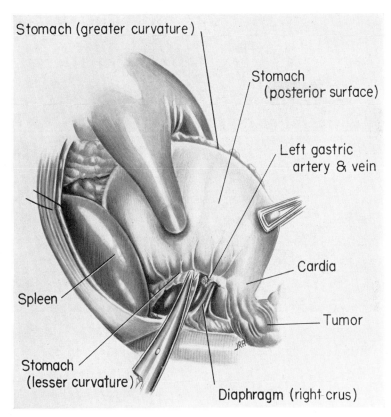

Fig. 128. Esophagectomy: Lower segment. Mobilization of the stomach: The gastro-lienal, gastrocolic and gastrohepatic ligaments have been divided; the attachments around the cardia and abdominal segment of the esophagus have been severed; the gastric ends of the severed left gastric vessels are shown. The stomach is rotated with the greater curvature uppermost, bringing the posterior surface into view.

the anastomosis is exactly circular. If a tab of omentum is available on the greater curvature, this should be swung up and sutured around the anasto-mosis for additional protection (Fig. 132, *A, B, C, D, E* and *F*).

ALTERNATIVE TECHNIC. In certain instances, when it is necessary to excise an unusually large portion of the stomach, leaving only a short distal frag-ment, an end-to-end esophagogastric anastomosis may be performed. Al-though this method may be somewhat more difficult technically and subject

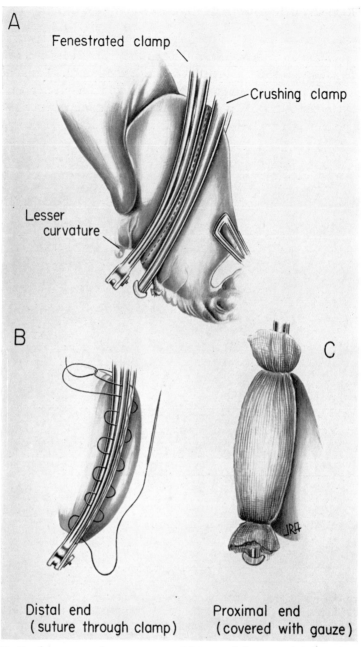

A

Fenestrated clamp

Crushing clamp

Lesser curvature

B

C

Distal end
(suture through clamp)

Proximal end
(covered with gauze)

Fig. 129. Esophagectomy: Lower segment. Division of the stomach below the group of lymph nodes surrounding the branches of the left gastric vessels on the lesser curvature near the cardia. *A*, The position of the clamps is shown. In practice when a clamp with limber fenestrated blades is employed as shown, the crushing clamp is not applied until after the through and through suture has been inserted. *B*, Details of the first suture, passed back and forth through the blades of the clamp but never over them. As soon as the lesser curvature end is reached, the clamp is released and the suture strand pulled out of the blade through which it passed last. *C*, Gauze cover of the proximal cut edge to minimize soiling the operative field.

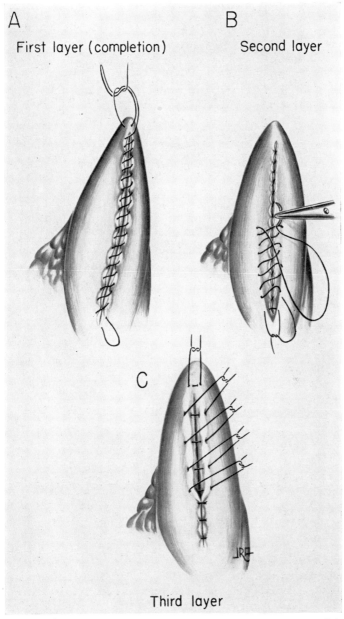

A
First layer (completion)

B
Second layer

C

Third layer

Fig. 130. Esophagectomy: Lower segment. Closure of the distal portion of the stomach. *A*, Completion of the first layer by over and over suture along the cut edges using the same strand of catgut as in Figure 129, *B*, ending at the starting point on the greater curvature. *B*, Second layer consisting of a Cushing right-angle stitch of fine catgut starting at the lesser curvature and ending at the greater curvature. *C*, Third layer of Lembert sutures using fine silk.

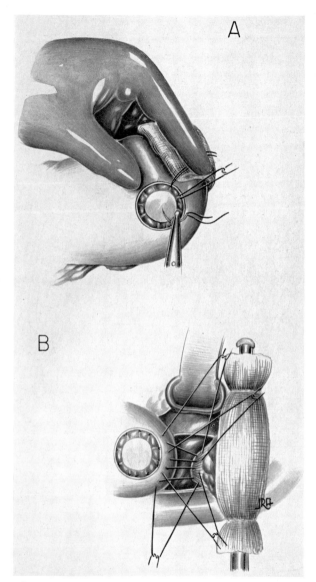

Fig. 131. Esophagectomy: Lower segment. Beginning of the anastomosis. *A,* Circular incision of the anterior wall of the stomach through the serosa and into the muscularis but avoiding severance of the intramural vessels. Suture ligatures of fine silk are being tied around the vessels which cross the incision line in anticipation of the excision of the contained disk of stomach wall. *B,* The anastomosis is begun with the outer layer of mattress sutures on the posterior aspect. Note that only one third of the circumference is sutured in the posterior portion. This is to avoid the inconvenience which might result from pulling the esophagus around too far at each end.

to greater danger of inadequate healing, it is sometimes preferable to performing a total gastrectomy or to leaving the turned-in distal segment and restoring continuity by esophagojejunal anastomosis. A large curved crush-

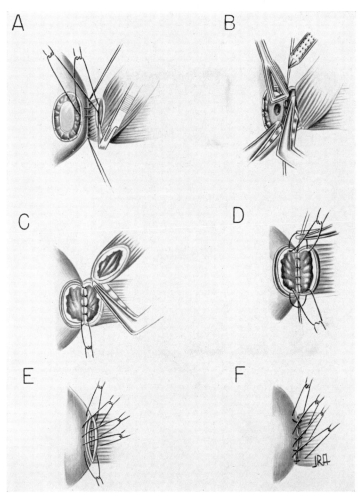

Fig. 132. Esophagectomy: Lower segment. Details of the anastomosis. *A*, Incision of the posterior muscular layer of the esophagus and beginning of the muscle edge to muscle edge approximation. *B*, Incision of the posterior portion of the mucosa of the esophagus and excision of the disk of stomach wall after aspiration of gastric contents with a trocar point suction apparatus. *C*, Posterior mucosal layer sutured and circumcision of the esophagus completed. *D*, Beginning of the anterior mucosal layer showing the manner in which the sutures are inserted so as to bring the knots on the intraluminal side. *E*, Anterior approximation of the muscle edges. *F*, Completion of the outer layer of mattress sutures.

ing clamp (Kocher) is applied, and near the greater curvature end a short straight clamp is put on to obviate the creation of a sharp angle at the end of the gastric remnant. The stomach is cut with a knife along these clamps so that the distal portion remains with its edges uncrushed. The open end of the distal portion of stomach is closed partially. The first layer consists of a continuous Connell suture of fine chromicized catgut, starting at the lesser curvature and extending to the point where the resulting opening has a

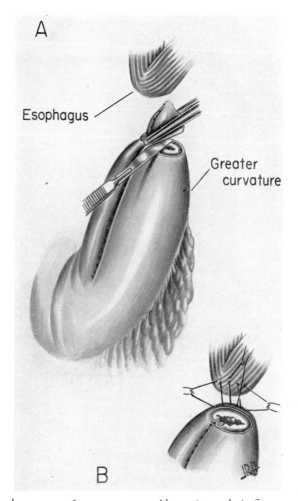

Fig. 133. Esophagectomy: Lower segment. Alternative technic for anastomosis by the end-to-end method. *A*, Closure of the end of the stomach partially completed, leaving a portion of the stomach on the greater curvature side open. Diagram shows the excision of the tip of the stomach necessary to prevent angulation at the site of anastomosis. *B*, Start of anastomosis. *Note:* The esophagus has not yet been cut across.

diameter which is approximately the equivalent of that of the esophagus. This corresponds to the portion outlined by the smaller clamp. Here the suture is tied. A second layer consisting of a continuous right angle stitch of the same material is inserted and an outer layer of Lembert sutures of silk is applied. All three layers are terminated before the greater curvature is reached, leaving an opening of adequate size for the anastomosis. The anastomosis between the esophagus and stomach is then performed in the same manner as described above (Fig. 133).

Special pains must be taken to secure a satisfactory approximation of the layers at the point where the sutures used to narrow the open end of the remainder of the stomach meet the suture line of the anastomosis. It is the possibility of failure to secure prompt healing at this point which makes

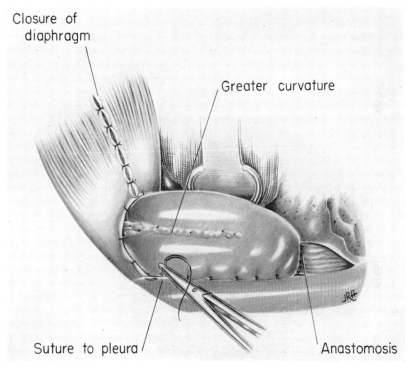

Closure of diaphragm

Greater curvature

Suture to pleura

Anastomosis

Fig. 134. Esophagectomy: Lower segment. Completion of the operation showing the location of the anastomosis at approximately the level of the inferior pulmonary vein, the method of fastening the stomach to the pleura over the descending aorta, and the closure of the diaphragm around the stomach. Note the absence of constriction of the stomach by the diaphragm.

this type of anastomosis more hazardous than that involving a circular opening in the stomach wall.

Tension on the anastomosis is prevented by fixing the stomach to the mediastinal pleura along the aorta with a row of silk sutures. The cut edges of the diaphragm are sutured to the stomach at an appropriate level below the anastomosis (Fig. 134). In fitting the diaphragm to the stomach, care should be exerted to avoid constriction. The opening through which the stomach is made to pass must be several times larger than the normal esophageal hiatus. The remainder of the diaphragmatic incision is then closed from the stomach wall to the costal insertion, using interrupted sutures of heavy silk (Fig. 134).

Before the closure of the diaphragm is completed, a solution containing 1 gm. of streptomycin and 100,000 units of penicillin in 30 cc. of saline is injected, one half in the upper abdomen and one half in the mediastinum and left pleural cavity. The usual closed catheter drainage is provided, using a Foley catheter brought out through the tenth intercostal space posteriorly.

Operation for Carcinoma of the Midthoracic Segment of the Esophagus; Partial Esophagectomy with High Intrathoracic Esophagogastric Anastomosis. As mentioned above, this procedure offers better palliation and greater prospects of ultimate cure than the Torek operation which it now supplants in the treatment of carcinoma of the midthoracic region of the esophagus. It is a natural development resulting from modifications of the technic used for the removal of carcinoma located at or near the cardia. By preserving the right gastric and right gastro-epiploic vessels and maintaining the continuity of the vascular communications along the greater and lesser curvatures and in the wall of the stomach itself, an adequate blood supply may be preserved so that the entire stomach can be mobilized without danger of necrosis. After this has been accomplished and the stomach has been cut across at the cardia, the fundus will reach as high as the apex of the chest and an anastomosis can be made at that level without danger of separation of the suture line. From the standpoint of the esophageal blood supply it is important to remember that the segment of esophagus between the aortic arch and base of the neck is almost entirely dependent upon the esophageal branches of the inferior thyroid arteries. Whenever, therefore, the high situation of the growth makes it necessary to mobilize the entire thoracic portion of the esophagus and to pull it from behind the aortic arch for a supra-aortic anastomosis, the level of division across the esophagus must be at some point above the superior surface of the aortic arch. In order to avoid the development of necrosis at the cut end of the esophagus, this rule must be rigidly observed, even if it appears that a greater useful length has been obtained as a result of such extensive mobilization.

After the thoracic and abdominal parts of the exploration have been carried out and the growth has been found to be suitable for resection, the freeing of the esophagus is completed from the diaphragm below to above the upper limits of the tumor. In the majority of instances this involves carrying the dissection up behind the aortic arch. Sometimes, however, a sufficient length of uninvolved esophagus exists between the growth and the aortic arch to make it possible to perform an anastomosis just below it. In a typical case the esophageal arteries from the descending aorta, the small esophageal branches of the bronchial arteries, and, with a high growth, the esophageal arteries arising from the aortic arch itself must all be divided.

The dissection between the hilus of the lung and the diseased area is often difficult. The freeing of an adherent tumor located behind the aortic arch is sometimes troublesome, but it can usually be accomplished by working from both above and below the arch. The dissection at this point may be facilitated by ligating and dividing the upper one or two left intercostal arteries as they arise from the aorta. This permits the aortic arch to be

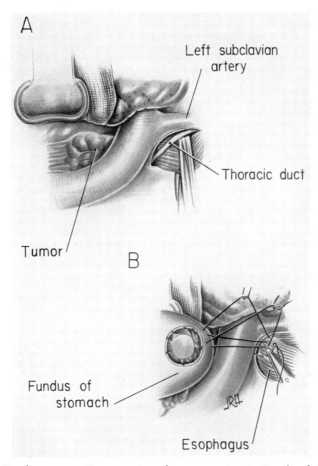

Fig. 135. Esophagectomy: Supra-aortic arch anastomosis. *A*, Details of the dissection behind and above the aortic arch, showing the thoracic duct as it crosses the esophagus above the arch. *B*, Start of the supra-aortic anastomosis; placement of the outer posterior layer of sutures.

drawn forward sufficiently to complete what might otherwise be an almost impossible dissection.

At the level of the superior surface of the aortic arch the thoracic duct is usually encountered as it crosses the esophagus to assume a more anterior location in the superior mediastinum whence it ascends into the neck (Fig. 135, *A*). If the thoracic duct is adherent and a section of it must be excised with the growth, or if it is traumatized to the point where leakage of chyle might occur, it must be ligated. If this is not done, a fatal outcome is almost certain to result from inanition due to the loss of chyle.

During the dissection of an adherent growth, the right pleural sac is often opened unavoidably. A portion of the mediastinal pleura and occasionally of the right lung itself may have to be excised. If the lung is cut across, the defect is sutured with a continuous suture of fine catgut. No attempt need be made to close the opening in the right pleural reflection because at the completion of the operation both lungs will be expanded by the positive pressure within the anesthesia system, and this expansion is maintained by the intrathoracic negative pressure after the wound has been made air-tight by closure.

After the dissection of the esophagus has been completed, the incision in the diaphragm is enlarged through the hiatus and the entire stomach is mobilized almost as extensively as in a case where a total gastrectomy is to be performed, with the vital exception that the right gastric and right gastro-epiploic vessels are preserved, together with the anastomotic arches along the curvatures. The continuity of the anastomotic arches along the lesser curvature depends upon the fact that the left gastric artery, with which the branches of the right gastric artery communicate to make a continuous channel, must be severed as close as possible to its origin from the celiac axis. (Fig. 138). Division of the stomach is carried out as close to the cardia as is consistent with the removal of the lymph nodes in that region. The distal cut edge of the stomach is inverted by the technic previously described. An alternative method, which can be used when the growth is so high that it is important to sacrifice no gastric vessels whatever, is to tie the esophagus 2 cm. above the cardia with a ligature of heavy silk and to invert the stump after transection by means of a purse-string suture in the stomach at the level of the cardia. Further reinforcement is provided by means of a layer of Lembert sutures. This method is unsatisfactory if lymph node metastases are present in the region of the cardia. Great care must be exerted in handling the stomach to avoid trauma to any of the intercommunicating anastomotic branches of the vessels in its walls, especially in the fundus where no extrinsic vessels exist.

The proximal cut end of the esophagus is covered by a rubber glove or a square of rubber tissue tied over it. The esophagus is then pulled up from behind the aortic arch and the stomach is brought up into the apex of the chest for the performance of an anastomosis (Fig. 135, B). The circular incision in the fundus of the stomach is prepared and the esophagogastric anastomosis is performed in exactly the same manner as in cases of carcinoma of the cardia. Because of the high level at which the anastomosis must be made, unusually long instruments are required.

At the completion of the anastomosis a suture of fine silk is placed on either side between the fundus and the adjacent edge of the incision in the pleural reflection over the superior mediastinum in order to hold the fundus up behind the anastomosis. The remainder of the stomach is fixed within the chest by means of a long row of sutures to the pleura overlying the thoracic portion of the descending aorta. The closure of the diaphragm about the stomach is completed as described previously (Fig. 134). The pylorus usually lies only a few centimeters below the diaphragm at the completion of the operation. The antibiotic solution is injected both above and below the diaphragm as already described.

Carcinoma of the Superior Mediastinal Segment of the Esophagus; Subtotal Esophagectomy with Intracervical Esophagogastric Anastomosis. The resection of a carcinoma in the superior mediastinal segment of the esophagus presents the most difficult technical problem of all possible locations. The high situation of the growth makes it necessary to transect the esophagus through its short cervical segment, thus removing almost the entire length of the esophagus. This entails the making of a separate cervical incision. Furthermore, it is necessary to provide a means of passing the completely mobilized stomach from the thorax into the neck where the anastomosis must be performed. This step may be completed in one of two ways. It is possible in some cases, if the stomach is not too large, to bring it up behind the aortic arch and into the superior mediastinum through the thoracic inlet in the bed from which the esophagus is removed. The employment of this method, however, involves the possibility of irreparable damage to the blood supply of the fundus of the stomach because of the amount of manipulation required or the possibility of ischemia of the fundus because of the constriction produced by forcing it through too small an aperture. Therefore, in the average case it is probably safer to create an artificial channel from the left thoracic cavity into the neck by excising the inner portions of the clavicle and the first rib as described below. It should be recognized that the exact details of this part of the procedure are not yet well established and may be modified subsequently as more experience is acquired.

The operation using the latter method consists of two steps performed in one stage as follows.

First Step; Dissection of the Esophagus and Mobilization of the Stomach. A standard thoracotomy incision is made on the left side resecting the eighth rib. If sufficient exposure is not available to reach the superior mediastinum, the seventh, sixth, and sometimes the fifth ribs may be divided posteriorly. The dissection is begun in the region of the tumor after incising the mediastinal pleura above the aortic arch and posterior to the left subclavian artery. If the tumor-bearing portion of the esophagus can be freed sufficiently to make it possible to perform a resection, the operation is continued by completing the dissection of the entire length of the thoracic portion of the esophagus. The freeing of the superior mediastinal segment presents no particular problem except that the thoracic duct must be identified as it crosses the esophagus just above the aortic arch. If the duct is invaded by tumor or is too adherent to be dissected free, or if it has been injured during the dissection, it must be ligated to prevent the development of a chylous hydrothorax after the operation. Below the aortic arch the esophageal arteries must be tied and cut. These arise from the aortic arch, the bronchial arteries and the descending aorta. In freeing the lower portion of the esophagus, the periesophageal lymph nodes must be included in the dissection insofar as possible. After the entire thoracic portion of the esophagus has been dissected free, the phrenic nerve is crushed and the diaphragm is incised from a point close to its costal insertion through the margin of the esophageal hiatus. This permits the complete mobilization of the stomach, which is carried out exactly as in the cases of esophagectomy for carcinoma of the midthoracic segment of the esophagus requiring a supra-aortic anastomosis.

After the mobilization of the stomach has been completed, the esophagus is tied and cut across just above the cardia, and the stump on the gastric side is inverted with a purse-string suture reinforced with a layer of Lembert sutures of silk. This technic is employed to avoid injury to any of the vessels of the anastomotic communications in the region of the cardia. A piece of rubber tissue or a rubber glove is tied over the proximal end and the esophagus is then pulled up and out from behind the aortic arch into the left pleural cavity so as to make its subsequent withdrawal into the neck somewhat easier.

The stomach is now drawn up as far as possible into the left side of the thorax behind the hilus of the left lung and lateral to the aortic arch. Fixation in this location is maintained by means of a series of interrupted silk sutures between the gastric wall and the mediastinal pleural surface which overlies the descending aorta. The fundus of the stomach is allowed to be free in the superior portion of the pleural cavity until the cervical portion of the operation is performed. The fixation sutures already applied prevent its falling down out of reach after the chest has been closed. The diaphragm is sutured to the stomach just above the pylorus and the remainder of the diaphragmatic incision is closed after injecting the antibiotic solution, as described in the section dealing with the technic of partial esophagectomy at lower levels.

A Foley catheter is led out through a small incision in the tenth intercostal space posteriorly. To complete the first stage of the operation the lung is expanded by the anesthetist and the thoracotomy incision is closed, using interrupted silk sutures in all layers.

SECOND STEP; PERFORMANCE OF THE INTRACERVICAL ESOPHAGOGASTRIC ANASTOMOSIS. After closure of the thoracotomy incision has been completed in the usual manner, the patient is turned on his back and an incision is made along the anterior margin of the left sternocleidomastoid muscle to the suprasternal notch and then downward over the upper portion of the sternum to the level of the second costal cartilage. The pectoralis major muscle is incised close to its sternal attachment and reflected laterally, at the same time severing its medial clavicular insertion. The sternal and medial clavicular insertions of the sternocleidomastoid muscle are severed and retracted laterally. The dissection is deepened in the space between the carotid

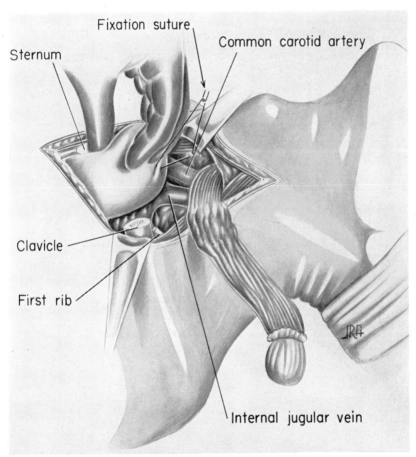

Fig. 136. Esophagectomy: Intracervical esophagogastric anastomosis. The esophagus has been pulled up from the mediastinum and brought out in front of the carotid artery. The fundus of the stomach has been drawn up from the left thoracic cavity through a channel created by the excision of the inner third of the left clavicle and a corresponding portion of the first rib. The suture shown is for the purpose of supporting the gastric fundus in its new position to avoid traction on the anastomosis which will be made in this instance on the posterior wall of the stomach.

sheath and the trachea to expose the esophagus, which is grasped with a forceps and pulled up from the mediastinum and out in front of the carotid sheath.

The medial half of the clavicle and a corresponding segment of the left first rib and costal cartilage are excised extraperiosteally. The clavicle should be cut with the Gigli saw. This produces a large opening from the base of the neck into the apex of the left pleural cavity through which the fundus of the stomach can be drawn easily and without danger of compression. The pleura is opened and the fundus is brought forward medial to the apex of the lung and pulled up into the lower portion of the neck through this channel (Fig. 136). A short linear incision is made in the posterior wall of the fundus close to its apex and an anastomosis consisting of three layers of interrupted fine silk (5–0) sutures is made. A careful approximation of mucosa to mucosa and muscle edge to muscle edge constitutes the inner and middle layers. The outer layer is of mattress sutures. Several sutures are used to fasten the fundus to the surrounding tissues of the neck to prevent tension on the anastomosis which, after its completion, lies in front of the carotid and internal jugular vessels. The wound is closed by suturing the lower end of the sternocleidomastoid muscle and the medial cut edge of the pectoralis major muscle to the sternum and placing a layer of fine silk sutures in the subcutaneous fat and another in the skin. Drainage is not employed.

SPECIAL CONSIDERATIONS RELATIVE TO THE TYPE OF LESION

The details of the operations required to resect segments of the esophagus at various levels have been presented from the viewpoint of the extirpation of carcinoma arising in that organ. Special emphasis is placed on radical extirpation including a large segment of the esophagus and all possible lymph nodes which may be within reasonable access to the surgeon. The limitations of surgery from the standpoint of radical excision have already been mentioned.

It should be borne in mind, however, that whereas a radical policy is not only justifiable but also highly desirable when dealing with a fatal disease such as carcinoma, the same attitude may not be applicable in the case of benign lesions. On the other hand, persons who develop intractable dysphagia or who require repeated instrumentation to keep a passageway open, and especially those who may be condemned to depend upon a gastrostomy for feeding, are often so unhappy and so uncomfortable that life offers a poor prospect and any reasonable risk becomes justifiable in the hope of a restoration to normal living. There are occasions, therefore, when the relatively radical procedures just described should be undertaken in order to rehabilitate the patient and to restore him to a happy and useful life. This applies particularly in the case of cicatricial stenosis resulting from ulceration at the cardia, found characteristically in the patient with a short esophagus and hiatus hernia, and in many cases of cicatrization from chemical burns of the esophagus. Brief reference will be made to the details of the application of the operation to these special problems.

Almost without exception the only types of benign inflammatory stricture of the esophagus which may require treatment by resection are those due to stenosis resulting from esophagitis with ulcerations and those resulting from chemical burns induced by the ingestion of sclerosing caustic solutions. In the former there is frequently a characteristic syndrome consisting of an underlying congenital anomaly with a short esophagus and hiatus hernia, the thoracic portion of the stomach resembling an inverted cone. Superimposed upon this anatomic arrangement there is esophagitis of the lower end just above the cardia and gastritis of the thoracic portion of the stomach. This leads to ulcerations of the peptic variety and ultimately to cicatrization and stenosis. There is also a high incidence of coexisting duodenal ulcer in this condition, sometimes also with stenosis. This fact must be kept in mind when a resection for stricture at the cardia is being considered. Separate surgical treatment for such a duodenal stenosis may be necessary before the proximal stricture is resected. Sometimes both conditions can be relieved at the same operation with a pyloroplasty to correct the former and a resection or an esophagoplasty to overcome the latter.

During the dissection required to free the lower esophagus and upper stomach in cases of this sort, it will be observed that the surrounding tissues of the mediastinum are exceedingly adherent, making the development of planes of cleavage more difficult than in the average case of noninvasive carcinoma. Most of the dissection in many cases must be accomplished with sharp instruments. When the time arrives for the transection of the esophagus, it is frequently difficult to determine the level where the pathologic changes merge with the normal esophagus. This is a matter of great importance, however, because it has been found in the cases of esophagitis that if the esophagus is transected too close to the diseased area, there is a decided tendency for the inflammatory process to spread proximal to the anastomosis. In this respect the lesion behaves much like regional ileitis or ulcerative colitis and a large proximal margin of normal tissue must be excised, even though the lesion is of an inflammatory and non–malignant nature.

Another important consideration in dealing with this disease is that it is complicated in a significant number of cases by the development of carcinoma. This is apparent from the observation that approximately 15 per cent of cases of carcinoma in the region of the cardia and lower end of the esophagus develop in the presence of a short esophagus and hiatus hernia. Therefore the surgeon should search for possible evidences of malignant change during the operation and plan the extent of his resection accordingly.

Because it is necessary to resect a large segment of both esophagus and stomach, it is necessary in the majority of instances to interrupt the continuity of both vagus nerves for technical reasons. In the case of the right vagus nerve which sometimes leaves the esophagus at a high level proximally, it is sometimes possible to preserve the major trunk. Moreover, in the majority of these cases, because of the hiatus hernia the left gastric vessels lie much closer to the diaphragm than in a patient with a normal anatomic arrangement. This also favors the preservation of the right vagus nerve by making it unnecessary, many times, to divide these vessels in order to swing the stomach up into the chest for the anastomosis. On both a theoretical and a practical basis, however, it is unwise to preserve this nerve because of the desirability of eliminating the acid-stimulating function of the vagus nerves in these patients who have a definite ulcer diathesis.

The effect of vagotomy, on the other hand, may be very troublesome in these patients because of the reduction in gastric peristaltic activity and the hypertonicity of the pylorus. This tendency to delayed emptying of the stomach can be overcome to some extent, at least in the absence of organic stenosis at the pylorus or duodenum, by dividing the gastrocolic and gastrohepatic ligaments as far as the region of the pylorus in exactly the same manner as required whenever an unusually high intrathoracic anastomosis is to be performed. This has the effect of interrupting some of the sympathetic nerve fibers whose activity might otherwise produce excessive tonicity of the pylorus. In cicatricial stenosis of the pylorus, obviously something more is required and the most effective procedure is a Heineke-Mikulicz pyloroplasty. This can always be done through the thoracic incision, although enlargement into the abdomen may be necessary occasionally to gain sufficient exposure.

Once the dissection has been completed and the mobilization of the stomach has been accomplished, the remainder of the operation proceeds in the manner already described.

Cicatricial stenosis from chemical burns of the esophagus presents similar difficulties which depend upon the nature and extent of the lesion. Also, in this condition there is usually marked evidence of periesophagitis and inflammatory fixation, making the dissection difficult. In fact, the freeing of such an esophagus is sometimes more difficult to accomplish than in any other type of disease in which a resection is required. It is difficult also to determine where the proximal dividing line between the normal and the diseased portions of the esophagus lies. This is almost invariably higher than one might guess by inspection and even by palpation. Reference to the roentgen film showing the pattern produced by the ingested barium mixture may be necessary in order to determine the correct level for transection. It should be remembered also that the proximal margin of the cicatrized area is almost invariably funnel-shaped. On the other hand, it is not necessary to cut across the esophagus any higher than the last normal tissue which lies just proximal to the lesion. This is a very important matter because of the necessity of conserving as much proximal length as possible in some of the cases of extensive injury.

It is important to remember also that in some cases of stricture resulting from ingested corrosive liquids, there is in addition to the esophageal injury a chemical burn of the pyloric end of the stomach. This is usually sharply localized at the pylorus but may occasionally involve some of the antral portion of the stomach as well. In a few such cases, although the ability of the patient to swallow may be temporarily maintained by means of bougienage, the inaccessibility of the pylorus allows the cicatrization to progress to the point of stenosis and ultimate obstruction. The surgical relief of the pyloric stenosis should be accomplished if possible by some procedure which will produce a minimum of shortening in order to preserve sufficient length and flexibility of the stomach for use later should an esophagectomy become necessary. The Heineke-Mikulicz pyloroplasty serves admirably for this purpose.

When with some patients it becomes obvious that bougienage must be abandoned, the possibility of performing a resection should be considered and the decision to operate made before the poor nutritional condition of the patient reaches the point where a preliminary gastrostomy must be established for feeding. It is possible thereby not only to shorten the interval of time before the definitive operation can be carried out, but also to avoid the inconvenience of having to close the gastrostomy during the performance of the procedure. Occasionally, however, a gastrostomy must be used and in that event several months should be allowed for the improvement of the patient's condition and the subsidence of the inflammatory reaction of the tissues about the gastrostomy site.

Ordinarily it is possible, even after a gastrostomy has been made, to mobilize the stomach sufficiently to carry out the usual procedure as described above with a partial or even subtotal esophagectomy and a primary esophagogastric anastomosis within the left thoracic cavity or actually within the neck. However, in those patients who have sustained an injury to the major portion or all of the esophagus and who have also developed a stricture of the pylorus which requires surgical relief with resultant foreshortening of the stomach, it may be necessary to use the jejunum for the restoration of continuity. When this is the case, the stomach is transected just distal to the cardia and the opening is closed in the manner described previously. The uppermost loop of jejunum is drawn up and prepared for use in the manner described originally by Roux. The vessels of the mesentery of this loop are studied and a series of the primary branches is singled out for ligation and division, preserving the continuity of the vascular arches and anastomotic communications in order to carry the circulation of the divided end of the bowel. The vascular pattern of the proximal portion of the mesentery which supplies the first twelve inches or more of the jejunum immediately beyond the ligament of Treitz is such that the vessels cannot be safely divided without danger of interfering with the nutrition of a portion of the bowel.

This area of the mesentery is therefore avoided and the transection of the jejunum is made about 12 to 14 inches distal to the ligament. The length of jejunum distal to this point which is needed to make the anastomosis with the esophagus is then determined by trial, and one or more branches of the superior mesenteric artery is divided beyond those already severed as required. After the necessary length of bowel has been prepared, the distal portion is pulled up through a short incision in the transverse mesocolon to a point as high as necessary in the chest. The edges of the opening in the mesocolon are sutured to the bowel where it passes through it. An anastomosis is made between the end of the proximal jejunal segment and the side of the distal segment several inches below the transverse mesocolon. Two or three layers of sutures of catgut or silk may be used.

After the intrathoracic esophagojejunal anastomosis has been completed or, in cases where this anastomosis is to be made in the neck through a separate incision, as soon as the bowel has been pulled up far enough into the chest, the diaphragm is closed around it in the same way as when the stomach is used. The lung is then expanded, a catheter is brought out through a lower intercostal space and the chest wall is closed.

A certain amount of coiling of the bowel cannot be avoided without dividing vessels which are important in the preservation of the vascular continuity through the anastomotic arcades. For this reason also it is not possible always, especially when the anastomosis is to be made at a high level, to avoid arching of the end of the bowel which is to be used. This may interfere with the performance of an end-to-end approximation. It is expedient under such circumstances to close the end of the distal jejunal segment and to make the anastomosis end-to-side at a point several inches away from the inverted jejunal end. Three layers of fine silk are used. The incision through the wall of the jejunum is linear. Sometimes, however, the anastomosis may be made end-to-end.

CARE OF THE PATIENT AFTER ESOPHAGECTOMY

At the completion of the anastomosis or, in the superior mediastinal segment group, after the stomach has been fully mobilized and the esophagus divided, 60 cc. of a solution containing 100,000 units of penicillin and 1 gm. of streptomycin are instilled, one half in the upper abdomen and one half in the mediastinum and left thoracic cavity. The administration of these agents is continued by intramuscular injection during the first five days after operation or until any suspicion of infection in the lungs or within the abdominal or pleural cavities or in the mediastinum has subsided. A satisfactory dosage is 0.25 gm. of streptomycin and 100,000 units of penicillin every six hours. Sulfonamides are no longer used.

Administration of oxygen by the intranasal method is employed during the first twenty-four hours. After that time it may be omitted in the average case. In the patients who have had a supra-aortic or intracervical anastomosis, the large incision required and the extensive dissection within the mediastinum, as well as the presence of almost the entire stomach within the left thoracic cavity, make the readjustment of the respiratory and circulatory functions more difficult; as a result the inhalation of oxygen may have to be continued at least intermittently for three to five days.

In the patients with an anastomosis low in the thorax, the Levin tube is left at the completion of the operation with its tip just proximal to the anastomosis in order to avoid the possible danger of necrosis at the suture line which might result from the pressure of the tube if it were passed through into the stomach. The amount of drainage obtained by continuous aspiration of the Levin tube is usually small and the tube can therefore be removed in the average case after twenty-four hours. However, in the patients who have a supra-aortic or intracervical anastomosis, because of the danger of sudden regurgitation of large amounts of gastric contents and the disturbances of the respiratory and circulatory functions which may result from the pressure of an overdistended intrathoracic stomach, it is preferable to overlook the possible disadvantages of the presence of a tube and to leave the Levin tube with its tip actually within the stomach at the completion of the operation. Continuous aspiration is then maintained for a period of three to four days before the tube is removed. Thereafter it may still be necessary to reinsert a tube temporarily if gastric dilatation should occur, but this is an infrequent occurrence.

The intrathoracic drainage catheter is removed after forty-eight hours. Subsequent removal of fluid by thoracentesis is rarely necessary when the antibiotics are used prophylactically. The reaccumulation of a large amount of fluid after the first effusion is over usually heralds the onset of empyema, a rare occurrence at the present time.

In patients 50 years of age or older the routine administration of quinidine and avoidance of the overadministration of fluid intravenously are applied as in any other patient of like age who is subjected to a major thoracic operation.

During the first few days the patient's requirements of food and fluid are maintained almost entirely by intravenous injection. By this means glucose, amino acids, vitamins and whole blood, if indicated, are administered, taking care always to avoid embarrassment of the circulatory system as mentioned previously.

The oral administration of fluids is begun after twenty-four hours, giving 30 cc. of water each hour. The second day after the operation 60 cc. of clear fluids, not including fruit juices, may be given hourly. It is unwise to increase this amount, however, on the third day or even, with some patients, on the fourth. By the fifth postoperative day liquids made with milk may be added and slightly larger amounts administered each hour. From that day on the amount and character of the feedings can be adjusted to suit the ability of the patient to take them. Gradually the amount per feeding is increased and the intervals between lengthened. The patient should not be urged to eat, however, until he feels the inclination to do so or at least until after the expiration of ten to twelve days, when the danger of damage to the anastomosis from overloading the stomach is not great. The majority of patients, however, are able to eat a soft solid diet divided into six small meals per day by the twelfth postoperative day.

The majority of patients who have had an esophagectomy are well enough to get up from bed on the second postoperative day. Many of them are allowed to begin ambulation on the first day after operation. A few patients, however, must be kept in bed four or five days before the readjustment of the respiratory and circulatory functions is sufficiently well established to allow greater activity. This rule applies almost exclusively to the patients with a growth which necessitates the performance of a high supra-aortic arch anastomosis or one within the neck.

THE MANAGEMENT OF THE LATE RECOVERY PERIOD

The majority of patients on whom an esophagectomy has been performed (excluding those whose growth lies in the cervical segment) are able to return home within two to three weeks after operation, depending upon the distance to be traveled and the possibilities of care at home. Then there is a period of readjustment which may present difficulties and lead to anxieties from which the surgeon should seek to protect the patient by explanation and advice.

In common with patients who have been subjected to a total gastrectomy, patients who have had operations of the sort described frequently complain that they do not regain a normal appetite. This may correct itself after weeks or months have elapsed, but in many instances the return of appetite is incomplete at best. This occurrence is associated with and possibly explained in part by the fact that many patients experience a functional delay in the emptying of the stomach. The interruption of the vagus nerves is a contributing factor because of the resulting diminution in the amplitude of the gastric peristaltic activity and because of the hypertonicity of the pyloric sphincter. The result is that the stomach remains partially filled much of the time. It is a common observation among these patients that they are able to eat a large breakfast, but that they have little appetite for their noonday meal and are able to accommodate hardly any of their supper. This functional difficulty is most pronounced in the patients with carcinoma of the cardia which requires excision of a large segment of the stomach. This of necessity leaves only a small distal portion which accommodates a limited volume of food. It has been observed, however, that pronounced examples of the inability of the stomach to empty after the performance of a partial gastrectomy and esophagectomy have become much less frequent than formerly and that the difficulty arises least often in patients who have had a high esophagectomy. A possible explanation for this is that the division of the gastrocolic and gastrohepatic ligaments is now carried all the way to the level of the pylorus in every case, thus probably interrupting many of the sympathetic fibers which would otherwise be overactive because of the absence of the vagus inhibition.

In evaluating the postoperative digestive function of these patients it should be kept in mind also that, except in the case of lesions high in the esophagus where the whole stomach is preserved, it is necessary to resect portions of the fundus of the stomach. This sometimes causes a very large reduction in gastric volume which further limits the ability of the patient to take food.

The inability of patients to handle large quantities of food during the first few months of their convalescence is sometimes so great that there is a progressive loss of weight. Such patients should be advised to take nothing but the most nourishing types of food and to avoid wasting valuable space on materials, either liquid or solid, which have a low caloric content. As time goes on, however, in the majority of instances the patient's capacity for food increases as the gastric remnant enlarges and the emptying time of the stomach approximates a normal rate. In spite of this it is unusual for the patient to regain his customary weight. More often he will gain only a few pounds. Many times he will be able merely to hold his weight at a reduced level without further loss.

Although it is frequently necessary to ligate the thoracic duct, particularly in the cases where the position of the growth requires a supra-aortic arch anastomosis, no disturbance of nutrition which can be attributed to this procedure has been observed. The nutritional status of such patients does not vary in any respect from that of those whose thoracic duct remains undisturbed.

A troublesome occurrence frequently observed is the tendency to regurgitation from the stomach if a recumbent posture is assumed soon after eating. All patients who have had the operation should be advised not to lie down during the first two hours after meals. In some patients it is never possible for them to lie on their right side without experiencing regurgitation.

Occasionally a patient may develop diarrhea which lasts sometimes a few days, sometimes several weeks before it subsides. This is probably caused by the disturbance of function resulting from bilateral vagus section. However, this phenomenon is observed in these patients much less frequently than among those who have had a vagotomy performed in the treatment of duodenal ulcer. Relief is obtained by means of the usual symptomatic treatment.

Recurrences of dysphagia are exceedingly unusual after esophagectomy with esophagogastric anastomosis. Cicatricial stenosis of the anastomosis is a rare occurrence. Treatment by bougienage is all that is necessary to overcome the difficulty if it should occur. Recurrence of carcinoma at the anastomosis is observed occasionally, but the majority of the patients who succumb to the disease die from the effects of distant metastases or local recurrence within the mediastinum, and retain their ability to swallow normally as long as they live.

Although a large portion of the left thoracic cavity may be occupied by the transplaced stomach, patients on whom an esophagectomy has been performed almost never experience any sensations which might make them aware of the presence of the stomach within the thorax. Gastric peristaltic sounds are occasionally heard, but they are more often noticed by other people than by the patient himself. Furthermore, after the immediate postoperative period of readjustment has gone by, there is rarely any striking dyspnea or evidence of circulatory disturbances.

CHAPTER 10

ABDOMINAL OPERATIONS PERFORMED THROUGH THORACIC INCISIONS

INTRODUCTION

The development of the technic of transthoracic or abdominothoracic approach to the upper portion of the abdominal cavity has broadened enormously the field of abdominal surgery, especially that having to do with the viscera of the left upper quadrant. Also it has been recognized recently that this approach is superior for the performance of a nephrectomy, particularly in cases of renal tumor, and for the exposure of the suprarenal gland. It provides the best exposure for splenectomy in the difficult cases and is useful in the performance of an anastomosis between the splenic vein and the renal vein. On the right side it gives good access to the vena cava and portal vein for the creation of an anastomosis between these two vessels.

The employment of the transthoracic approach for the performance of these operations has a threefold advantage. The first is the superiority of the exposure of the area where the lesion lies in comparison with the difficult or limited exposures obtained through the classical abdominal or flank incisions. Under some circumstances, notably in carcinoma of the stomach invading the lower end of the esophagus, this advantage is so great that it converts what would otherwise be an inoperable case into one which is favorable for surgery. The second advantage lies in the fact that because of the lateral recumbent position of the patient there is little or no necessity to handle the intestines, particularly the small bowel. The effect of gravity comes to the aid of the surgeon and walling off with pads of gauze is not necessary. The shock-producing effect of manipulation of the viscera is thereby avoided. The third advantage, which depends to some extent upon the second, is the fact that since there is no necessity for handling the majority of the abdominal viscera and since relaxation of the abdominal musculature is not required to obtain an adequate exposure of the operative field, it is possible to perform the entire operation with a relatively light level of anesthesia. Therefore, by using a transthoracic incision a long and difficult procedure can be carried to completion without any evidence of shock to the patient. Using gastric surgery alone as an example, the relative absence of shock in patients whose operation is done through a transthoracic incision as compared with those who are operated upon through an abdominal incision is striking.

An important use of the thoraco-abdominal approach is in the surgery of trauma. With patients who have sustained penetrating wounds of the upper abdomen or lower portion of the chest, the possibility that both body cavities may have been involved makes it advantageous to explore through a thoraco-abdominal incision. The wide exposure thus obtained makes it possible to deal with injuries to the lung, esophagus, heart or pericardium, stomach, liver, spleen, the splenic or hepatic flexures of the colon, or the upper small intestine at one and the same time. On the contrary, patients who are suspected of having a ruptured spleen, as the result of a crushing injury or a blow upon the upper abdomen, should be explored abdominally because of the possibility that a tear of the mesentery or a rupture of the small intestine may also have occurred. Such injuries are more readily found and dealt with through a laparotomy incision.

TRANSTHORACIC GASTRIC SURGERY

Incision

The vast majority of transthoracic operations upon the stomach can be performed through a low left standard thoracotomy incision resecting the ninth rib. If the exposure thus obtained is insufficient, the incision can be made thoraco-abdominal by cutting across the costochondral arch opposite the ninth intercostal space and incising the lateral musculature of the abdominal wall in the direction of the thoracic incision. This method of enlargement has been described (Chap. 3). The necessity for this maneuver arises chiefly in certain cases of carcinoma of the stomach which require a total gastrectomy, particularly when the mesentery of the upper loop of the jejunum is so short that it must be elongated by division of vessels or when it seems preferable to use the Roux type of anastomosis.

Under certain circumstances, particularly when the case is presumed to be inoperable, it may be advantageous to start the incision in the upper left quadrant of the abdomen, extending it obliquely toward the costal margin at the ninth intercostal space. If the previous suspicion of inoperability is confirmed by exploration through this short incision, nothing further is done. If the growth is resectable, the incision is readily converted into an abdominothoracic one by cutting the costochondral arch and extending it into the ninth intercostal space.

The diaphragm must always be incised except when only an abdominal exploration has been done. With benign lesions and with carcinoma requiring total gastrectomy, in which the abdominal segment of the esophagus is not involved by the disease, it is unnecessary to carry the diaphragmatic incision completely through the esophageal hiatus. In every instance when the esophagus must be severed several inches above the cardia, complete incision is required. In the latter group it is desirable to crush the left phrenic nerve in the chest so as to eliminate the tug upon the portion of the stomach or jejunum which lies in the embrace of the diaphragmatic incision after completion of the anastomosis.

Gastric Operations in Which the Transthoracic Approach Is Preferable

Transthoracic operations upon the stomach may be classified under two headings depending upon the indications for the use of the thoracic approach. The first category comprises those procedures in which the transthoracic (or thoraco-abdominal) approach is preferable or mandatory, such as the local excision of benign tumors of the fundus, partial gastrectomy for localized lesions near or involving the cardia, and extensive lesions which require a total gastrectomy for their complete removal. These will be described in turn.

Excision of Benign Tumors of the Proximal Half of the Stomach. The proximal portion of the stomach is a frequent site of benign intramural tumors, the majority of which are leiomyomas or neurofibromas. For their removal a limited excision of the portion of the gastric wall from which they arise is sufficient. In the majority of instances excision of an elliptical or wedge-shaped section of the stomach through all layers, including a generous margin of normal tissue around the base of the tumor, provides adequate insurance against the possibility of local recurrence in the few cases where sarcomatous changes may be detected by histologic examination.

The exposure is obtained in the usual manner, using a transthoracic incision with a limited incision of the diaphragm. Occlusive clamps are not used. In order to prevent soiling of the operative field, the fluid contents of the stomach should be removed by aspiration as soon as the lumen is opened. The defect which remains in the stomach after the tumor has been excised may be closed in any of several ways, depending upon the preference of the surgeon. A convenient method is to use a continuous suture of chromicized catgut inserted in such a manner as to invert the cut edges of the gastric wall (Connell technic), followed by a second layer of Lembert sutures of fine silk or catgut. A somewhat better method, especially from the standpoint of the prevention of postoperative bleeding, involves the use of three layers. The first layer consists of a continuous Connell suture of catgut to invert the mucosa only. The second layer (also of catgut) is an over and over continuous suture to approximate the edges of the muscularis. The outer layer comprises a row of interrupted Lembert sutures of silk or fine catgut.

Sometimes the growth is attached so close to the margin of the cardiac orifice that it is impossible to perform a limited excision of the gastric wall without encroaching upon the lumen at that point. Resort must be made under these circumstances to the performance of a resection involving the tumor-bearing area in the stomach, the cardia and a short length of the lower esophagus. The easiest and safest method of restoring continuity is by end-to-side esophagogastric anastomosis after closing the open end of the stomach. This technic has been described (Chap. 9).

Closure of the thoracic incision, including the incision in the diaphragm, is made in the usual manner. Even in such a simple operation as this it is wise, for reasons already presented, to provide closed suction drainage of the left pleural cavity. This rule applies in all types of operation upon the stomach performed through the thoracic or combined thoraco-abdominal incision.

Resection of the Proximal Portion of the Stomach with Esophagogastric Anastomosis (Proximal Partial Gastrectomy). This procedure is used in those cases of carcinoma of the upper portion of the stomach which are not so extensive as to require a total gastrectomy, in cases of benign tumor arising close to the cardia, and in certain cases of benign gastric ulcer situated in the proximal portion of the stomach. Benign gastric ulcers are sometimes of enormous size, often with penetration into the pancreas or occasionally the left lobe of the liver, and cannot always be distinguished clinically from the ulcerating type of carcinoma.

The essential details of the technic of the operation have already been described in Chapter 9 under the discussion of resection of the lower end of the esophagus. The identical method is used for lesions near the cardia, no matter whether they arise in the stomach or in the esophagus. The difference consists only in the level of transection of the two organs. In lesions of the lower esophagus near or involving the cardia, only a relatively small segment of the stomach need be excised. The patient is then left with a fairly large distal segment of stomach. On the other hand, in lesions which arise within the stomach, a large portion of the stomach must be removed, but more of the esophagus can usually be preserved so that an esophagogastric anastomosis can still be made. However, the patient is left with a much diminished gastric volume. In the latter group of patients the use of an end-to-end anastomosis may be the only satisfactory manner in which union of the esophagus with the distal remnant of the stomach can be effected, although in the majority of instances the end-to-side technic can be carried out. The technical details of both types of anastomosis have been described (Chap. 9) and will not be redescribed here.

Total Gastrectomy. The incision is made according to the principles outlined previously. Complete division of the diaphragm is necessary only when the lesion has extended into the esophagus so far that transection must be made at or above the level of the hiatus. Since in the majority of instances the operation is performed in the treatment of carcinoma, the description of the technic will be directed toward the management of such a case.

Once it has been decided on the basis of a thorough exploration of the abdominal cavity that the growth is resectable, a survey of the local extent of the disease should be made in order to plan the steps of the procedure. In many cases removal of the entire stomach with short segments of the esophagus and duodenum together with the entire omentum, as much as

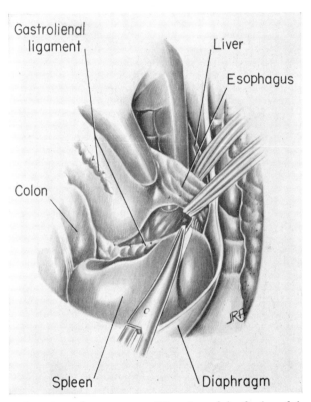

Fig. 137. Transthoracic total gastrectomy. Dissection of the fundus of the stomach and abdominal portion of the esophagus; division of the gastrolienal ligament. *Note:* The incision of the diaphragm in this instance does not extend through the esophageal hiatus.

possible of the gastrohepatic ligament, and the lymph nodes around the duodenum and in the region of the origin of the left gastric artery is sufficient. In other cases, because of local invasion by the growth or the necessity for sacrificing important arteries, it may be necessary to remove the spleen in addition or to excise with the stomach portions of the liver, the transverse colon, the pancreas, the left suprarenal gland and the diaphragm. Splenectomy with or without partial pancreatectomy is frequently necessary as an accompaniment of total gastrectomy. Excision of a portion of the liver and resection of a segment of the colon are required less frequently. On occasion all of these additional maneuvers must be included in the same operation. The decision in each instance should be made before the dissection is begun.

Technic. In the uncomplicated case the operation is begun by freeing the omentum from the colon. For this purpose the transverse colon is drawn

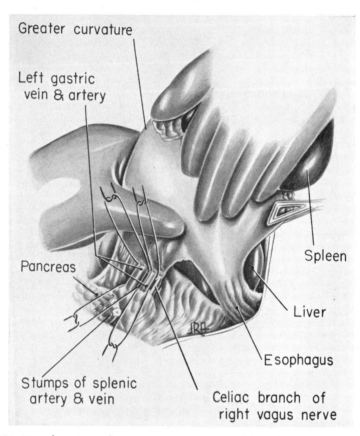

Fig. 138. Transthoracic total gastrectomy. Exposure of the left gastric artery and vein for ligation and division along the superior margin of the pancreas. The stomach is turned up, exposing the posterior surface to view. *Note:* In this patient it was necessary to remove the spleen and the distal two thirds of the pancreas with the stomach. The sutured proximal end of the pancreas and the ligated stumps of the splenic artery and vein are shown. The terminal branch of the right vagus nerve was observed in this case as shown.

out through the lower end of the incision. The omentum is held up by the assistant and the colon is held by the surgeon so that the relatively avascular omental attachment can be exposed for division with the scissors. The few small vessels encountered are secured with small hemostatic forceps for ligation at an appropriate moment. By this maneuver the lesser omental cavity is entered. This facilitates the division of the omental attachment between the spleen and the splenic flexure of the colon and the gastrolienal ligament. At this point the left gastro-epiploic artery and vein and later the vasa brevia of the stomach are cut and ligated. The small retroperitoneal surface of the fundus of the stomach adjacent to the diaphragm is exposed and the abdominal segment of the esophagus is freed of its peritoneal covering. A strip of Penrose tubing is passed around the esophagus and held with a hemostatic forceps for traction purposes (Fig. 137). Several small retrogastric and retro-esophageal blood vessels which are always encountered in this region must be divided. These blood vessels are a posterior gastric branch of the splenic, branches from the superior suprarenal and inferior phrenic arteries and from the lowermost esophageal vessels. This step frees the cardia posteriorly.

The next step is to divide the upper portion of the gastrohepatic ligament which contains one or more anastomotic vessels from the ascending branches of the left gastric artery. Suture ligatures are used to secure these vessels after division. The greater curvature of the stomach with the omentum attached is swung up over the proximal edge of the incision and the pedicle of the left gastric vessels is exposed for division (Fig. 138). Here provision should be made for the excision of the large and important group of lymph nodes which is so frequently involved by metastatic implants from the tumor. By careful dissection along the superior border of the pancreas the left gastric vein can be isolated as it enters the splenic vein, where it should be tied. The corresponding artery can be identified and ligated close to its origin from the celiac axis, avoiding at the same time any injury to the splenic and hepatic branches. Also, in this area it is usually possible to identify the termination of the right vagus nerve near the celiac plexus (Fig. 138). After the nerve and vessels are severed, the stomach can be drawn upward a distance of several inches to gain better access to the duodenum. With the stomach held up, the right gastric and right gastro-epiploic vessels are cut and ligated (Fig. 139).

In complicated cases which require a wider excision including all or portions of adjacent viscera, the dissection is carried out somewhat differently. The invasion of the spleen or pancreas by tumor or the presence of lymph node metastases around the origin of the splenic artery necessitates the performance of a splenectomy, often with a partial pancreatectomy as well. Under these circumstances, the spleen is held up and the peritoneal reflection lateral to the splenic hilus is incised. The dissection is carried medially in the retroperitoneal tissues over the left kidney and suprarenal gland, reflecting the splenic vessels and the tail of the pancreas. Occasionally a portion of the left suprarenal gland may have to be removed with the growth, but more often the gland is uninvolved and merely the branches of the left superior suprarenal artery have to be severed. As the stomach, spleen and pancreas are turned forward en masse, the splenic vessels come into

13

view. The artery can be traced along the superior border of the pancreas to its origin, near which it is tied and divided. The vein, which is usually found lying behind the pancreas, is tied and cut at a convenient level. If only the spleen is to be removed, the tail of the pancreas must be reflected from the hilus of the spleen, dividing several branches of the splenic vessels to

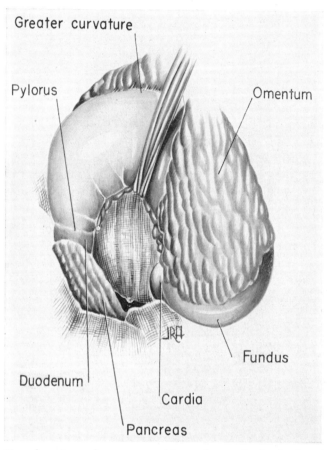

Greater curvature

Pylorus

Omentum

Fundus

Duodenum

Cardia

Pancreas

Fig. 139. Transthoracic total gastrectomy. Stomach completely freed with all vessels ligated and cut. The entire omentum remains attached to the greater curvature after separation from the colon. The esophagus and first portion of the duodenum are ready for transection. *Note:* In this patient it was not necessary to remove the spleen or any of the pancreas. The restoration of continuity in this case was by esophagoduodenal anastomosis (see Fig. 140).

accomplish this. If the tail of the pancreas is adherent or invaded, it must also be removed along with the spleen and the stomach. A transverse wedge-shaped incision is made across the body of the pancreas as far as necessary away from the growth but avoiding the superior mesenteric vessels which lie behind the pancreas close to its head. The wedge-shaped incision leaves a deep groove which makes it easier to suture the cut edge without having the sutures cut through the pancreas as they are tied. The end is closed with one row of interrupted interlocking mattress sutures. If the pancreatic duct is identified, it can be ligated independently. If it is not seen, the interlocking

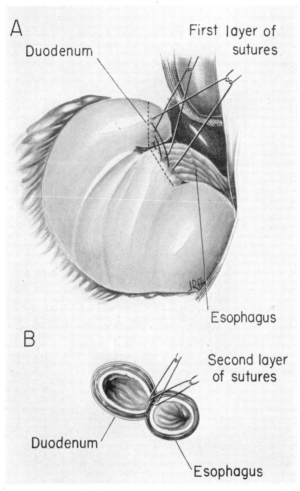

Fig. 140. Transthoracic total gastrectomy. Restoration of continuity by esophagoduodenal anastomosis. *A*, First step: Placement of the outer posterior layer of sutures (mattress). *B*, Appearance of the esophagus and duodenum after complete transection. The first posterior layer of sutures has been tied and cut. The middle layer of sutures to approximate the muscle edges is being inserted. The mucosal layer remains to be put in for the completion of the posterior aspect of the anastomosis. The layers of the anterior aspect will then be inserted in reverse order as in esophagogastric anastomosis (see Fig. 132).

sutures are certain to occlude it. The sutured end of the pancreas is then buried in the retroperitoneal areolar tissues overlying the kidney by means of several interrupted sutures. From this point on, the operation proceeds as in an uncomplicated case (Fig. 138).

If in addition the transverse colon is involved or if, in order to circumvent the growth, it is necessary to interrupt and ligate the middle colic artery, a segment of this portion of the colon must be resected. To accomplish this a pair of short straight crushing clamps is applied at the proper place both proximal and distal to the segment to be removed; the bowel is then cut with the electric cautery between each pair of clamps, leaving the isolated segment attached to the mass of tissue which is to be removed. The proximal and distal ends of the colon are covered with pads of moistened gauze and left for ultimate anastomosis after the completion of the rest of the procedure.

The next step is the transection of the duodenum, but before this is done one must decide whether the duodenum or the jejunum is to be used for the anastomosis. In approximately 10 per cent of the cases it is possible to perform an end-to-end esophagoduodenal anastomosis, but this eventuality depends upon the presence of an unusually mobile duodenum and complete lack of carcinomatous invasion of the lower end of the esophagus. The mobility of the duodenum may be improved by incising the peritoneal reflection lateral to the second portion, thus swinging the entire duodenum and head of the pancreas toward the midline. In the majority of patients, however, it is necessary to use the jejunum.

Anastomosis by Esophagoduodenostomy. When conditions are favorable for anastomosis with the duodenum, the two organs are drawn close together, leaving the stomach attached, and an outer posterior layer of fine silk mattress sutures is inserted (Fig. 140, *A*). After all have been placed, they are tied in turn and the last suture at each end is held by a hemostat. The intervening sutures are cut. A right angle clamp is applied to the esophagus distal to the level of intended transection and usually also to the duodenum between the pylorus and the level of anastomosis. Using a knife with a bent blade, the muscularis of both the esophagus and the duodenum is incised, avoiding the mucosa, and the muscle-approximating middle layer of fine silk sutures is introduced and tied. The mucosa of each organ is then incised in turn and the contents of the proximal esophagus and of the duodenum distally are aspirated. The posterior mucosal sutures are inserted next and tied. The division of both the esophagus and the duodenum is then completed, using the right angle scissors.

Sometimes it is more convenient, especially in the presence of a large heavy tumor or when more than just the stomach is being removed, to perform this step of the procedure before inserting the posterior mucosal layer (Fig. 140, *B*). The anastomosis is finished by carrying each layer of sutures around to complete the anterior aspect. The anterior layers are inserted in reverse order, proceeding from the mucosa outward to the final inverting layer of mattress sutures. The duodenum is held in its new position by means of several fine silk sutures, fixing it to the peritoneum over the pancreas or occasionally to the inferior surface of the diaphragm. With the

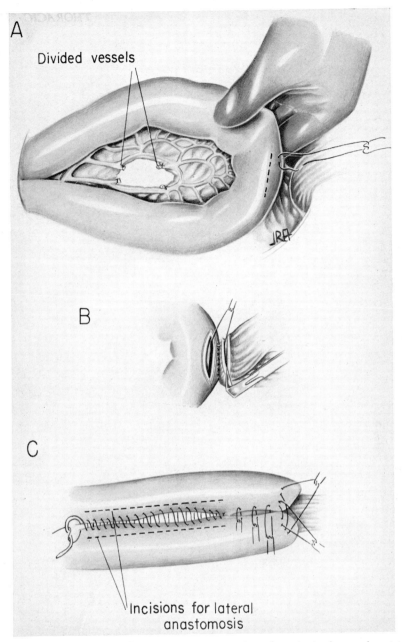

A

Divided vessels

B

C

Incisions for lateral
anastomosis

Fig. 141. Transthoracic total gastrectomy. Restoration of continuity by esophagojejunal anastomosis (end-to-side). *A,* Method of elongating the jejunal mesentery by ligation and division of one or more jejunal arteries close to their origins from the superior mesenteric artery. The corresponding veins are likewise interrupted. The correct position for the line of incision for the anastomosis is shown on the jejunum. *B,* Posterior aspect of the anastomosis. The outer layer has been completed; the muscular layer is being started. *C,* The esophagojejunal anastomosis has been completed with three layers all around. The jejunal loop is shown folded together to cover this anastomosis, and the position and length of the large jejunojejunostomy are indicated.

completion of the anastomosis, the operation is finished. The fact that only one anastomosis is required constitutes one of the many advantages of this method.

Anastomosis by Esophagojejunostomy. An esophagojejunal anastomosis can be made either end-to-side (Fig. 141) or end-to-end by the so-called Roux technic (Fig. 142). The choice between the two methods rests somewhat upon the preference of the surgeon, but to a greater extent upon the anatomic factors prevailing in each individual patient. In the majority of instances either method is satisfactory; however, when because of the extent of invasion of the lower esophagus by the growth it is necessary to transect the esophagus at a high level, often above the diaphragm, it is sometimes difficult or impossible to use the end-to-side technic without resorting to the elongation of the jejunal mesentery by dividing some of its vessels. This maneuver may be necessary also when the mesentery of the proximal jejunum is unusually short, even though a satisfactory length of esophagus may be available. Under these conditions the Roux Y-type of anastomosis is sometimes preferable to the end-to-side. Either method is satisfactory from the functional standpoint, but, as will be pointed out, the end-to-side anastomosis can be modified in such a manner as to make it possible for the patient to consume a larger volume of food at one time than when the end-to-end method is employed. Furthermore, the latter technic is somewhat more difficult to use successfully. When correctly made, neither type of anastomosis should be complicated by the formation of a stricture or leakage from the suture line.

The adoption of either method of performing an esophagojejunal anastomosis implies that the duodenum must be divided and closed as a preliminary step. The technical details of this portion of the operation may be varied to suit the preference of the surgeon. The duodenum may be cut across proximal to the jaws of a right angle clamp, thus avoiding spilling of its contents, or it may be severed and closed without the use of a clamp. In the former method a continuous through and through suture of catgut may be inserted behind the jaws of the clamp which is then removed. A second layer consisting of a continuous Lembert suture of fine catgut or of interrupted sutures of silk or catgut is then inserted. As a further protection against leakage a third layer of interrupted sutures, preferably of silk, should be used to roll the inverted end over against the peritoneal covering of the pancreas.

Esophagojejunostomy by the End-to-side Technic. Many times the proximal loop of the jejunum can be brought up to the end of the esophagus with ease. On the other hand, the approximation may be impossible without relaxing the pull of a short mesentery. To accomplish this the loop which is to be used for the anastomosis is held up and the vascular pattern of its mesentery observed. It will be discovered in every instance that by dividing from one to three jejunal branches close to their origin from the superior mesenteric artery, together with the accompanying veins, the pull will be immediately released, making it possible to draw the loop several inches higher than before. By dividing as many vessels as necessary it is possible to advance the jejunum a relatively long distance into the thorax, often as high as the level of the inferior pulmonary vein. It is not necessary to close the resulting aperture in the mesentery (Fig. 141, *A*).

Two precautions must be observed in carrying out this maneuver. The first and most obvious is to interrupt the vessels close to their origin so as to preserve the continuity of the anastomotic vascular arches in the mesentery, distal to the point of ligation. The other is to avoid using the highest jejunal loop just beyond the ligament of Treitz because at that level the vascular arches are either inadequate or are finally lost in favor of a type of vascular pattern more closely resembling end arteries with a minimum of inter-communication. Interruption of any vessels at this level may lead to the development of a localized area of necrosis of the bowel proximal to the anastomosis. In practice the site chosen for the anastomosis is usually at least 8 to 10 inches distal to the ligament of Treitz.

The loop of jejunum may be drawn up either in front of the transverse colon or behind it through an opening made in the transverse mesocolon. The advantage of the former location lies in the fact that the possibility of herniation of small intestine through the opening in the mesocolon is completely eliminated, while that of the latter obviously is the fact that sometimes a somewhat shorter loop can be used.

The anastomosis is made in three layers, using interrupted sutures of fine silk in exactly the same manner as in the performance of an esophagogastric anastomosis, except that a linear incision is used in the jejunum instead of excising a circular portion as is done in the gastric cases (Fig. 141, *B*). When the esophagus is not invaded by tumor and the level of transection can therefore be below the diaphragm, the anastomosis is usually placed on the antemesenteric surface of the bowel at the apex of the loop. The loop is suspended with a row of sutures to the crura of the diaphragm behind the anastomosis and another row between the jejunum in front of the anastomosis and the surface of the diaphragm near the anterior margin of the esophageal hiatus. When the esophagus has been divided above the diaphragm, the anastomosis is placed on the anterior surface of the jejunum just beyond the antemesenteric border. At its completion it will be observed that the jejunum then has a tendency to fold upon itself as a result of the forward movement of the two arms of the loop which can be sutured together in such a way as to surround the anastomosis completely (Fig. 141, *C*). The loop is suspended within the chest by means of several sutures fixing it to the edges of the incision in the mediastinal pleura.

No matter what the details of the esophagojejunal anastomosis may be in any given case, it is always advisable to perform an entero-enterostomy between the proximal and distal arms of the jejunal loop in order to insure proper function. This is done by a side-to-side approximation without the use of clamps. Two layers of sutures suffice. Interrupted silk or, if time is a factor as it often is at the end of a long operation, continuous fine chromicized catgut may be employed. This anastomosis should be placed close to the bottom of the proximal arm of the loop near the ligament of Treitz. A highly desirable modification of this portion of the procedure consists in making the jejunojejunostomy unusually long (Fig. 141, C). Instead of the customary 2 or 3 inches it may be elongated to 6 or 8 inches. This has the disadvantage that it prolongs the operation, but if the condition of the patient warrants the expenditure of this additional time, it is worthwhile from the functional point of view because the long intercommunicating opening thus produced makes it possible for the patient to consume a larger volume of food at one time. As a result he can eat with more comfort and at less frequent intervals.

When the loop has been passed up behind the colon, the peritoneal edges of the opening in the transverse mesocolon should be sutured to the loop so as to avoid leaving any apertures through which another loop of small intestine might pass. Several sutures of fine silk usually suffice. The level of fixation of the mesocolon should be near the upper limit of the enteroenterostomy or even above it.

Esophagojejunostomy by End-to-end Anastomosis (Roux Technic). There is nothing about the use of the Roux technic of esophagojejunal anastomosis in cases of transthoracic total gastrectomy which differs essentially from the application of the method in the abdominal approach, except that a larger dissection and freeing of the mesentery of the distal segment is necessary when the esophagus must be transected at some point within the chest. This involves the ligation and division of a larger number of jejunal arteries, but if the usual precaution of cutting the vessels close to their origin so as to avoid interference with the continuity of the vascular arcades in the mesentery is observed, an adequate circulation can usually be preserved all the way to the end of the bowel where the anastomosis is to be made. The color of the end should be observed from time to time; if an adequate blood supply has not been preserved, as determined from discoloration beyond the termination of the active circulation, the precarious end of bowel should be trimmed away and discarded no matter how long it may be. When the proper length of healthy bowel has been freed, the anastomosis is begun. It matters little whether the esophagojejunal or the jejunojejunal anastomosis is made first. For the former, two layers consisting of an inner to join the mucosa edge to edge and an outer of mattress sutures to invert the first layer are usually sufficient. Because of the precariousness of the blood supply of the jejunal end, a third layer is usually omitted unless the approximation produced by the first two layers is not entirely satisfactory. The jejunum is suspended in the usual manner by means of a few fine silk sutures to the mediastinal pleura. These must be placed with infinite caution to avoid injury to any of the jejunal vessels. If the bowel has been brought up behind the colon, the opening in the transverse mesocolon must be closed. The jejunojejunal anastomosis is made end-to-side at any convenient point using two layers of sutures (Fig. 142).

At the completion of the anastomosis, the usual dose of penicillin and streptomycin solution is inserted and the diaphragm is closed. If the anastomosis lies within the chest, an opening of sufficient size must be left to prevent

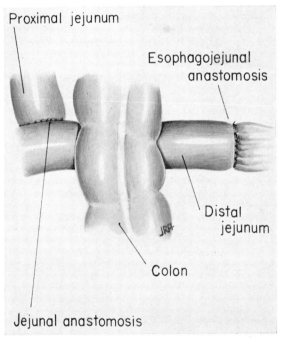

Proximal jejunum

Esophagojejunal anastomosis

Distal jejunum

Colon

Jejunal anastomosis

Fig. 142. Transthoracic total gastrectomy. Restoration of continuity by esophagojejunal anastomosis (end-to-end, Roux technic). The distal arm of the divided jejunal loop has been drawn up through an opening in the transverse mesocolon for the esophagojejunal anastomosis. The jejunojejunostomy lies below the mesocolon.

encroachment upon the jejunum where it passes through. The edges of the diaphragm are sutured to the bowel at several points. Closed suction drainage of the chest should be provided by a Foley catheter. The lung is reexpanded and the chest wall is closed.

Transthoracic Gastric Operations Ordinarily Performed Through Abdominal Incisions

The second category of gastric operations which may be performed through a transthoracic approach includes those procedures which are ordinarily carried out through the usual abdominal incision but which for any of several reasons may have to be performed through the chest. These include partial gastrectomy for lesions in the distal half of the stomach, gastroenterostomy and gastrostomy.

Resection of the Distal Portion of the Stomach with Gastrojejunal Anastomosis (*Distal Partial Gastrectomy*). This operation is frequently spoken of as "sub-total gastrectomy," a term which is obviously inaccurate and misleading because of the fact that, with rare exceptions, a relatively large segment of the proximal portion of the stomach is not removed. The occasion for performing it through a transthoracic or abdominothoracic incision is usually in the rare case of carcinoma of the stomach in which the roentgen examination has erroneously suggested that the lesion extends so far toward the cardia that a total or proximal partial gastrectomy is indicated, whereas on exploration the upper half of the stomach is discovered to be uninvolved. The technical details of the procedure need not be discussed since, with the exception of the incision, they do not differ from the usual operation as performed through an abdominal incision. It should be mentioned, however, that the thoracic approach provides such ready access to the upper portion of the stomach that the securing of the vessels on the curvatures and the transection of the stomach can be carried out with greater ease than in some instances when the operation is performed abdominally. In some patients it may be necessary to enlarge the incision across the costochondral arch.

Gastrojejunostomy. A gastrojejunostomy can be performed through a transthoracic incision just as readily as through the abdomen. The occasion for its performance is almost always as an adjunct to a vagectomy done through the chest. The indications for supplementing a vagectomy with a gastrojejunostomy need not be discussed here. Because the surgeon is likely to be more familiar with the topography of the viscera as observed through the abdomen, he should be careful to make the correct adjustment of the relations of the stomach and the proximal jejunum to each other before the anastomosis is actually begun. In the average case of this sort, drainage of the pleural cavity is not necessary.

Gastrostomy. In certain patients who have a carcinoma of the esophagus which is discovered at exploratory thoracotomy to be inoperable, it is desirable to perform a gastrostomy because of the completeness of the obstruction. This can be done either through the thoracic incision or, after closing the chest, through a separate laparotomy incision. The former course obviates the necessity of turning the patient from his side to his back and re-preparing and redraping for a different approach. If the decision is made to proceed through the thoracotomy incision, a short incision is made through the diaphragm if this has not already been done as a part of the exploration. The stomach is drawn out and the gastrostomy is carried out according to whatever method the surgeon may prefer. A rubber tube may be inserted, but the Spivak modification of the Janeway technic gives the most satisfactory results. After the catheter has been inserted into the stomach or the living tube has been constructed from the anterior gastric wall, the catheter or gastric tube is drawn out through a short incision over the upper portion of the left rectus muscle. The anterior wall of the stomach is sutured to the peritoneum of the abdominal wall on each side of the small incision and the diaphragm is closed. Closure of the thoracic incision is made in the usual manner.

After-care

The principles of postoperative care following the performance of an esophagectomy, as set forth in Chapter 9, are applicable for patients after transthoracic gastric surgery. The details of feeding obviously must be varied to comply with the needs of the individual patient and to conform with the type of operation performed.

SPLENECTOMY

A thoracic or thoraco-abdominal incision provides the best exposure of the spleen which can be obtained. The superiority of this approach is most obvious during the removal of a large spleen which is adherent to the diaphragm or when the vasa brevia are unusually short and inaccessible through the usual abdominal incision.

The single exception to the use of the thoracic approach for splenectomy is the case of traumatic rupture of the spleen. In this instance the possibility that injuries to hollow viscera elsewhere in the abdomen may have occurred makes it preferable to use a laparotomy incision.

For the transthoracic approach to the spleen the incision may be either thoracic or thoraco-abdominal. In the former the chest may be opened through the ninth intercostal space (in young patients) or through the bed of the ninth rib (if the patient is older). In older patients the ninth or tenth intercostal space may be employed also, with extension into the lateral abdominal muscles. In practice it is advisable to use the tenth intercostal space in order to avoid the disadvantages of cutting the costochondral arch. In a large number of patients, however, the cartilage of the tenth rib is unattached so that the ninth space may be employed. The diaphragm should be incised widely in the direction of its fibers but not into the esophageal hiatus. Because of the ease with which a wide separation of the anterior portion of the wound edges is obtained, a somewhat shorter diaphragmatic incision can be made when a thoraco-abdominal incision is used than with a strictly thoracic approach.

The details of the technic employed in the actual removal of the spleen need little comment. The wide exposure provided by the incision makes it relatively simple to deal with the adhesions between the upper pole and the diaphragm. After these have been severed, the peritoneum lateral to the splenic hilus is incised and the spleen is swung forward and medially. The gastrolienal ligament is then cut and separate ligatures are placed on the vasa brevia. The omental attachment at the lower pole of the spleen is severed,

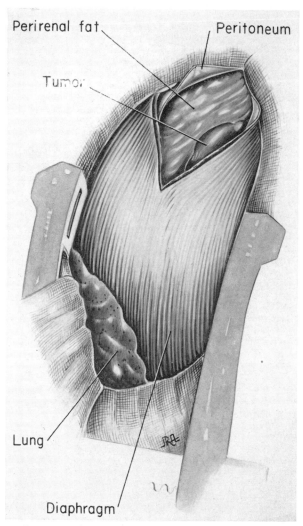

Fig. 143. Transthoracic nephrectomy for renal tumor. Incision through the tenth inter-costal space on the right side with enlargement into the oblique muscles of the abdominal wall below the costal margin. The beginning of the incision into the diaphragm is shown.

taking pains to avoid injury to the splenic flexure of the colon which some-times lies unusually close to the spleen. The splenic artery and vein are within easy reach and can usually be ligated individually. The tip of the tail of the pancreas should be avoided.

After the spleen has been removed, all bleeding points are secured with ligatures. The edges of the diaphragm are approximated with a single row of heavy silk sutures and the wound is closed in the usual manner after expanding the lung. Drainage of the pleural cavity is not necessary.

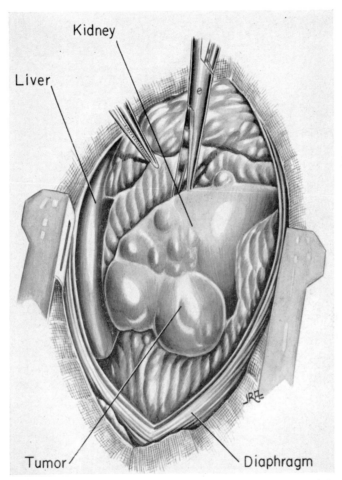

Fig. 144. Transthoracic nephrectomy for renal tumor. Further stage of the operation illustrated in Figure 143, showing wide exposure of the diseased kidney after completion of the diaphragmatic incision.

ADRENALECTOMY

A thoracic or thoraco-abdominal incision made exactly as for the removal of the spleen is of great value in the extirpation of tumors of the suprarenal gland. The technical details of the operation, once the incision has been made, depend upon the circumstances in each individual case and do not require further comment.

NEPHRECTOMY

A recent development in the field of urologic surgery is the adoption of the thoraco-abdominal incision for nephrectomy. As experience accumulates, it begins to be apparent that the exposure provided by this incision is

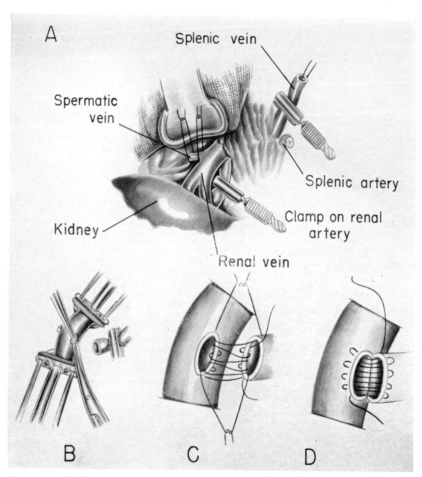

Fig. 145. Transthoracic approach for anastomosis between the end of the splenic vein after removal of the spleen and the side of the left renal vein. Exposure obtained through a left abdominothoracic incision into the tenth intercostal space with partial incision of the diaphragm: details of exposure and anastomosis. *A,* Exposure obtained. *B,* Method of temporary occlusion of the renal vein using the Linton modification of the Bethune lung tourniquet. *C,* Posterior aspect of the anastomosis. *D,* Posterior aspect of anastomosis completed; anterior suture being inserted.

often superior to that obtained with either the classical flank incision or the transabdominal approach. The reasons for this are obvious to those who have used it. They are principally that the kidney is easily and quickly approached and that the exposure of the renal artery and vein is direct and unobstructed.

The most striking evidences of the advantages which result from the use of a thoraco-abdominal incision are observed in patients with large renal tumors or very adherent kidneys and in those with scoliosis when there is marked encroachment upon the space available in the flank. The only important contraindication to the use of this method is the presence of an active pyogenic infection which might lead to wound sepsis and empyema.

The incision should be made through the tenth intercostal space with suitable extension into the lateral muscles of the abdominal wall. The diaphragm must be incised a short distance in the direction of its fibers. If an unusually wide exposure is required, the tenth or eleventh rib may be resected and the incision made through its bed. The method is applicable in either the right or the left side (Figs. 143 and 144).

Except for the remarkable ease with which the structures of the renal pedicle may be reached, the details of technic employed in the removal of the kidney do not differ essentially from those employed in a nephrectomy performed through the classical incision. If drainage is required, the drains are brought out through the flank and the incision is closed tightly. With this exception the principles involved in the closure are the same as for every other thoracic or thoraco-abdominal incision.

ANASTOMOSIS BETWEEN SPLENIC VEIN AND RENAL VEIN OR BETWEEN PORTAL VEIN AND THE VENA CAVA

A low thoraco-abdominal incision such as may be employed in the performance of a nephrectomy is ideally suited to the cases of portal hypertension which require the creation of a venous shunt for the relief of bleeding from esophageal varices. In the case of a splenorenal anastomosis the incision is made on the left side. With a portocaval anastomosis it must obviously be made on the right. The tenth intercostal space with adequate extension into the abdominal muscles provides an excellent exposure.

The technical details of these interesting and important operations may be sought elsewhere (Fig. 145).

CHAPTER 11

SURGERY OF THE DIAPHRAGM

INTRODUCTION

The development of thoracic surgery has provided a new impetus for the treatment of conditions of the diaphragm which were formerly either not operated upon or only imperfectly treated through an abdominal approach. At the present time, with the single exception of hernia in the sinus of Morgagni, every surgical intervention having to do directly with the diaphragm can be more easily and more effectively accomplished through a thoracic incision. Intratracheal inhalation anesthesia is required to provide control of the expansion of the lung while the chest is open. A standard thoracotomy incision is used. The choice between the intercostal and rib resection technics rests with the exigencies of the case and the preference of the surgeon. For a discussion of these details reference should be made to Chapter 3. In the majority of instances the best exposure of the diaphragm is obtained through the bed of the eighth rib or through the eighth intercostal space. Closure of the incision is made in the customary manner. Except under unusual circumstances it is not necessary to drain the pleural cavity. If, on the other hand, there is reason to believe that the lung may have been torn or otherwise injured as a result of the necessity for freeing adhesions to the thoracic wall, or if as a result of recent inflammation the adhesions are unusually vascular, it is wise to provide drainage through a catheter by the method already described in Chapter 2.

CONGENITAL DEFECTS

Although the etiology of certain of the conditions, the treatment of which is to be described, is not thoroughly established, it is convenient to group them together under the heading of congenital defects.

Eventration

There is rarely any occasion to operate for the correction of the condition known as eventration of the diaphragm. Patients who have involvement of one entire side of the diaphragm do not as a rule experience any symptoms from it and surgical treatment is only occasionally attempted. If it seems wise to correct the situation which results from the unusually high position in the chest occupied by the thinned-out diaphragm, the diaphragm can be altered to an appreciable degree even though it cannot be made to function in a normal manner. This is accomplished by means of a series of plicating sutures of heavy silk placed in such a fashion as to shir up the flabby structure, reducing its expanse and thereby diminishing the size of the dome-shaped curve. The same result may be obtained by overlapping the diaphragm, thus producing two folds, each of which must be sutured with medium heavy silk. In either case the repair may be strengthened and made more permanent by weaving over the silk suture line several strips of fascia lata obtained from the uppermost thigh of the patient. A fascia stripper of the Wilson type introduced by an assistant through a short incision just above the lateral aspect of the patient's left knee provides a ready method of obtaining the strips while the operation is in progress.

Localized small areas of eventration of the diaphragm are sometimes encountered but are rarely the cause of symptoms. They are usually seen at operation, either as an incidental finding or as a result of mistaking them for tumors or herniations. Elimination of the bulging area may be readily accomplished as previously described by the method of plication or by overlapping and suture.

Defects Resulting from Failures of Fusion

In all of the conditions grouped under the heading of defects of fusion there is a localized aperture at some point in the diaphragm through which the abdominal contents may protrude into either the pleural cavity or the mediastinal space. With one exception and possibly a second, these conditions may be classified as true hernias because of the presence of a peritoneal sac which prevents the abdominal viscera from lying free in the pleural cavity after they protrude through the opening. This distinction is necessary in order to understand the principles of the operations to be described. The embryologic aspects, though interesting, are not a subject of concern in this work.

Pleuroperitoneal Sinus (Sinus of Bochdalek). Although this condition may exist in either side of the diaphragm, it is usually the subject of surgical intervention only on the left because of the fact that on the right the liver prevents the passing through of any of the hollow abdominal viscera. The defect is usually in the muscular portion of the diaphragm not far from the periphery. It is not, strictly speaking, a hernia because of the lack of a sac of peritoneal covering. In this condition, therefore, as well as in traumatic rupture of the diaphragm, the herniated abdominal viscera lie uncovered within the pleural cavity. These are the only conditions in which this finding is ever observed.

The repair of a pleuroperitoneal sinus is a relatively simple matter. A standard thoracotomy incision is made. The abdominal viscera are usually not adherent and can be pushed into the abdomen easily. Once this is accomplished, the defect can be closed in one of two ways. In the first, the edges of the opening are merely approximated by means of a series of sutures of heavy silk. This closure may be reinforced with a second layer of silk sutures of the Lembert type to invert the sutured edges or by means of a strip of fascia lata. The second method of closure is to overlap the edges, with fixation in their new position by means of two rows of sutures, one along the edge

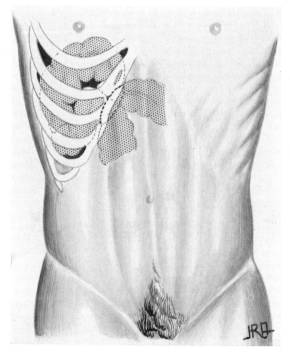

Fig. 146. Sinus of Morgagni hernia. Diagram illustrating the characteristic location of the hernia orifice which results from failure of attachment of the diaphragm to the costal cartilage of the seventh rib.

which lies against the inferior surface and the other along the edge which lies on the superior surface of the diaphragm. This method of closure is strong and rarely requires reinforcement. In either case, however, if greater security seems to be necessary, a strip of fascia lata may be inserted.

Parasternal Hernia (Hernia of the Sinus of Morgagni; Hernia of the Space of Larrey). A hernia through the parasternal space, commonly called the sinus of Morgagni, provides the only occasion where an abdominal approach is usually superior to the transpleural exposure. The condition can be corrected, however, from within the thoracic cavity. On the other hand, in some instances it is necessary to enlarge the abdominal incision across the costal arch into the chest to make the operation successful (Fig. 147). This type of hernia may be encountered on either the right or the left side of the sternum, but it seems to be more frequent on the right (Fig. 146).

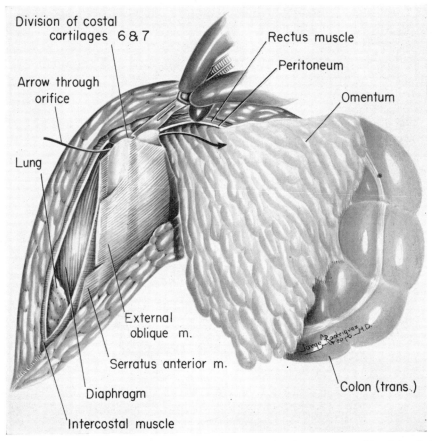

Fig. 147. Sinus of Morgagni hernia. Exposure obtained by the extension of the abdominal incision across the costochondral arch into an intercostal space to make an abdominothoracic approach. In this patient the colon and omentum were incarcerated within the hernia sac and could not be pulled down into the abdomen until the incision was enlarged. Release of the constriction at the orifice of the sac was only partially successful because the contents were adherent in the sac. Bimanual manipulation consisting of pushing from above and pulling from below was necessary to reduce the hernia into the abdomen as shown. The adherent viscera were then dissected free and the sac was excised.

A subcostal incision may be used, but because of the possibility that it may be necessary to enlarge it into the chest, it is preferable to make the incision longitudinal over the upper portion of the rectus muscle, parting the fibers of the muscle to gain access to the peritoneum in the location of the hernia. The abdominal cavity is entered and the hernia opening into the

chest is visualized. In the average case the herniated abdominal viscera, usually
the colon and omentum and occasionally a portion of the stomach, may be
pulled back easily into the abdomen, leaving the edges of the defect free. It
is sometimes possible, by exerting traction, to pull the peritoneal sac down
so that it can be excised, thus denuding the unattached portion of the edge
of the muscular portion of the diaphragm. It is not necessary, however, to
insist upon this step because an adequate closure of the opening can usually
be made, leaving the hernia sac within the chest. This does not appear to
cause complications or postoperative symptoms. A series of sutures of heavy
silk is used to fasten the free edge of the diaphragm to the edge of the lower-

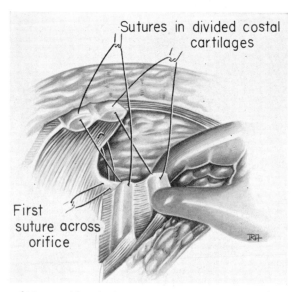

Fig. 148. Sinus of Morgagni hernia. Same patient as in Figure 147. The opening is shown
after retraction of the wound edges and excision of the peritoneal sac of the hernia. The defect
in the diaphragm was closed partly by sutures pulling the muscle edges together, one of
which is shown, and partly by fixing the free edge of the diaphragm to the lower rib cartilage after the divided cartilages had been reapproximated by the sutures shown in the
drawing.

most costal cartilage, and nothing more is required except to close the abdominal incision in the usual manner.

Sometimes the contents of the hernia are so firmly adherent that it is impossible to reduce them into the abdominal cavity or to effect a reduction
en masse by turning the sac inside out. In that case, in order to make a satisfactory repair it is necessary to enlarge the incision into the thorax, thus con-
verting it into an abdominothoracic approach. This step is accomplished by
extending the incision over the costal arch and obliquely upward and outward to the anterior axillary line. The cartilage is cut with a knife or heavy
scissors and the appropriate intercostal space is incised as far as necessary to

obtain access to the hernia sac. Division of the cartilage is the most necessary part of this maneuver (Fig. 147). Occasionally, however, it is possible to avoid cutting the arch by merely making an incision through the intercostal space. In this manner, with the aid of a rib spreader, the hernia sac can be opened and its contents freed or mobilized by dissection and invaginated into the abdomen. Once the sac and its contents have been dealt with, the repair can be made essentially as described above. In closing the incision, the ribs are held in position by means of pericostal sutures of chromicized catgut. Heavy silk sutures or wire may be used to hold the ends of the severed cartilage together (Fig. 148). The peritoneum is closed and finally the muscle, fascial and skin layers are approximated in the usual manner.

Failure of Crural Attachment. Another condition which results from the failure of embryologic elements of the diaphragm to become properly fused to their appropriate attachments is the defect which results from the absence of one of the crura. This rarely encountered condition gives rise to an unusually large form of herniation through the incompletely formed esophageal hiatus. The principles of repair are essentially the same as for any pronounced hernia in this area, but before this can be accomplished, the unattached portion of the diaphragm must be fixed in some manner to the vertebral column. This maneuver may tax the ingenuity and resourcefulness of the surgeon, but by using long instruments it is possible to sew the muscle edge to the fascial investment of the vertebral column with heavy silk sutures. From this point on the steps of the operation are exactly the same as in the repair of the usual hiatus hernia. It is difficult to conceive how this condition could be adequately corrected through an abdominal incision.

Hiatus Hernia

Herniation through the esophageal hiatus is the condition which is the most frequent indication for surgery of the diaphragm. Two anatomic variations are encountered. By far the more frequent is the so-called short esophagus type. Much less frequent is the type spoken of as para-esophageal. In order to explain the principles upon which the success of the operation depends, a description of the anatomic characteristics is given in each instance before the treatment is described (Fig. 149, *A*).

Short Esophagus Type (Sliding). (Fig. 149, *A*). In the majority of instances of hiatus hernia the cardiac end of the stomach is pushed up through the relaxed esophageal hiatus, carrying with it a portion of the fundus as the condition becomes more pronounced. As the herniated portion of the stomach rises higher and higher it pushes upward, allowing the esophagus to retract to an extent equivalent to the amount of upward displacement of the cardia. Thus the esophagus appears to be short when observed by roentgenographic studies and at operation. However, in the majority of

A, Sliding (Short Esophagus)

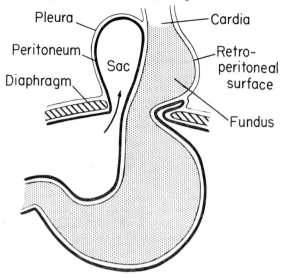

Pleura — Cardia

Peritoneum — Sac — Retro-peritoneal surface

Diaphragm — Fundus

B, Parahiatal (Para-esophageal)

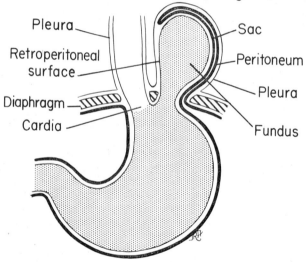

Pleura — Sac

Retroperitoneal surface — Peritoneum

Diaphragm — Pleura

Cardia — Fundus

Fig. 149. Diagram illustrating the anatomic relations of each of the two types of hernia which may occur in the region of the esophageal hiatus of the diaphragm. *A,* Usual type, often spoken of as the "short esophagus type." Note (1) that the cardia and adjacent portion of the stomach are pushed upward through the hiatus into the chest, the esophagus rising with the stomach but (with the exception of a true congenital shortness) not actually short; (2) that such a hernia is a sliding hernia of the upper part of the stomach which comprises one side of the hernia sac. *B,* Infrequent type, commonly called "para-esophageal." A better term is parahiatal because there is a strand of tissue sometimes consisting of a few bundles of diaphragmatic muscle which holds the cardia down below the hiatus of the diaphragm. The hernia orifice comprises a defect in the diaphragm beside the hiatus, sometimes almost a part of it. Through this a peritoneal sac passes with the stomach or other viscera pushing up from below.

instances, the esophagus, although apparently short, will stretch to its normal length as the hernia is reduced. On the other hand, in a very small percentage of patients the esophagus is congenitally short. Patients with this condition have had since birth an abnormal arrangement of the viscera of the upper portion of the alimentary canal, characterized by an esophagus which may be no longer than one half to two thirds of the length of the mediastinal space and a transposition of the cardia and cardiac end of the stomach into the lower mediastinum. This condition is from the first congenital, whereas the ordinary case of hiatus hernia is actually acquired, although it may develop because of a congenital weakness of the hiatus.

It is of great importance in the understanding of the condition and the requirements of its surgical repair to realize that hiatus hernia of the so-called "short esophagus" type (excluding the rare cases of congenitally short esophagus) is actually a sliding hernia similar in mechanism to a sliding hernia of the cecum in the inguinal canal. As in the latter condition the herniated viscus, in this instance the stomach, makes up one side of the hernia sac which in hiatus hernia lies in front of the stomach with extensions around each side. If a cross section were made through the hernia sac, it would have the shape of the letter U, with the stomach lying inside of the curve.

TECHNIC OF REPAIR. Before the patient is anesthetized a Levin tube should be introduced into the stomach. After the usual left thoracotomy incision has been made and the lung is retracted, an incision is made through the mediastinal pleura. Usually the herniated stomach and the sac can be seen through this pleural reflection. The diaphragmatic attachment of the pulmonary ligament is severed so as to give free access to the margin of the hiatus. The phrenic nerve is crushed to abolish diaphragmatic contractions. A strand of heavy silk is then passed through the edge of the diaphragm at the apex of the hiatus. This is held by an assistant to improve the exposure. The lower esophagus with the adjacent vagus nerves and the hernia sac and herniated portion of the stomach are freed by blunt dissection. A few small mediastinal blood vessels and occasionally one or more lower esophageal veins must be divided. The crura of the diaphragm which are now easily visualized are freed of areolar tissue by one or two sweeps of the finger, sometimes assisted by the scissors. These preliminary steps prepare the field for the repair which consists of two important maneuvers.

The first measure essential to the repair of a hiatus hernia is the elimination of the peritoneal sac. In an uncomplicated case with a sac of moderate size this is accomplished by infolding and plication, using as a rule a single row of sutures placed circumferentially (Fig. 150, A). These sutures should not include the wall of the stomach. If enough sutures have been inserted and if they have been correctly applied, this row will suffice to hold the hernia in a state of complete reduction with the cardia below the rim of the hiatus.

Occasionally with a rather large sac, a second row should be inserted. This is illustrated in Fig. 150, *B*.

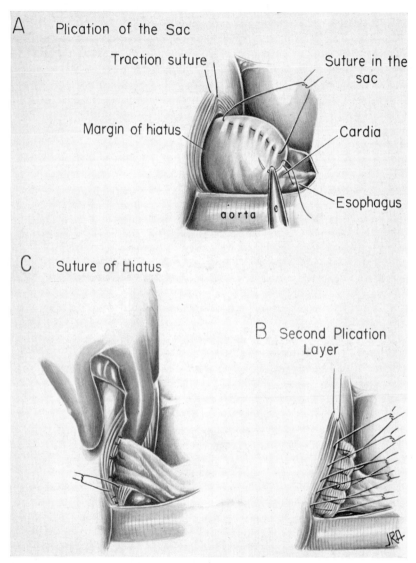

A Plication of the Sac

Traction suture

Suture in the sac

Margin of hiatus

Cardia

aorta

Esophagus

C Suture of Hiatus

B Second Plication Layer

Fig. 150. Hiatus hernia. Method of dealing with a small sac by plication. *A,* Manner in which the plication sutures are inserted. It should be noted that they include only the peritoneal reflection and not the wall of the stomach beneath. (To make this clear reference should be made to Fig. 149, *A.*) *B,* In some cases a second layer of plication sutures is required as shown. *C,* Placement of sutures in the diaphragm to narrow the hiatus to the proper size (see text, page 328).

If the sac is unusually large, as when the major portions of the stomach and sometimes loops of intestine and portions of omentum have been forced through the hiatus in advanced cases, it is usually necessary to remove it (Fig. 151). To accomplish this either of two methods may be employed. In the first method the entire procedure is performed above the diaphragm. The sac is dissected free and excised, leaving the edges of the peritoneum at its base to be approximated with a row of silk sutures placed close together

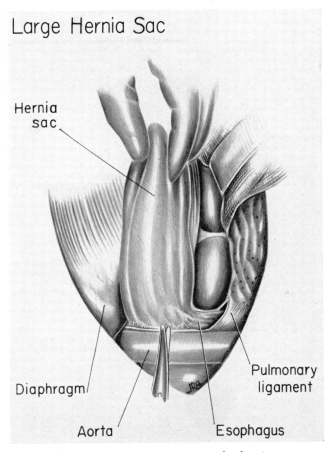

Fig. 151. Hiatus hernia. Large sac requiring excision. The drawing represents the appearance of the sac after its contents, consisting of a portion of the stomach, the transverse colon and the omentum, had been reduced into the abdomen. The relation of this sac to the anterior surface of the cardiac end of the stomach is the same as in the case shown in Figure 150, *A*. The difference lies only in the size.

(Fig. 152). Occasionally it may be possible to transfix and tie a large portion of the sac with a single ligature. The remainder is then obliterated by plication in the usual manner.

Under unusual circumstances, when the reduction of a large hernia is difficult or when it is impossible to hold the viscera below the diaphragm while the repair is being carried out, the second method of surmounting the

Large Sac   Method I

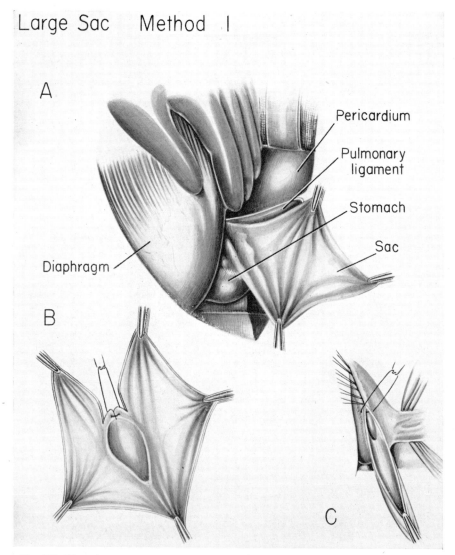

Fig. 152. Hiatus hernia. Large sac, repair method one. Removal of the sac within the chest and without counterincision in the diaphragm. *A,* The emptied sac held in readiness for opening and excision. Note its relation to the stomach. *B,* The opened sac showing the hernia orifice at the neck of the sac and the start of the excision by cutting along the margin of the orifice with closure of the aperture using ordinary silk sutures. *C,* The excision of the sac and closure of the opening are almost complete. It is to be noted that after the excess of the sac has been removed in a case such as this, one or more layers of plication sutures may still be required to maintain an effective reduction of the hernia (see text).

difficulty is used. A short counterincision is made in the muscular portion of the diaphragm several inches away from the hiatus. Through this the herniated viscera are pulled back into the abdomen. As this is done, the peritoneal sac is likewise drawn down and invaginated so that it is almost completely eliminated so long as the stomach is held firmly within the

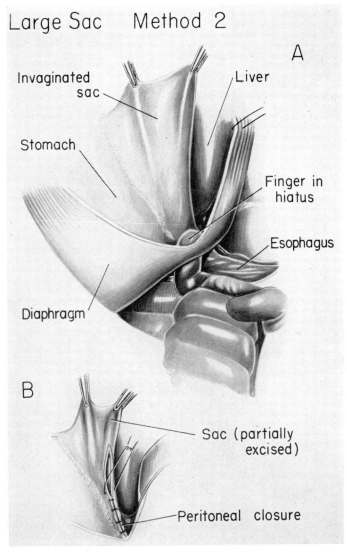

Fig. 153. Hiatus hernia. Large sac, repair method two. *A*, A counterincision has been made through the diaphragm away from the hiatus and the sac invaginated and drawn down into the abdomen where it lies in front of the upper anterior surface of the stomach. *B*, Excision of the sac and closure of the peritoneum from within the abdominal cavity. *Note:* The counterincision is then closed and the remainder of the repair of the hernia is completed from the thoracic side.

abdomen. Permanent ablation of the sac under these conditions can be accomplished from the abdominal side either by plication or by excision and closure of the defect (Fig. 153). Further reinforcement should be obtained from the thoracic side by a row of sutures placed in the retroperitoneal fascial layer.

The second important measure to be accomplished in the repair of a hiatus hernia is the narrowing of the hiatus to a proper size (Fig. 150, C). This should be made small enough to prevent a recurrence of the herniation and still not so small that it might constrict the esophagus. Heavy silk is used and the sutures are placed across the hiatus on each side of the esophagus. Because the long axis of the hiatus is usually oblique, pointing toward the dome of the diaphragm, the sutures are actually right anterior and left posterior in relation to the esophagus, rather than strictly anterior and posterior. The correct size of the opening which should remain after the narrowing has been completed may be estimated by inserting the index finger beside the esophagus in the posterior portion of the hiatus where there is no obstruction resulting from the ablation of the peritoneal sac. If, with the Levin tube inside the esophagus, the finger can be accommodated easily without much encroachment on the esophagus, there will be no danger of constriction and yet a degree of narrowing sufficient to produce the desired result will have been attained. The repair may be further reinforced by an additional suture of fascia lata obtained from the left thigh, but this step is rarely necessary.

When in the repair of a hernia of unusually large size it has been necessary to make a counterincision to maintain reduction while the repair is accomplished, the closure of this additional incision is made by means of interrupted silk after the viscera have been replaced within the abdomen. Under certain circumstances it will be found that there is a tendency for the muscle to tear as the silk sutures are tied. This occurs either because of the obesity of the patient or because the abdominal cavity in the case of an unusually large hernia is too small to hold all its contents, some of which have been lying for many years in the thorax. When this situation arises, the attempt to close with silk should be abandoned and one or more strips of fascia lata should be employed instead. This material is strong and, because of the large breadth of the strips, does not cut through the muscle fibers.

Once the hernia has been repaired, the edges of the mediastinal pleura are drawn together and reattached to the diaphragm with a few sutures of fine silk, the strand of silk used for traction is withdrawn, and the chest wall is closed in the accustomed manner (Fig. 154). Drainage of the left pleural cavity is employed only if there is a possibility that the lung has been injured while separating adhesions or if there is reason to expect a larger serosanguineous effusion than normal.

Special mention should be made at this point of the infrequent situation where the esophagus is congenitally short and the cardiac end of the stomach lies transposed within the mediastinum. This type of hernia cannot be cured in the anatomic sense. The esophagus cannot be elongated and the cardia cannot be reduced below the diaphragm. Nevertheless the symptoms can be relieved in many patients who have this condition if the hernia sac is dissected free from the stomach and either infolded by plication or excised in order to eliminate the pinching of the peritoneum by the edges of the hiatus. The operation is completed by narrowing the hiatus to the appropriate size, but no attempt to alter the location of the cardia and stomach or to displace the diaphragm upward need be made.

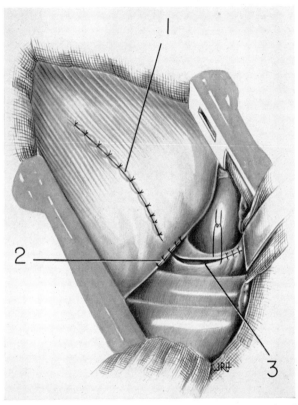

Fig. 154. Hiatus hernia. Appearance of the region after the repair has been completed showing (1) the sutured counterincision in the diaphragm (only in certain cases with a large sac); (2) the reapplication of the diaphragmatic pleura to the margin of the hiatus; and (3) closure of the lengthwise incision in the pleura.

Para-esophageal (Parahiatal) Type. (Fig. 149, B). In the relatively rare type of hiatus hernia usually referred to as "para-esophageal," the cardia does not rise above the level of the diaphragm and as a result the esophagus retains its normal length and position. The only part of the stomach which participates in the hernia, at least until the condition becomes far advanced, is the fundus. As the hernia enlarges, more and more of the stomach, including the body and sometimes even the antral portion, is pushed up into the chest. The cardia, however, remains fixed below the diaphragm and often in advanced cases actually lies beside the pylorus which is drawn to the left by the ascent of the fundus and body of the stomach. It is characteristic of this condition, also, that as the hernia enlarges, the stomach rotates and ultimately lies with its greater curvature uppermost at the top of the hernia sac, giving rise to the popular term "upside-down stomach."

Another important difference between the para-esophageal and the so-called short esophagus types of hernia is that the former is not a sliding hernia. The sac in this variety consists entirely of a protrusion of the peritoneum through the aperture, and the stomach lies free within it.

The reason for the difference between the two varieties lies in the fact that in the para-esophageal type a narrow portion of the muscle, often consisting of only a few bundles of fibers, remains between the hernia and the esophagus, whereas in the majority of instances all the bundles are pushed aside to make way for the protrusion of the hernia through the hiatus. Thus although the hernia orifice may be wide and the sac exceedingly large, there remains in effect an esophageal hiatus of relatively normal size. The para-esophageal hernias are therefore technically not hiatus hernias. It is more nearly correct from the anatomic point of view to call such a hernia parahiatal than to speak of it as para-esophageal.

In some instances a combination of both types may be observed in the same patient with a large parahiatal sac and a small sliding hernia through the hiatus.

TECHNIC OF REPAIR. Although hernias of the parahiatal type comprise some of the largest herniations through the diaphragm which may be observed, they are usually more easily repaired than those of the sliding hiatus type. The sac can usually be freed readily and unless the contents are incarcerated, the stomach or other viscera which lie within are easily reduced into the abdomen. The sac can then be excised. It is a frequent occurrence to find that after it has been freed completely, the sac can be transfixed and ligated in as satisfactory a manner as in many cases of inguinal hernia. The defect in the diaphragm is then closed with heavy silk. The operative technic in every other respect resembles that employed in the usual type of hernia.

DEFECTS RESULTING FROM INJURY

Traumatic Rupture. This condition is encountered more frequently on the left side than on the right. The rupture may be localized and in the periphery of the diaphragm, or it may be large, irregular in shape, and may often extend completely across the diaphragm into the esophageal hiatus. Unless the operation for its repair is performed soon after the injury, the abdominal viscera which were forced through the opening into the thorax are likely to become adherent to the raw edges of the torn muscle. In the pleural cavity, however, they lie free and are almost never adherent to the lung or pericardium. It is a striking sight on opening the thoracic cavity to observe the stomach, loops of intestine, and all or a portion of the omentum lying uncovered beside the lung within the chest.

In patients who are operated upon soon after the accident, a search should be made for rupture of the spleen and evidences of injury to other abdominal viscera. In many early cases the signs and symptoms of an injury to an abdominal organ, particularly the spleen, provide the indication for immediate operation. In others, when the abdomen does not participate in the injury, the most frequent decision is to postpone surgery. The operation is therefore performed at a time of election. These considerations are important in planning the correct surgical approach. Obviously if there is the possibility that a hollow viscus may have been injured, a laparotomy provides the best access to all the organs which should be explored. The decision whether to suture the lacerated diaphragm at the same operation in cases of severe injuries to the intestines must be based on the circumstances in each instance. If only the spleen has been injured, the ruptured diaphragm can be sutured at the time of the splenectomy if the condition of the patient permits. If there is doubt, however, this part of the procedure should be postponed. If one can be certain in a case of ruptured diaphragm that there is no real prospect of an injury to the intestines, the operation can be carried out most easily and expeditiously through a thoracic incision which can be enlarged if necessary by extending it across the costochondral arch into the muscles of the abdominal wall.

When the injury is not recent and there is no reason to investigate the lower abdominal viscera, the best approach is without question through the lower thorax. In the majority of instances this situation prevails, so that the occasions for employing the abdominal approach are unusual.

TECHNIC. A standard thoracotomy incision is made through the eighth intercostal space or the bed of the eighth rib, depending on the age of the patient and the circumstances of the case. The abdominal viscera are freed of any attachments which may have resulted from adhesions to the edges of the rent in the diaphragm and pushed down into the abdomen. When the accident is a recent one, a search is made for other injuries such as rupture of the spleen and lacerations of the lung, liver or stomach. These are dealt with in the appropriate manner.

The opening in the diaphragm is closed with interrupted sutures of heavy silk and, if necessary, the closure can be strengthened further by interweaving a strip of fascia lata as may occasionally be done in the repair of a hiatus hernia.

Temporary diaphragmatic paralysis induced by crushing the phrenic nerve close to its termination in the diaphragm is usually advisable to favor unobstructed healing. The lung is then expanded and the chest wall is closed. Closed catheter drainage is advisable, at least in cases of recent injury where a large amount of serosanguineous effusion is to be anticipated.

Penetrating Wounds. Lacerations of the diaphragm are frequently observed as a part of the complicated injury produced by penetrating wounds of the lower chest. There are almost invariably other serious injuries to the lung, liver, spleen, kidney, stomach or colon, or even the small bowel. These must be dealt with according to the exigencies of the case. The repair of the diaphragmatic injury under these circumstances assumes a minor importance and is carried out in the same manner as repair of a traumatic rupture. The principles outlined above should be followed.

THERAPEUTIC PARALYSIS OF THE DIAPHRAGM

Therapeutic paralysis of one side of the diaphragm can be accomplished by crushing or cutting the homolateral phrenic nerve at any appropriate level in its course through the neck or mediastinum. When postoperative inactivity of the diaphragm is desired as an adjuvant part of the surgical procedure, as for example to assist in the obliteration of the pleural space after pneumonectomy or to avoid tugging upon the stomach after esophagectomy, the phrenic nerve is crushed with a hemostat at some point within the chest. A convenient site for crushing is the terminal portion of the nerve where it leaves the surface of the pericardium to enter the diaphragm. If regeneration of the nerve is to be prevented, as after pneumonectomy, it is desirable to crush the nerve at each of several levels within the chest, such as in the upper mediastinum, in the middle of its course within the thorax, and close to the diaphragm.

When paralysis of one side of the diaphragm is required as an independent procedure, the phrenic nerve is interrupted at a convenient point within the neck. This operation is a simple one requiring for its performance merely an accurate knowledge of the topographic anatomy of the cervical region.

Technic. Local anesthesia induced by infiltration of procaine hydrochloride solution (1 per cent) into the skin and subcutaneous tissues is used. An incision approximately 3 inches long is made about 1 inch above the clavicle and roughly parallel with that bone. The midpoint of the incision should lie over the posterior margin of the sternocleidomastoid muscle (Fig. 155). The subcutaneous fat and the platysma muscle are divided, exposing the sternocleidomastoid muscle beneath the anterior half and a pad of fat and deep fascia beneath the posterior half of the incision. The posterior margin of the sternocleidomastoid muscle is freed by dissection and a small retractor is inserted. The edge of the muscle is displaced medially a short distance, exposing the deep cervical fascia which covers the anterior scalene muscle. At first the muscle is not visible but it can be identified by palpation with the finger. A pair of curved scissors is used to open and spread apart the deep fascia and overlying fat, whereupon the thin glistening fascial investment of the scalene muscle is seen. Immediately beneath this membrane and directly on the anterior surface of the muscle lies the phrenic nerve. It cannot be mistaken for any other nerve in this area because of the fact that it crosses the anterior scalene muscle in an oblique direction to assume a more and more medial position the lower it descends in the neck.

If the above procedure is followed, the only difficulty which may be encountered results from the occurrence of an anomalous course of the nerve, which may lie along the medial border of the muscle or may sometimes be

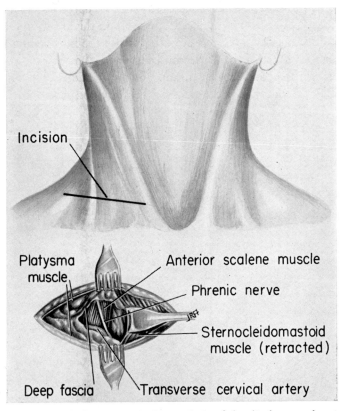

Fig. 155. Intracervical phrenicotomy for paralysis of the diaphragm, showing the line of incision and the exposure of the nerve at the point where it is to be interrupted by the technic described.

actually embedded among the muscle fibers. Likewise the possible presence of accessory branches should be kept in mind. By careful dissection these difficulties can usually be resolved by finding the aberrant trunk or discovering the presence of anomalous branches.

If the surgeon is uncertain about the identity of the nerve trunk which he believes to be the phrenic, he has merely to grasp it gently with a forceps, whereupon the twitching of the diaphragm and the pain over the top of the shoulder which the patient experiences will reveal the fact that the correct nerve has been isolated.The nerve is then injected with procaine hydrochloride solution to render the conclusion of the operation painless.

If a temporary paralysis of the diaphragm is sought, the nerve is merely crushed thoroughly with a hemostatic forceps for a distance of about ½ inch along its length. Whenever a permanent interruption of the nerve is desired, the nerve is cut and the distal end is grasped securely with a straight hemostatic forceps which is then rotated several turns, winding up a considerable length of the distal segment of the nerve upon its jaws. When a sufficient length of the nerve has been drawn up in this manner, the trunk is cut and the lower end allowed to drop back into the mediastinum. By this means a long segment of the nerve can be avulsed, thereby precluding with certainty any subsequent regeneration. This operation of phrenic nerve exeresis, though widely used at one time, is rarely performed in the present day.

After the nerve has been crushed or a section of it removed, as the case may be, the incision is closed with a layer of fine suture material in the platysma muscle and a second layer in the skin. For the latter purpose, especially in young women, a subcuticular suture may be chosen to avoid the unsightly appearance of stitch holes in the skin.

There is no special problem in the after-care of the patient.

INDEX